LOVE, MONEY, DUTY

GENDER AND CULTURE

GENDER AND CULTURE

A SERIES OF COLUMBIA UNIVERSITY PRESS

Nancy K. Miller and Victoria Rosner, Series Editors
Carolyn G. Heilbrun (1926–2003) and Nancy K. Miller, Founding Editors

For a complete list of books in this series, see the Columbia University Press website.

LOVE, MONEY, DUTY

STORIES OF CARE
IN OUR TIMES

RACHEL ADAMS

Columbia University Press
New York

Columbia University Press
Publishers Since 1893
New York   Chichester, West Sussex

Library of Congress Cataloging-in-Publication Data
Names: Adams, Rachel, 1968– author.
Title: Love, money, duty : stories of care in our times / Rachel Adams.
Description: New York : Columbia University Press, [2025] |
Series: Gender and culture | Includes bibliographical references and index.
Identifiers: LCCN 2024036418 (print) | LCCN 2024036419 (ebook) |
ISBN 9780231218085 (hardback) | ISBN 9780231218092 (trade paperback) |
ISBN 9780231562065 (ebook)
Subjects: LCSH: Caregivers. | Care of the sick. | Medical care. | Child care.
Classification: LCC RA645.3 .A33 2025 (print) | LCC RA645.3 (ebook) |
DDC 362/.0425—dc23/eng/20241112

Cover design: Julia Kushnirsky
Cover image: © Janine Antoni. Courtesy of the artist and
Luhring Augustine, New York.

GPSR Authorized Representative: Easy Access System Europe—Mustamäe tee 50,
10621 Tallinn, Estonia, gpsr.requests@easproject.com

CONTENTS

CARE: FOURTEEN AXIOMS

An axiom establishes the assumptions, both descriptive and ethical, that underpin an argument. In the interest of putting my own assumptions on the table, I start with this highly subjective and nonexhaustive list of assertions. Some readers will recognize this form as inspired by Eve Kosofsky Sedgwick's landmark study *Epistemology of the Closet*, where she used a set of axioms to articulate the otherwise implicit terms of the project that would lay the foundation for queer theory.[1] Likewise, I believe it is worth bringing my own values and priorities to light so that they can be discussed, debated, and reimagined when necessary. In case of emergency, break glass and run with them.

Axiom 1: The need for care is universal among human animals, although its norms are historically and culturally specific. All human animals are born dependent and require care through infancy and childhood. Most will require care at other points in their lives. Layered over the undeniable needs of the body are social determinations of who counts as dependent, what it means to need care, who will provide it, and on what terms. These norms have varied over time and from one culture to another. Activities that seem caring to some might be perceived as oppressive by others; what passes for care in one time or place might seem neglectful in another. Differences in perception of care's quality and value may vary from one group to another or from person to person.

Axiom 2: All human animals—and all living beings—are interdependent, but some are more dependent than others. Liberal societies equate personhood with independence, a principle that obscures the reality of our shared interdependence. No human animal can survive without some form of dependence on others. To recognize the universality of interdependence does not mean that all persons have the same level of need. Some categories of person, like children, people with disabilities or debilitating illnesses, and those with age-related frailties, require a considerable amount of care in any context. Others, like women, people of color, or the poor, have been rendered dependent by social structures. Interdependency is situational; it is not an identity but a fluid spectrum ranging from the status we call "independence" to total dependence on others for all aspects of survival.

Axiom 3: Care is a relationship that is usually asymmetrical and may be nonreciprocal. Care can be an activity, a feeling, or an ethic, but it is always relational and rarely equivalent. Assuming the uneven distribution of dependency, we recognize that some people will inevitably need more care than others and that some will give more than they receive. No person can give care without having received it, but care is hard to quantify. How it is measured and valued varies, ranging from financial compensation to expressions of gratitude or recognition to signs of growth to bare survival. Sometimes even the best care results in decline or death; sometimes it is invisible and unacknowledged. The nature and extent of care any one person is capable of giving is similarly varied. Rarely if ever are the capacities of care giver and receiver equally matched.[2]

Axiom 4: Caregiving is a form of work. Care is work—which I define as an activity requiring cognitive, affective, or physical effort to achieve a purpose or result—regardless of whether it is paid or unpaid, voluntary or forced. Sometimes an effort is obvious, as when caregiving involves lifting, cleaning, moving, or preparing. Sometimes it is subtle, as when it involves waiting, watching, or withholding, activities that require mental or emotional exertion, even if imperceptible to others.

In some circumstances, inaction can be just as important to caring as an activity. In some places and times, care has been seen as a vital form of labor contributing to the well-being of family and society. Sometimes it is recognized with a job title and salary. At other times, it has been seen as an instinctual behavior, a natural proclivity of some classes or identities. When caregiving is naturalized, its status as work is obscured. It is further obscured in modernity, when work has been more narrowly defined as the capacity to engage in paid labor even as the majority of care work continues to be unpaid.

Axiom 5: It is work to be cared for. To say that a person "receives" care implies passivity, being done to. It is possible to be cared for in a state of unconsciousness, such as during sleep, a coma, or unresponsive wakefulness syndrome. However, in the majority of caring scenarios, the recipient participates in some way. To say that care is received does not specify anything about the demeanor of the cared-for, who might be appreciative, resistant, or anywhere in between. Sometimes the work involves accepting care even when it feels shameful or unwanted, and sometimes it involves protest. Recognizing the effort involved in accepting care helps reframe the care relationship as a negotiation among participants—each acting according to their capacities—rather than an active giver and a passive recipient.

Axiom 6: There is no natural predisposition to care associated with particular races and genders; however, the work of caregiving is disproportionately distributed to women and people of color. There is a long history of identifying women and nonwhite people as inherently good caregivers and an equally long and contradictory history of identifying nonwhite people as inferior caregivers. Often attributed to biology, these assertions direct the assignment of such social roles as wives, mothers, daughters, nurses, and servants. They justify the asymmetrical distribution of caring responsibilities in the family and beyond. When the occupant of such a role is disinclined to care or acts in ways described as careless, they are perceived as unnatural or perverse.

Axiom 7: Ideally, care is given and received with generosity, kindness, gentleness, and compassion, but it may also include such negative emotions as boredom, anger, resentment, and hostility. Some argue that care counts as such only when it combines good intentions with actions that benefit and sustain the recipient. This potentially worthy ethical ideal is impossible to fulfill in reality. Feeling and action do not always align and cannot be forcibly reconciled. The good will associated with caring about a person or thing does not always lead to caring action. Caring actions can be necessary, even when unwelcome to the provider or the recipient. Care can be given with neutral or even bad feelings, particularly when it is obligatory. It can be received even when undesired or resisted. Mothers care for children while feeling bored and frustrated; nurses work through exhaustion and disgust; partners recoil at the vomit or shit of a beloved. The same activities may be administered with sincerity on one day and a performance of feeling on another.

Axiom 8: Care involves the production of affect, the submerged undercurrents of feeling generated by interactions among people. The sociologist Arlie Hochschild is credited with coining the term "emotional labor" to describe work that requires a demeanor and attempts to evoke feelings in others.[3] Emotions are internally generated by an individual, who is aware of experiencing them, whether or not they are visible in bodily disposition. Care is also an affect, meaning it includes not only conscious feelings but also those registered at the level of autonomic processes like temperature, heart rate, digestion, and stress level. Affect is also shared. It is not bounded by individual bodies but an ambience that emanates among people, implicitly communicated through gesture and expression. Caregivers and receivers generate affect together, sometimes the good or bad feelings of one communicated to the other, sometimes collectively producing an atmosphere that encompasses multiple parties in a shared environment.

Axiom 9: Caregivers possess special knowledge about disgust, desire, and vulnerability. Caring intimately for another person's body may require wrestling with and overcoming aversions to taboo substances and activities. Caregivers can become familiar with the smell, sight, and tactile sensation of other people's shit, blood, urine, and vomit. Sometimes, care that involves intimate bodily processes is best supplied by a family member; sometimes, it is less emotionally fraught to have a professional care worker deal with such effusions. Distributing the work of cleaning and maintaining the ailing body to paid caregivers may be a way to preserve the quality of time spent with a beloved family member. Sometimes, familiarity with bodily processes can shade into callousness toward dependent others. But it can also yield strategies for maintaining dignity in the face of dependency, as well as knowledge about how bodies communicate needs in a language other than words. In an ideal world we would value such knowledge and skill by compensating it accordingly and by recognizing the wisdom of experienced caregivers.

Axiom 10: Care is a process, a set of actions that do not necessarily develop toward a predictable outcome or goal. It is often redundant, inefficient, and slow. An activity is caring when it responds to a need. Needs are not efficient; they often cannot be addressed on a schedule; and they do not always align with a caregiver's time, energy, or patience. Sometimes care work leads to a socially valued result, and its progress can be measured: a typically developing child arriving at adult maturity or a sick or injured person convalescing to health. Reaching desired outcomes can make care rewarding, but care is not a failure when it results in maintenance, decline, or death.

Axiom 11: The roles of care giver and receiver are fluid and may change over the course of a day or a lifetime. Independence and dependency are legal categories, but care giver and recipient are not fixed roles or identities. Caring activities and needs lie on a spectrum with infinite possibilities. One person can and usually does occupy the roles of care giver and recipient simultaneously, as well as switching positions repeatedly over the course of a day. Those who are obligated or paid to give care also need care themselves. They too began life in dependency and may be dependent in the future. Such role reversals may feel right and natural, but they may also be exceedingly difficult, such as when illness or accident renders an able-bodied person dependent. Some who are gifted caregivers resist being cared for, and some accustomed to the care of others may be grudging or awkward care givers.

Axiom 12: Care involves the potential for desire. Intimate acts may be tinged with eroticism and also carry the risks of sexual violation, since care inevitably involves imbalances of power. When bodies are vulnerable, exposed, and in need, when attention to the body is tender, intimate, soothing, or painful, exchanges of care sometimes stir desire in givers or receivers. Some who give or receive exceptional amounts of care enjoy what Elizabeth Freeman calls "medical kink."[4] Desire is not bound to politics or standards of appropriate behavior, although this does not ever justify nonconsensual action toward another. Dependent people are especially vulnerable to sexual assault, even as they may suffer from a deficit of social or physical intimacy. Caregivers often do their work in privacy and isolation, where they too are at risk for sexual violence.

Axiom 13: Caring begins in an intimate encounter between a giver and a recipient, but caring relations are embedded in and sustained by networks of people and institutions. The kind of care addressed by this book originates in and always entails an exchange between a dependent person and a caregiver, whether parent and child, siblings, life partners, patient and health provider, or a person with disabilities and a paid assistant. The success of those exchanges has something to do with the temperaments and values of the individuals involved but is also directly related to the strength of the networks or webs in which they are suspended. Often these webs are invisible, concealing unpaid caring labor that subsidizes the socially valued contribution of productive, wage-earning workers. Sometimes they become hypervisible, as when a sick caregiver upends the functioning of an entire family or a pandemic puts the world's activities on pause, creating new forms of dependency in the process. Art and literature can conceal or naturalize care webs but can also be an important resource for making them visible.

Axiom 14: Care has its own temporalities that may differ from standard clock time or modern measures of work, productivity, and development. The time of care is dictated by the needs of the body, which cannot always be disciplined according to the clocks, schedules, and markers of normative progress so important to the modern world. Care is not always productive. Sometimes it involves being present while doing nothing at all. Usually it is slow, its course meandering, uneven, or regressive. Sometimes it is urgent, requiring the interruption of productive or planned activity. This makes care an uneasy fit with a modern economy reliant on standard measures of productivity and effort and structured around established schedules and routines. In contrast to the linear, forward-moving temporality of modernity, care time is often repetitive, delayed, backward, slowed down, or speeded up. Paid care is often compensated in units of time and effort, although such accounting has little correspondence to what matters most to the actual work of care: a gentle touch, attentive listening, being present. These qualities help explain why care is so undervalued, as well as its radical possibilities. Care has the potential to upend the values, norms, and practices that govern capitalism and our modern social and political systems.

ACKNOWLEDGMENTS

One way to read this book is as an extended acknowledgment of all the people who have cared for me and my family, allowing me time and space to write. Even as I follow convention, confining my gratitude to this section, I hope that reading will draw attention to my incredible good fortune at the broad, deep, and usually invisible webs of care that enable me to do my work.

I have written this book in the company of my colleagues at Columbia University and Barnard College, who support me with friendship and interest in my work. Among the many, special recognition goes to Chris Baswell, Monica Cohen, Sarah Cole, Sayantani DasGupta, Rishi Goyal, Arden Hegele, Jean Howard, Laura Kaufman, Ana Paulina Lee, Monica Miller, Hazel May, Victoria Rosner, and Maya Sabatello. Denise Cruz deserves a sentence of her own for being a remarkable friend, colleague, and leader. Kat Chen was my student and teacher, an excellent proofreader who inspired me with her brilliance and creativity. Thanks to Olivia Breibart for introducing me to the work of Janine Antoni, which illustrates the cover of this book.

Support from Columbia University also enabled me to develop a community of colleagues beyond the university, first through the Future of Disability Studies project, funded by the Center for the Study of Social Difference, and then the Disability, Culture, and Society seminar, supported by the University Seminars program. Among the members of that wonderful group, I am especially appreciative of Chris Baswell, Christina Crosby, Julia Rodas, and Lotti Silber. I thank Julia and Lotti for friendship that extends well beyond the time and place of those groups.

Outside of my own university, I am sustained by a wider web of colleagues. Among the group I cherish, these people have made a particular contribution to my work on this book: Sari Altschuler, Michael Bérubé, Sara Blair, Emily Bloom, Leslie Bow, Liz Bowen, Russ Castronovo, Sarah Ensor, George Estreich, Jonathan Freedman, Chris Gabbard, Faye Ginsberg, Sarah Hendren, Scott Herring, Eva Feder Kittay, Janet Lyon, Jordana Mendelson, Nancy Miller, Tahneer Oksman, Rayna Rapp, Julia Rodas, Talia Schaffer, Lotti Silber, David Serlin, Cristobal Silva, and Ben Reiss.

I might have survived the pandemic without the Ladies of Zoom, but much the worse for it. Thank you for all of it, Laura Kaufman, Hazel May, and Victoria Rosner.

I hope that my notes convey the extent of my debt to the many scholars who have written about care before me. But beyond those references, I acknowledge more directly my gratitude to Christina Crosby, Beth Freeman, Eva Feder Kittay, Laura Mauldin, and Talia Schaffer.

I am grateful to Victoria Rosner and Nancy Miller for included me in their series, Gender and Culture, and for tireless encouragement, feedback, and friendship at every step of my work on this project. Philip Leventhal was a generous and loyal interlocutor for years before I even thought of the idea for this book, and I am so glad it gave me the occasion to work with him. Rob Fellman was a patient and attentive copy editor.

A fellowship at the Heyman Center at Columbia University gave me time to get a good start on this book, which was also supported by a Guggenheim Fellowship that had long been high on my bucket list. The cost of this book's production was generously subsidized by a grant from the Columbia University Seminars' Schoff Publication Fund. Portions of chapter 4 were previously published in an article in *Gender in American Literature and Culture*, edited by Jean Lutes and Jennifer

Travis. Portions of chapter 5 were published in an article in a *Journal of Medical Humanities* special issue, *Caregiving, Kinship, and the Making of Stories*, edited by Mark Osteen and Carol Schilling. I thank the editors of those publications for the opportunity to work through ideas important to this project.

Janine Antoni, Leon Borensztein, Therese Frare, Nathan Gray, and Paul Karasik were generous in allowing me to use their artwork. Thank you to Ben Schwartz for his helpful interventions.

Naomi Kovacs, Melanie Brazil, and Angela Grullón allowed me to share their stories. Thanks to Michelle Sagan at the NDSS for providing a photograph.

It would take a whole book to thank all of the caregivers who have made it possible for me to write, but Angela Grullón and Nancy Mello deserve special mention.

I thank my extended family—Adams, Connolly, Cray, Kovacs, Martell, Myerhoff—for the many ways they hold me up in a wide-ranging web of care. I also count Jenny and Lev Eisenberg as treasured members of my chosen family. Noah and Henry inspire me to care bigger and deeper even as they hamper my writing about it. Jon Connolly is my interdependency, a remarkable life partner, coparent, and caregiver. He does not like to be written about, but he knows how often I use the singular pronoun when I really mean we.

LOVE, MONEY, DUTY

INTRODUCTION

Why Care?

Because Dr. Laura Evans Saved Craig Spencer's Life with the Help of 119 Others."[1] This entry—number eight of *New York* magazine's 2014 "Reasons to Love New York"—is a study in care. A two-page grid of 120 portraits recognizes the collaboration among hospital staff ranging from the chief of medicine to mail delivery and janitorial services. It pictures care as asymmetrical—one patient required the attention of over a hundred—but also reciprocal—Spencer is a doctor who was infected with Ebola virus while caring for the sick during an outbreak in Guinea; in turn, he received care when he became sick. He would continue to serve patients after his return to health. Spencer's story is site-specific. It is about the human and technological resources that can be marshaled by a well-financed institution in the wealthiest country in the world. Hospital care is coordinated, distributed, and hierarchical. The photo grid draws attention to such hierarchies while also making some effort to disrupt them. The first two rows are illustrative. On top is a series of middle-aged male-appearing subjects whose names and jobs are listed beneath. Their titles indicate positions of authority such as chief of medicine, chief of pathology, medical director, and associate director. The subjects in the row just beneath all appear to be people of color. Two are male- and five female-appearing. Their names and jobs are also listed beneath, all with the title of nurse. The majority of workers in the bottom rows of each page, with occupations involving security, transport, and waste disposal, appear to be nonwhite (figures 0.1–0.2).

The story is geographically specific, featured in a magazine devoted to all things New York City. Spencer is an American citizen who had access to the abundant technological and human resources of a major hospital in the United States. The story celebrates the excellent care that contributed to his survival. (Not pictured: the thousands of West Africans who died alone and untreated during the epidemic.) Care is also historical. Since I clipped this story from the magazine (at that point still circulating largely in print), it acquired an ironic cast in light of a global pandemic that would bring the same wealthy hospital to its knees, its ravages reflecting the same interdependencies as well as the asymmetries intimated by the 2014 portrait.

Back in 2014, the story caught my eye because it seemed a novel way to recognize the care networks that sustain a single human life. At that point, I was starting to write about the fault lines in our current systems of care. I appreciated the portrait's symbolism—each carer an individual and a participant in a collaborative system—and its prominence, since I believed that care work—so often done in private and without acknowledgment—needed more recognition. In 2014 I probably could have predicted that it would take me a long time to write this book, given the many obligations of care and work I was juggling but never that, in the spring of 2020, I would start to write the introduction just as a global pandemic was making the problem of care unexpectedly timely, urgent, and visible. Care at its best is invisible, allowing us to feel independent even as we are sustained by a network of interdependencies. It is that thing we prefer not to think about until it is absolutely necessary. It is always somebody else's problem, until it isn't.

Why care? The three terms in my title—love, money, duty—are meant to be a provisional answer to this question. But I hope they feel insufficient, demanding stories to fill the outlines with meaning and specificity. This book relies on stories to better understand our complicated feelings about giving and receiving care, the systems and institutions we have built to facilitate it, the many ways they are failing us, as

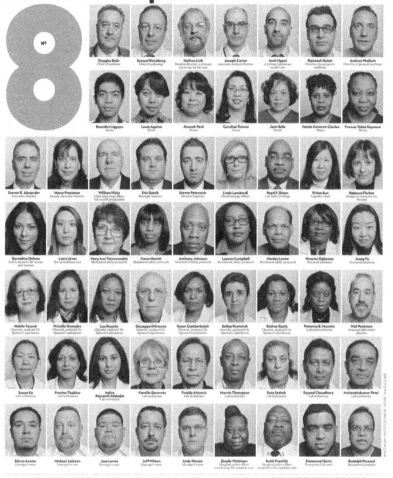

Photographs by Christopher Anderson

FIGURE 0.1 The design of the first page of the grid from *New York* magazine's 2014 "Reasons to Love New York."

Source: Christopher Anderson, Bellevue Hospital Staff, *New York Magazine*.

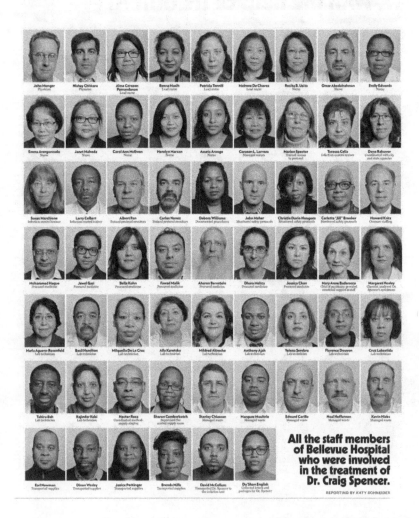

All the staff members of Bellevue Hospital who were involved in the treatment of Dr. Craig Spencer.

REPORTING BY KATY SCHNEIDER

FIGURE 0.2 The second page from *New York* magazine's 2014 "Reasons to Love New York."

Source: Christopher Anderson, Bellevue Hospital Staff, *New York Magazine*.

well as, sometimes, examples of success. It is not about the COVID-19 pandemic, but that global crisis gave its subject an unexpected patina of relevance. The book I have written draws from my personal experiences, but it is also a work of scholarship that comes from many years of studying a slower, less visible, but far more pervasive crisis in our attitudes toward and structures of care for dependent persons and those who provide for them. As a cultural critic, I am trained in narrative analysis, and I see narrative as a vital resource for accessing lived realities—particularly the realities of those who are different from us— but also expressing inchoate fears, anxieties, and desires that might be obscured by more straightforward sociological or historiographic methods. Narrative—a broad term I use to describe stories in media ranging from literary fiction to memoirs to comics, films, videos, visual arts, and blog posts—can illuminate problems with our current systems of care, why we fear and shun dependency, and how we devalue the work of caregiving. More hopefully, this book draws attention to the art of interdependency—the ingenuity and resourcefulness of dependent people and their caregivers—and challenges the panicky rhetoric of catastrophe evoked by the growth of dependent elderly and disabled populations. It is not the only way to arrive at these insights, but it is a good one and the one I know best.

I define care as the intimate and necessary labor required to sustain those who are dependent, activity that is always imbricated with others dispersed across time and space. It is the immediate work, both paid and unpaid, of providing physical and emotional sustenance to those in need and unable to provide for themselves. Those exchanges are nodes in a network of interdependencies that sometimes manages a functional, if tenuous, balance and is sometimes strained to the breaking point. In keeping with my subject, I have tried to read with care, a critical posture that is flexible, creative, and receptive to marginal, obscure, and minor details. This is more an attitude than a method. I argue that the social and political failures of modern care arrangements start with a failure of imagination. Stories are a portal to the imagination, a rich fund of shared knowledge and feeling about caring and being cared for, dependency and dependency work. Stories are not going to solve all of our problems, but they have the potential to expose them and to begin the work of rewriting social scripts that stigmatize dependency and devalue care work.

With a bracing dose of humility, I also try to write with awareness of the many things stories cannot do: wash the dishes, pay for childcare, hold someone who is crying. They don't raise the salaries of home nursing aids, provide universal health care, or redistribute wealth. Much as they expose, stories also conceal, sometimes erecting thickets of denial or redirection. Even the most moving stories can fail to produce change, and sometimes stories prompt action that undermines the interests of those in need. Yet I find that when I share my personal stories alongside those I have collected, readers and listeners feel prompted to think and talk in new ways about their own needs for care and their work as caregivers. These conversations persuade me that the work is worth doing. Critical care is both my book's approach and its subject: being critical means reading with an eye to analysis, understanding, and assessment, but I also see care as critical in that it is the most necessary and precious of resources required to sustain individuals, species, and life itself. We fail to appreciate it at our peril.

THEORIES OF CARE

Care is work, an attitude toward others, and an ethical ideal. Reading with care, this book uses the affordances of narrative to examine its subject from many different angles rather than being guided by a single theory or ethical model. It relies on a rich tool kit of theoretical work available to readers who want to pursue questions of care in a systematic and conceptual way. (Those who are primarily interested in particular stories and the wisdom they impart might choose to skip this section, since many of its key insights will be embedded in the discussions to come.) In its approach to care, this book stands at the intersection of moral philosophy, disability studies, health humanities, literary criticism, critical race studies, and feminist and queer theory. The field most actively engaged in delineating an ethics of care is moral philosophy. The turn to care represented a pivot from a more traditional focus on the actions of individual, autonomous people and toward the consideration of interdependency and social relatedness. Care ethics also challenged a core premise of modern social contract theory, which posits that a just society is built on consensual agreement among equal, rational, and autonomous agents.[2] Instead of taking the free-standing individual as its model subject, care ethics emphasizes a spectrum of relationships that are overlapping, asymmetrical, and particular. In place of abstract universals, care is specific, local, and embodied. It involves emotions and needs at least as much as reason. It often operates affectively, via currents of feeling produced between and among participants in an exchange, rather than contained by discrete bodies or subjectivities. Instead of defining personhood in terms of capacity for reason, philosophers of care see it as relational, with people bound together by shared vulnerability and interdependence. Once we recognize that all lives begin in dependency and that no person would survive to adult independence without others, care becomes the most universal and primary of human activities.

Having acknowledged care as a bedrock for all human life, we also have to recognize the gendering of caring responsibilities. We hardly need scholars to point out that in most societies the majority of care work is done by women, who have been seen as more naturally predisposed to such caring virtues as nurture, generosity, and empathy and have also been obligated to care by their social status as daughters, wives, and mothers. Feminist thought, with its attention to gender roles, embodiment, and the emotions, has been essential to developing the philosophies of care that underlie my approach throughout this book.[3] Some feminists have taken the gendered associations of care as an opportunity to elevate women's activities, priorities, and moral sensibilities.[4] Others have taken the mother-child bond as a basis to claim the social and ethical importance of care. For these thinkers, the universal dependency of infants and children makes them a paradigm for the necessity of care to survival and thriving.[5] Nel Noddings names women's instinctual and ethical impulse to care "the maternal factor."

Sara Ruddick proposes "practices of mothering" as the foundation for a politics of nonviolence and "maternal thinking" as an approach that recognizes the intellectual and physical work of caregiving.[6] Eva Feder Kittay argues that the universal experience of being "some mother's child" is a more just and inclusive foundation for personhood than the social contract because it points to our shared origins in the fundamental caring relations required to sustain human life. Instead of being guided by mutual self-interest, a model of personhood grounded in the experience of being mothered looks to relationships "forged through the care of a vulnerable dependent, and to the value that this relation imparts both to the one cared for and to the caregiver."[7] These thinkers affirm the value of caregiving while also providing a framework for rethinking personhood in terms of mutual need and interconnection rather than a property of discrete, rational individuals.

I find the case for an ethics centered on care and women's work of undeniable philosophical significance. Just because women are often assigned to caregiving roles, however, does not mean there is an inherent connection between women and care. Nor do I take mothering as an ethical ideal because doing so risks obscuring the burdens shouldered by actual mothers and the negativity that sometimes colors actual mothering activity. Idealizing the mother-child bond makes it too easy to use the biological aspects of reproduction as evidence that it is the proper and natural function of those assigned female gender at birth. Idealization makes it easy to castigate real mothers for being bored, frustrated, impatient, or otherwise imperfect caregivers or for distributing care of their children to others. Grounding theories of care in the mother-child bond can also subordinate or deny the contributions of non-female-identifying caregivers to the work we call mothering. And it can influence how we think about care for dependents who are not children, causing us to infantilize care recipients and devalue the work of care providers. For these reasons, I recognize the importance of mothering as a starting point for exploring its many contradictions as a paradigm for care.

The image on the cover of this book, a photo of Janine Antoni's *Umbilical* (2000), reflects aptly on the complexities of mothering care.

Its title evokes the biological connection between a fetus and the maternal body, but its form bespeaks the more mediated relationship between a child and a maternal figure. The sculpture is a spoon cast from the artist's family silverware, with an impression of her own mouth at the bowl, the inside of her mother's hand at the handle. As an object, it captures a moment of relation and fixes it in place. Mother and child, hand and mouth, flesh and metal, *Umbilical* suggests that care is a social practice and a physiological necessity, an intimate bodily relationship that is also always mediated by culture. I appreciate that Antoni focuses on the spoon, which is typically the first utensil used in feeding but has also become a potent metaphor for the limited energy possessed by some people who are ill or disabled. Although Antoni's sculpture was cast before Christine Miserandino wrote her contagious 2003 essay, "Spoon Theory," the concept adds resonance to an artwork that has everything to do with embodiment, sustenance, and the uneven distribution of dependency and care.[8] *Umbilical* thus crystallizes this book's intention to approach care as a form of embodied labor that is at once fundamental and mediated, a relation that can be intimate and sustaining, but also a source of oppression and constraint.

Caring is also a disposition. Some are more inclined to be caring than others, and a caring temperament does not always align with caring responsibilities. I recognize the penchant to care as a spectrum. Much like gender, it is shaped by character and proclivity, as well as the environment. Among philosophers of care, there is considerable disagreement about whether there is a necessary correspondence between caring activity and the attitude with which it is given. Some argue that an activity is caring only if it is given or received in a spirit of generosity and attunement. Care is not simply a set of gestures or an external demeanor but a feeling and a relationship among people.[9] Noddings describes care as an attitude of responsiveness, mutual recognition, and commitment, in which caring about must be aligned with caring for.[10] Grace Clement includes concern for the other in her definition of care.[11] However, Joan Tronto sees disposition as distinct from practices, arguing that it is possible (if not desirable) to engage in caring action without a caring attitude.[12] Others acknowledge that sometimes caring activity may coexist with bad feelings like resentment, hostility, and anger. Once again mothers—inhabiting a social position defined by the obligation to care—are a case in point. Ruddick writes, "What we are pleased to call 'mother-love' is intermixed with hate, sorrow, impatience, resentment, and despair; thought-provoking ambivalence is a hallmark of mothering."[13] Adrienne Rich recognized the negativity in mothering in her feminist classic *Of Woman Born*, asserting, "Every woman has known overwhelming, unacceptable anger at her children."[14] Sarah LaChance Adams focuses on "maternal ambivalence," acknowledging some "mothers' simultaneous desires to nurture and violently reject their children."[15] The potential for frustration and rage associated with mothering extends to other caring relationships, especially those in which work is unevenly distributed. Selma Sevenhuijsen argues that care has a "shadow side" that includes "conflict, aggression, ambivalence and discord."[16] The excellent title of Ellen Nakano Glenn's book, *Forced to Care: Coercion and Caregiving in America*, captures the tension that arises when activities thought to be selfless and instinctual are performed under duress, often with little or no compensation.[17]

Narrative is especially good at representing ambivalence; mixed feelings are fertile ground for telling stories about how the external gestures of care can coexist uneasily with the sensations and thoughts generated by an individual subject and the affect that emerges from the relationship of participants in a caring exchange. While moral philosophy delineates the ideals we should aspire to, narrative goes for a fuller spectrum, accessing currents of shame, resentment, hostility, and boredom that may flow beneath even the most tender exchanges. Even the most artful, intentional, and chosen interdependencies run into dissonance, tension, rupture. When I read with care, I am attuned to those moments of particular harmony or dissonance among the entangled strains of feeling and doing. I read because I want to better understand the circumstances that generate caring feelings and activities, how participants in a caring exchange may be aligned or out of sync, and how different narrative forms are equipped to capture an ambiance of care. I am not looking for only the best examples, although I am thrilled to come across instances of care that works for all involved. Care is an art because it is unsystematic, often difficult, messy, and exhausting. Certainly, care can have joys and rewards, but to think critically, to "stay with the trouble" as Donna Haraway memorably puts it, requires that we also attend to its more negative valences.[18] In the interests of staying with the trouble, this book includes actions tinged with feelings of frustration, animosity, and protest in its definition of care. Staying with the trouble means recognizing that care is not always given or received with grace and appreciation; that sometimes it involves manipulation, coercion, or domination; and that sometimes good care coincides with bad feelings.

It is one thing for the participants in a caring exchange to feel bored, hostile, or detached and another to act on those feelings by being neglectful or causing injury to another. The same qualities of dependency, vulnerability, and frailty that make care necessary also make it potentially dangerous; the imbalance of power involved when one person gives care that is essential to the survival of another is always open to abuse. Caregivers can be good or bad; the care they provide can be better or worse. But when an action inflicts harm, it is no longer caring. The philosopher Christine Kelly recognizes that for some people with lifelong dependencies, particularly those living in institutional settings, "care and help are intricately interwoven with violence, oppression, and harm."[19] Harm may take the form of physical assault, sexual violence, or emotional abuse, or it may be subtler and harder to see, especially when victims have limited ability to communicate. It is possible to receive maintenance care while being deprived of desired sociability, compassion, or warmth. Actions described as caring may be designed to or have the unintended effect of control or discipline. Uma Narayan describes colonial settings where a discourse of care justifies paternalism, a complaint echoed by many people with disabilities and their advocates.[20] Those who provide care are also vulnerable to abuse. Sometimes care work can be dangerous or exploitative, especially when care workers do not have access to the care they need to thrive. When I chose materials for analysis, I did not look for idealizations of care but rather those that allowed me to explore and understand its many varieties. The chapters to come will explore the porous boundaries between care and domination, where care masks or bleeds over into harm and coercion.

Care is an attitude, but it is also work in the broadest sense, meaning activity that requires an expenditure of energy. "Caregiving is cleaning up after the news crews have left," writes Kate Washington in a brilliant essay about caring for her husband with cancer, "scrubbing the hidden black mold years later, becoming ill from the contaminated floodwaters."[21] Her bleak metaphors depict effort that is important and necessary but feels joyless, exhausting, and unrewarding. Describing care in terms of "cleaning up" and "scrubbing," Washington emphasizes that care is labor. It is often unseen and unrecognized, repetitive and unglamorous. It may be dangerous. The caregiver can be sickened or injured as a result of her efforts. Although associated with women and such typically feminine virtues as gentleness, warmth, and patience, it can require strenuous exertion like lifting and moving bodies or equipment, making nursing among the most dangerous modern professions.[22] And although it is associated with women, care work is also often performed by men, who tend to be overlooked in philosophy and sociological research on care.[23] But care work also has an affective dimension that the sociologist Arlie Hochschild calls the "emotional labor" involved in evoking a feeling in others.[24] "While you may also be doing physical labor and mental labor," she explained in a 2018 interview, a job requiring emotional labor means "you are crucially being hired and monitored for your capacity to manage and produce a feeling."[25] Describing the production of feeling as "labor" emphasizes the effort it requires without denying that it may sometimes entail more genuinely felt expressions of compassion and kindness. Good care workers tend to the physical needs of dependents while also projecting more inchoate qualities like patience, attention, and generosity. These qualities are performed with the intention of eliciting corresponding feelings in the care recipient. But the work is asymmetrical in that the giver's emotional labor is expected, whereas no such response is required of the dependent subject. Affective work is all the more paradoxical in an economy structured around wage labor. Compassion cannot be documented on a time sheet, measured in units of effort, or quantified with any of the typical gauges used to record and compensate labor.

Sometimes the best care involves doing nothing, knowing when to hold back. It is best when imperceptible, seemingly effortless. Not doing is also a form of work. Care may require putting self-interest aside, deferring or ignoring one's own feelings when they conflict with the more urgent needs of another. The home care worker in Rebecca Brown's short story collection *Gifts of the Body* tends to people dying of AIDS, who sometimes lash out at her with anger or sarcasm.[26] She feels their hostility but knows to bite her tongue. She knows not to dash their hopes of recovery or their plans for the future, no matter how unrealistic. She can sense when it is more caring to sit quietly with them on the couch than to bustle around cleaning and cooking. Rarely do such performances of care fit neatly into an hourly or daily schedule. They are most effective when unseen. In her graphic memoir about the AIDS epidemic, *Taking Turns*, the nurse M. K. Czerweic describes waiting for the elevator, exhausted after clocking out of a long shift, when a sick patient calls out, asking her to hold him.[27] She has no choice but to return and offer comfort. She does not feel a dramatic emotion, whether that would be resentment or the uplifting awareness of her own generosity. There is no good way to quantify the expenditure of time and feeling in a paycheck or performance review. She is simply worn out, doing what must be done. Her comic creates a record of a gesture that would otherwise be unseen and unremembered.

When my father was dying, I sat and held him in the middle of the night. I would like to say that I experienced attunement, absorbed in those last hours together and fully attentive to his needs. What I remember most was being desperately thirsty and uncomfortable, perched on a metal stool by the chair where he slept because it was too painful to lie down. I thought about this book and all the ways my caregiving fell short of the ideals laid out by philosophers and bioethicists. I imagined myself somewhere else, writing about my discomfort after it was over, turning it into something generative even as I affirmed the virtues of work that is not always productive, goal oriented, profitable. It was oppressively hot; I watched the clock.

Care is so often linked to the term "giving" that it can masquerade as a voluntary act of generosity. Anthropologists associate gift giving with an economy in which exchanges are personalized and relational.[28] Giving connotes a transfer, in a spirit of generosity and good will, with no expectation of reciprocity. The very idea that care is "given" complicates its association with work, paid or unpaid, so it is unsurprising that care is largely absent from Marxist theories of labor, which focus primarily on work that can be exchanged for wages. Feminists have complicated that view, arguing for a concept of labor that includes the unpaid work of social reproduction involved in caring for home and family and done primarily by women. Behind every seemingly independent individual engaged in an economically productive activity recognized as "work," Marxist feminists point to the uncompensated labor of numerous others, mostly women and people of color, that subsidizes the capitalist economy.[29] Recognizing care as work draws attention to the unpaid labor of maintaining the family, the social unit that reproduces and sustains successive generations of wage laborers. But it also brings into focus the paid caregivers like nannies, home health aides, and elder companions who are among the most poorly compensated and unappreciated of all workers. Their low salaries are also a subsidy that enables other workers—more recognizably skilled, credentialed, gifted—to leave their own dependents behind to do better-paying and more prestigious jobs outside the home.[30]

Conceiving care as work draws attention to the deep irony, made visible during the COVID-19 pandemic, that the jobs we consider most "essential" are often among the least dignified and lowest paying, if they are paid at all. During the pandemic, the obscure hazards of care work became glaringly visible in the divisions between who could shelter in place and who remained on the job, which subway lines were empty and which still crowded with passengers, the populations that survived infection and those that were disproportionately devastated. All too often, the work of caring for those we love most—our children, elderly parents, ill and disabled friends and family members—is considered "unskilled labor" and compensated accordingly. Meanwhile, parents of young children and the guardians of dependent adults feel overwhelmed by the cost of care. Something is terribly wrong when parents, people with disabilities, the frail elderly, and their loved ones bend under the expense of paid care while care workers barely eke out a living.

It is a bitter irony when the needs of dependents and their families are pitted against those of care workers. I experienced it firsthand when the agency that manages my son's Medicaid benefits asked me to protest proposed wage increases for care workers. Without added government funding, the organization argued, it could not afford to pay workers (at the time earning just above minimum wage) unless it cut their hours or laid them off altogether. Had it not really happened, this would seem like the stuff of absurdist political satire. It is hard to think of a standoff between any more devalued groups than Medicaid recipients and their home health aides, two classes of people that are far more alike than different. The stigma of dependency borne by the cared for is communicated, by association, to those who do the labor of caregiving, resulting in what Kittay calls "secondary dependency."[31] Even when not disabled themselves, paid care workers are rendered dependent by the lowly associations, meager wages, and dangers of the work they do. Although shared hardships can lead to conflict, they can also be the ground for solidarity and mutual recognition.

In an added dose of irony, feelings of identification or sympathy have made it harder for care workers to self-advocate as individuals or to organize, as have workers in other professions.[32] The emotional labor involved in care is incommensurate with overt displays of animosity. The performance of caring feelings can, over time, become genuine, especially when care is greeted with appreciation, gratitude, or thriving. Caregivers often develop emotional bonds with dependents that include not just a sense of duty but also loyalty, admiration, and love. This is particularly true for those who work in private homes as nannies, companions, personal assistants, or home health aides. Dependents are not bosses in the same way as managers who run factories and corporations. Children are inherently vulnerable, as are long-term dependents. Adults with disability-related dependencies are more than twice as likely to live in poverty than their able-bodied peers, despite the impression given by the implausible films *Me Before You, The Upside*, and its French inspiration, *The Intouchables*.[33]

The shared vulnerability of care givers and receivers means that they tend not to have the kinds of adversarial relations that arise among more conventional employers and employees. Traditional protest strategies like strikes, sick-outs, or work slowdowns are unrealistic in situations where the employer is a vulnerable person who might suffer harm or even death in the absence of care. As a result, labor organizers have had to imagine unconventional strategies for protest. The historians Eileen Boris and Jennifer Klein see this challenge as an opportunity, and they describe how its successes have expanded the tactics of organized labor. "Precisely because the work of care rests on trust and attentiveness, home care offered the possibility of a unionism that could define the employment relationship as non-adversarial," they write. "Consumers and caregivers would act together on shared interests and respect the needs of each for dignity, autonomy, and security. In the process, such coalition politics opened up a space for the self-activity and politicization of tens of thousands of low-wage women."[34] Given the nature of the work, any successful organization of home caregivers must preserve the good relationships between care workers and dependents, employees and consumers.

But real change to our care systems will require a broader shift in attitudes, a recognition of the ways care subsidizes work that we consider to be productive, and—in an even more utopian vein—a shift in the kinds of work we value and honor. Any equitable outcome must recognize the social and political significance of giving and receiving care, respecting the dignity of both dependents and dependency workers. A society that recognizes the true value of care would require adequate financial compensation for caregivers, as well as their dependents, and would finance it upstream to avoid the kinds of impasses confronted by our Medicaid agency. The narratives explored in this book provide ample evidence that in the United States we do not currently live in such a society, and they attest to the high costs of uncaring or, as is more often the case, caring in the context of extreme inequity. Occasionally, they also offer hopeful glimpses of environments and social arrangements that enable more just and sustainable exchanges of care.

Another way to describe care work is to say that it is queer. I have found queer theory—often in alignment with disability studies—a valuable resource for explaining the intimacies, social configurations, and temporalities of care giving and receiving.[35] At the most obvious level, queer theory has helped me understand the imbrication of care with sexuality and desire, as well as gender. Modern care arrangements are also rooted in a concept of family that queer critics see as heteronormative and essentialist.[36] Queer theory denaturalizes family by distancing it from biology, generational hierarchy, and capitalist productivity. It creates the conditions of possibility to rethink traditional understandings of kinship that obligate women to caregiving roles and assume biological or legal family to be a primary and consistent wellspring of unpaid care work. Queer families are chosen families that may be organized around atypical assemblages of gender and generation.[37] They may model more salutary and flexible caregiving configurations, but they may also bear the brunt of heteronormative assumptions about the definition and conduct of family.[38] Queer theory understands the current social order as historical and thus subject to change. It uses the future to imagine how we could be otherwise. Beyond its attention to gender and sexuality, queer theory questions the capitalist imperatives of productivity, growth, and progress. Care rarely serves these interests, and sometimes it actively undermines them. Queer theory is primed to recognize the value in care, even when it results in death or decline or the absence of progress. In more general terms, it can help identify alternative ways to measure the worth and contribution of care work and the interdependencies it occasions.

In dialogue with disability studies, queer theory has been especially useful for conceptualizing the temporalities of care. Clock time marches forward in predictable units. But for dependent people, time is more subjective and unpredictable. It may be organized around their needs or the stamina of their caregivers, it may move more quickly or slowly depending on context, and it may often be spent in seemingly unproductive activities like waiting or resting. Some adult dependents are beholden to institutional care, which endeavors to manage the competing temporal demands of hourly work and daily shifts, the coordinated activities of dependents and care providers, and the needs of particular bodies. Time that an employer might consider "wasted" or "lost" might be experienced by a dependent person as the most meaningful time in a day or as just living on. Sometimes workers have to steal or misuse their paid time in order to provide good care. They become guerilla caregivers who break rules, thwart their employers' instructions, and do whatever else they can to make the cared-for happy, comfortable, and empowered. Sometimes the care giver and the cared-for experience time in radically different ways.

Care is a basic need, regardless of whether the future is bright; indeed, it is often most necessary and intense when there is no future except imminent loss and death. Queer critics have been especially wary of normative understandings of the future that assume a standard path of development with goals like "maturity," "independence," or "settling down." Lee Edelman decries the association of futurity with the figure of the child, which, he argues, implicitly upholds the norms of reproductive heterosexuality.[39] Kathryn Bond Stockton offers the concept of "growing sideways" to describe how queer children deviate from the straight and narrow trajectory toward normative, heterosexual maturity.[40] More recently, Maggie Nelson has made the case for expanding these concepts. Atypical temporalities are not exclusive to queers, she notes, given how the escalating crisis of climate change has so dramatically thrown the notions of generations, futurity, and development out of whack.[41] Time is now queer, perhaps prompting us to live more care-fully in the present, complicating how we hope or plan.

Disability studies uses a similar concept: the term "crip time" describes the misfit between atypical bodyminds and the schedules and rhythms set by those who are fit, healthy, and normatively abled.[42] Queer/crip time may be recursive, uneven, sideways, or backward. It speeds up and slows down depending on experience and environment. People with disabilities, like queers, know what it is to skip over, delay, or hurry predictable developmental milestones. They attest that a good life does not require being on time, checking off boxes in the expected order, or arriving at a predetermined outcome. Crip time cannot be harnessed to standard measures of productivity, growth, or accomplishment. Lest this sound too celebratory, crip time comes with evident liabilities. People with disabilities, like queers, are highly attuned to the losses and exclusions experienced by those who set their own clocks. They use the metaphor of "spoons" to describe time in terms of packets of available energy, which vary from person to person, day to day, only becoming apparent when there aren't enough to go around. Queers and crips are frequent protagonists in the narratives explored by this book because they know firsthand what it is to run afoul of clock time. They miss out and get passed over; they are labeled slow, unproductive, inefficient. But in its ideal form, caring in queer/crip time means respecting differences of pace and perception, promoting the flourishing of those who live by alternative clocks and calendars, and adequately compensating workers whose effort cannot be measured according to standard timesheets. Queer/crip caring can also be generative, creating new strategies for living in interdependency and creative forms of storytelling to recount them.

Because this book is concerned with care that is necessary but that a person in need cannot provide for themselves, people with disabilities are its most frequent point of reference. While the importance of care to the queer community is well established, some may find the association of disability and care to be more controversial.[43] In the modern world, dependency is a stigma especially damning to disabled people, who are cast as burdensome and tragic. The movement for disability rights has long been organized around calls for independence, blaming environmental barriers rather than the vulnerabilities of particular bodies.[44] Activist voices lead by insisting on all that people with disabilities can do with the proper accommodations. The Independent Living Movement that emerged in the 1970s described care as a form of "benign oppression,"[45] its very name signaling an aspiration to shake off the help of others. Advocates pointed to a long history in which care has been used to control or disempower people with disabilities.[46] But as we will see in the next section, history also tells us that dependency was not always the stigma it has become in the modern era. Instead of downplaying the fact that some people with disabilities need extra care, this book takes them as paradigmatic figures of the uneven interdependency of all living beings. When we center the frame of analysis on the fact of our shared vulnerability, people with disabilities and their supporters become a resource, modeling how dependency can coexist with dignity, sometimes honing interdependency to an art. On the flip side, people with disabilities have insight about the expense and indignities of being dependent in a world that values independence, self-reliance, and personal freedom. Their hardships and achievements are a form of embodied knowledge that can help us better understand and, perhaps, reimagine the status of care in our society.

It is also useful to distinguish "independence" from related terms like "autonomy" or "sovereignty," all of which make frequent appearances over the course of this book. Although "independence" and "autonomy" are often used synonymously, the latter can coexist with various forms of dependency, which would be antithetical to the former. For those who are dependent, autonomy is the opportunity to direct the circumstances under which care is given, expressing preferences and making choices to the extent that one is capable. Although the U.S. Constitution makes no mention of autonomy, the United Nations Convention on the Rights of Persons with Disabilities' list of "human rights and fundamental freedoms" includes "respect for ... individual autonomy including the freedom to make one's own choices."[47] Chapter 5 will complicate the notion of "individual autonomy" by looking at cases where satisfying one individual's desires and needs may impinge on those of another. It explores how writers with extreme forms of physical disability negotiate care they need for dignified survival with caregivers, who have their own claims to personhood and autonomy. "Sovereignty" is a related concept, having more to do with self-government than action. In the arena of politics, it typically means possession of power and authority; however, the anthropologist Danilyn Rutherford introduces the notion of "sovereignty of vulnerability," which recognizes the agency that dependent people exert in their capacity to elicit the care they need or want. Although people with the most significant levels of dependency might seem to lack sovereignty, she asserts that "they institute a web of obligations when they demand a response."[48] Rutherford comes to this understanding by applying a bracing dose of Derridean philosophy to the case of her non-verbal but highly communicative daughter with autism. She writes vividly of environments where Millie exerts this kind of authority and invites us to imagine "alternative worlds" where the sovereignty of vulnerability is recognized and valued.

When Rutherford writes of the "alternative worlds" that might be or might have been, she calls for a visionary act, akin to the "disability worlds" that Faye Ginsberg and Rayna Rapp describe hopefully as "projects of cultural creativity and reinvention."[49] It is a challenging theoretical puzzle for philosophers to rethink such fundamental concepts as personhood, dependency, and the meaning of a good life. To produce a corresponding shift in collective attitudes will also entail powerful feats of imagination and feeling. This book begins with the assumption that any change in beliefs, cultural practices, or institutions of law and society requires an underlying reorientation of how we imagine the value of a life, its need for sustaining care, and its interconnection with other lives. Aesthetics is my gateway to the imagination. In a well-known formulation, Jacques Rancière connects aesthetics to politics, with his description of "aesthetic acts" as "configurations of experience that create new modes of sense perception and induce novel forms of political subjectivity."[50] In other words, art can motivate shifts in feeling that guide how we act in the world. Aesthetics is especially salient to the disabled body, which tends to disrupt the feelings and perceptions of those in its vicinity, triggering such sensations as fear, disgust, solicitude, pity, or curiosity. With disability in mind, Tobin Siebers writes that aesthetics "defines the process by which human beings attempt to modify themselves, by which they imagine their feelings, forms, and futures in radically different ways, and by which they bestow upon these new feelings, forms, and futures real appearances in the world."[51] These accounts of aesthetic activity as an endeavor to galvanize the senses, perceive the environment differently, and communicate new perceptions to others inform my recognition of narrative and visual forms as a resource for deepening and potentially transforming how we understand the meaning and value of care. When I refer to the "art of interdependency" or "artful care," I mean to emphasize not only the ways that caring relations have been represented in creative expression but also the creativity and resourcefulness of dependents and caregivers who have figured out how to do interdependency with panache.

As I looked for perspective on the arts of care, I turned to narrative because of my training as a literary and cultural critic. Narrative is not the only place to go, but it is the one I know best. Across the wide and varied range of questions I have posed over my career, I've found narrative a rich point of access into the nuances of a shared cultural imagination, a loose term I use to describe the storehouse of images, stories, beliefs, and other points of reference available to those who inhabit the same time and place. Care may be hard to document in billable hours or a job description, but it can be represented. And the narratives explored in this book attest to the varied forms that authors and artists have used to depict experiences and perceptions of caring and being cared for. A narrative representation can communicate silence, absence, vacancy, as well as presence. The insights that narrative provides are not as straightforward as the hypothetical examples or thought experiments favored by philosophers and bioethicists. I am drawn to accounts that are thickly textured and sometimes contradictory, capable of revealing ambivalence, conflict, and difference. Reading with care, I look for what is unsaid, as well as what is manifest, the ambiance communicated among people or an environment, as well as any direct account of time, place, and event. I will often use the terms "narrative" and "story" interchangeably. Narrative is the more precise term for representational choices that give shape and meaning to the raw material of lived or imagined events. But "story" has a colloquial ring to it that often feels more appropriate to describing the way people communicate experience to one another.

I am not the first to claim that narrative representation is fundamental to understanding care. The philosopher Maurice Hamington writes, "Care is most adequately reflected in the stories of people's lives, where more is brought to light than the rules or outcomes of a given situation. Those interested in care would do well to investigate literature as well as first-person stories to discover the degree to which care flows through everyday experience."[52] We tell stories to explain the origin and importance of our needs, commitments, and resources. Personal stories of those involved in giving and receiving care are a form of embodied knowledge, which can also be communicated in fiction and other narrative forms. Stories are especially valuable to understanding the particular and context-specific dimensions of care. But stories are more than reflections of lived reality. Their forms may communicate meanings that enhance, complement, or contradict more explicit content. Stories can be deceptive, multivalent, or otherwise unreliable. Multiple tellers may see things differently, and one telling may invite competing interpretations. There is also meaning in the unsaid, the gaps, silences, and omissions that break up a narrative flow. Whereas philosophers often prefer the representative case, writes Amelia De Falco, "literature is elaborate, specific, and interpretively enigmatic enough to express the multiple, often irresolvable dilemmas of care, the simultaneous impossibility and necessity of responding to the needs of others."[53] For De Falco, "literature" refers to narrative fiction in print. I take the lead provided by these critics and run with it, adding diversity by drawing examples from such media as novels and short stories, life writing, visual arts, journalism, essays, films, and theater. Across these varied forms, I explore not only how narrative contributes to and reinforces cultural biases that see dependent bodies as ugly, wasteful, and burdensome but also how it intervenes to reshape prevailing understandings of dependency and care work.

Along the way, I will also tell stories of my own. I hope these will enliven the work of critical analysis but also ground my claims in situated knowledge that comes from my own experience. My standpoint includes my role as a teacher and a writer but also a person who has been both a recipient and a provider of care. Like all human animals, I am, in the words of Kittay, "some mother's child," although my mother died when I was very young, so I have few memories of being mothered. Good care is, by definition, forgettable, but I have memories of care's absence. This vacancy has profoundly shaped my experience of being a mother, a role I eagerly assumed but that has never felt natural or the least bit intuitive. Much of my thinking about care has been forged while parenting my children, including a son with multiple disabilities that make him exceptionally dependent. *Raising Henry* was the title of my last book, but it is also the theme of this one, which has been inspired, hampered, and forcibly squeezed into existence by our life-altering interdependency.

Writing a memoir also made me especially aware of what narrative cannot do. A reviewer for this book manuscript described it as having "almost CBT-like faith in the possibility of exposing the unpleasant economic, intersubjective, and historical details of caregiving." Their words made me realize that I need to be more upfront about the limits of my archive and my methods or risk sounding hopelessly naïve and optimistic. I am well aware that narratives can lie and misdirect and also can have no notable impact at all. Hearing other people's stories *might* stir us to new insights or even action but not necessarily toward solving the social problems they expose, since they can just as easily inspire denialism, magical thinking, or complacency. Narratives are not going to create a more functional welfare state, provide respite to exhausted care workers, or give dependent people the support they need to thrive. Nonetheless, I am convinced that it is worthwhile to practice a reading method that finds traces of care (or its concerted erasure, also a trace) absolutely everywhere in the cultural narratives that give meaning to our lives, as well as a set of stories that make care work central. I felt this might be true when I started to write, and it has only become more evident when I have opportunities to present my work on this book. Stories reflect and propagate our eagerness to listen, tell, and deliberate a central problem of our time: Why care?

CARE: A BRIEF AND PARTIAL
HISTORY AND A POLITICS

My first axiom bears repeating: *The need for care is universal among human animals, although its norms are historically and culturally specific.* We cannot understand problems of the present without knowledge of the past. While care has a longer association with sorrow, concern, and burden, its connotation as a sustaining activity, "charge, oversight, attention, or heed with a view to safety and protection," first arose in the English language in the 1400s.[54] In a preindustrial social order where most people were subjects rather than citizens, care was the obligation of the ruling class toward those below. Dependency was the norm, with relationships founded on mutual reliance between powerful men and their subordinates. The hierarchy of feudal society was replicated within individual households, where each person had an assigned role. Wives, children, and servants were socially and legally beholden to the family patriarch, who was duty-bound to protect and provide for them. I don't want to romanticize: it goes without saying that such societies made inequalities of class and gender seem natural and right. Yet care was distributed in ways that allowed the contributions of men and women alike to be considered work that was valuable and necessary to the survival of family and society.[55] Who gets classed as dependent, and what it means to care for them, has varied over the course of history. Nancy Fraser and Linda Gordon argue that "dependency" is an ideological term whose shifting meaning tracks changing "assumptions about human nature, gender roles, the causes of poverty, the nature of citizenship, the sources of entitlement, and what counts as work and a contribution to society."[56] I would add health and ability to this list and note that the value and assignment of caring responsibilities are directly related to definitions of dependency at any given time.

Conceptions of dependency and care changed in the era of industrialization and the introduction of wage labor, which sharpened social divisions, reinforcing the separation and gendering of public and private, work and domestic life, paid and unpaid labor. New democracies in the United States and Europe made ownership of one's labor the avenue to rights and political representation. Independence, once associated with possession of land or wealth, was redefined as the capacity to work, meaning that it was within reach of all able-bodied white, male citizens. As paid labor was valorized over domestic activities, the time-consuming, physically taxing maintenance of the home, including care of dependent children, the elderly, and disabled, became increasingly invisible as work. "Work" became an activity done predominantly by men, especially among more privileged classes, where women did not seek paid employment outside the home. Under this new regime, dependency, which had once been the norm, became a stigma associated with economically marginalized groups such as paupers, single women, and nonwhite people, and it took on moral associations with weakness, inability, and poor character.[57] These changes set the stage for the modern problems of care that are the primary focus of this book.

Another important development in the history of care is the rise of the welfare state, which made citizens' well-being an important responsibility of government. In its more generous versions, most obviously in Western Europe, welfare benefits extended to all citizens, while in other cases, like that of the United States, they were available only to needy groups like the poor, sick, and disabled.[58] Early welfare programs in the United States entrenched the stigma of dependency by separating "entitlements" for the elderly and unemployed—understood to deserve the support of a system to which they had contributed—from "aid" for the dependent poor—seen as getting something for nothing. Those who qualified for social security were called "claimants," worthy recipients whose benefits were intended to forestall the dependencies that otherwise befell the elderly.[59] Where initially many U.S. welfare programs were targeted toward white recipients, over the course of the twentieth century dependency became increasingly racialized, its stigma heightened by the association with women of color, particularly Black women. The figure of the slatternly, promiscuous welfare queen was born in a 1976 campaign speech delivered by Ronald Reagan, who promised to stem the wasteful flow of money to women who were lazy and undeserving. Under the presidency of Bill Clinton, welfare reform limited payments and made them contingent on the recipient's efforts to find work.[60] "Workfarist" policy increasingly channeled women of color into care work, which was readily available and considered "unskilled labor" that could be done by even the least-qualified employees. A double standard of care guided this stingy welfare state, affirming more affluent women for staying at home to raise their children while obligating poor mothers to work, even if the majority of their income went to pay other people to watch their children.[61]

The redistribution of care responsibilities was high on the initial agenda of second-wave feminism, which sought to increase the numbers of women in the workforce but also to recognize domestic chores as work and distribute them more equitably among members of a household. Feminist conversations reframed housework and childcare not as the natural domain of women but as drudgery performed under duress. In *The Feminine Mystique*, Betty Friedan decried the tedium of suburban domestic life and its unrewarding parade of endless, redundant chores.[62] Adrienne Rich's poem "Snapshots of a Daughter-in-Law" described an aging beauty, her mind "moldering like wedding cake / heavy with useless experience," and the fed-up housewife "banging the coffee pot into the sink."[63] One obvious solution to this gender trouble was to require men to do their share. The soundtrack of the popular 1972 children's album *Free to Be You and Me* included the song "Housework," which reasonably suggested that the hated but necessary burden of domestic chores could be lessened if everybody in the family did their part. Another feminist innovation was "wages for housework," a short-lived international movement that advocated pay for all forms of care work.[64] It would prove easier for women to find paid work outside the home, however, than to create policies that paid them to stay at home or to more equitably distribute the responsibilities of unpaid care.

It was both a sign of feminist success and of changing economic imperatives when the 2000 U.S. Census first reported a majority of families listed both parents as wage earners. But as increasing numbers of women entered the workforce, conversations about care fell out of the mainstream feminist agenda, particularly in the United States. Instead of demanding that men do an equal part of household chores and dependent care, women who worked more often did double duty or hired other women to clean their homes and care for their children.[65] Feminist priorities also turned away from those who did care work for a living, especially those employed informally in other people's homes.

More recently, the political agendas of feminists, BIPOC, and organized labor have realigned to advocate for domestic workers, including
care providers, who continue to be among the most poorly compensated and undervalued of all workers.[66]

The history of modern care is further shaped by the professionalization of medicine and development of medical technologies. Until the
late nineteenth century, most health care occurred at home, where the sick
and disabled were tended to by women in their own families, sometimes under the direction of a local healer. The emergence of profes-
sionalized medicine meant that health care increasingly fell under the
purview of trained doctors. Some new procedures required special
equipment that could only be administered by professionals in designated environments.[67] Hospitals rose to new prominence as settings for
surgery, medical care, and healing. However, the hospital's status as the
primary space of health care would be short lived since extended stays
are extremely expensive. By the time of the Great Depression, the U.S.
government was already seeking to relieve hospitals of financial burden
and overcrowding by relocating care for the elderly, disabled, and
chronically ill to the home. In a period of widespread unemployment,
returning medically fragile dependents to their homes had the added
benefit of creating jobs for visiting nurses, as well the first cohort of
paid companions and home health care workers.[68]

The "rehoming" of health care was further hastened toward the end
of the twentieth century, as medical devices became more portable
and user-friendly.[69] Care that once required bulky equipment could
increasingly be administered at home. Complex machinery became small,
compact, and mobile, simplified for use by patients or their caregivers.
Computerization allowed consumers' vital information to be transmitted to medical experts without a professional intermediary.[70] I got a
taste of the brave new world of home health care technology when we
briefly tried a CPAP for Henry's sleep apnea. The machine arrived in a
typewriter-sized case containing a small control box with a flexible
tube connected to a mask that would strap over the nose and mouth.
After a quick lesson, I found myself in charge of operating, cleaning,
and maintaining this sophisticated medical device, which was designed

to keep his airway open during sleep and also transmit information about nighttime breathing patterns to his doctor. It was easy enough to work, but there was no instruction in how to persuade Henry to use it properly, and this is where my home nursing abilities failed. I had some success at getting him to wear the thing. I called it "the Gonzo mask," after the beaked blue daredevil he loved from *The Muppet Show,* and wrote him a homemade book about how to use it. He was game and got used to the strange feeling of air whooshing into his nose and mouth. He even fell asleep wearing it. But soon after, he would take the mask off to shift into his preferred sleeping position. The machine that so effortlessly sent data to Henry's doctor also communicated with our insurance company. After about a month, they reported that he wasn't wearing the mask for the required four-hour minimum and declined to pay for us to keep the machine.

I can't say I regretted the loss of this time-consuming addition to our bedtime routine. I never got around to learning the machine's cleaning and maintenance requirements, which would have added to my list of caregiving chores. Absent the CPAP, Henry's sleep apnea has not been disabling enough to seek further treatment. But it gave me a glimpse of what it means to be responsible for a medical device that takes up space and requires the regular attention of family or other unpaid caregivers. Forget about enlisting the help of a teenaged babysitter or kindly neighbor who offers to drop in to watch your kid once in a while. To be sure, in many households such equipment keeps vulnerable people alive and allows them to be included as part of a family and community. Some have welcomed the autonomy, ease, and portability it provides. No doubt others find using and maintaining elaborate medical technology at home a crushing burden. It's ugly and time consuming, and can limit the options for nonspecialized caregivers. There is no question of its utility for hospital management, which has economized by discharging patients who were sicker and more medically involved to their homes or to outpatient facilities, offloading much of their care onto unpaid family and friends.[71]

The rehoming of care also extends to death and dying. In an illustrated op-ed, the cartoonist-doctor Nathan Gray observes that more

Americans are dying at home than in a hospital for the first time since the early twentieth century. Hospice care—which prioritizes comfort and quality of time at the end of life—was once a small-scale movement built on idealistic principles. But it has become increasingly widespread in the United States, often administered in the patient's own home. Home hospice makes good business sense, saving money on staffing and freeing up hospital space.[72] It is also popular with consumers, many of whom embrace the idea of dying at home, cared for by loved ones in a familiar environment. Sometimes hospice fulfills its promise of a good death, but the realities of dying at home can be exhausting and disruptive to caregivers. "Seeing the brutal realities of caring for a sick loved one at home has sobered my enthusiasm for sending people home to die," Gray writes.[73] The current system relies heavily on unpaid labor. His illustrations depict traumatized family members, the upheaval of domestic space and routines, and limited access to professional advice or care. In one panel, he listens somberly while a tearful caregiver confesses her burnout. They stand outside, suggesting that the space of her own home has become oppressive and inhospitable (figure 0.3).

My own experience of home hospice was far from ideal. My dying father was examined by a visiting nurse who prescribed medications for his pain, ordered a hospital bed and some oxygen, and then left. Her job was to direct his care but not to provide it. We had questions. When my stepmother called the helpline, she got a recording. No actual human was available to advise us, even over the phone. This made us uncomfortable, so we started the whole process over with a different hospice provider. Friends rearranged the furniture to accommodate a bed in the dining room, while the intimate work of tending to my father fell to my stepmother, my sister, and me. None of us had the slightest experience with care at the end of life. After my father died, the hospital bed and oxygen tanks sat in the dining room for days—a reminder of his suffering and far-from-peaceful end—until they could be picked up by a short-staffed supply company. I still wonder what it would have been like if other people had been there to take responsibility for cleaning, tending to the space, and managing pain. Maybe I would have been more present, attuned to the significance of a momentous life event.

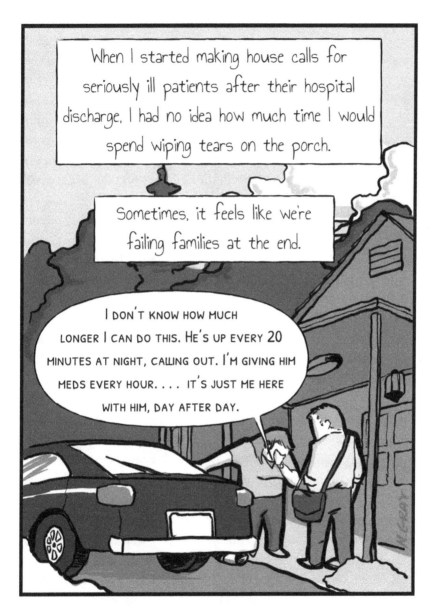

FIGURE 0.3 A frame from Dr. Nathan Gray's graphic op-ed about dying at home shows a visiting doctor witnessing the burdens of caring for a gravely ill person. The toll it takes on caregivers inspired him to write this comic.

Source: Nathan Gray op-ed, "So You Think You Want to Die at Home?" (2020). © Nathan Gray.

But maybe I am idealizing a more institutional environment. Maybe it would have diminished death, rendering it impersonal and sterilized. Maybe I want to rationalize an experience that should be mysterious and will always be difficult, regardless of where it happens. Is it better for those of us who live on to know that we respected my father's wish not to be in the hospital, or to have avoided the fear, mess, and emotional strain of caring for a dying person? There is no way to answer such questions, except to say that they exemplify the contradictions of interdependency, care, and work in the modern world that are the subject of chapters to come.

Not all adult dependents are sick or dying, and the care they require may not be medical. Many people with intellectual disabilities are healthy but not what most would consider "independent." Their care has followed a similar historical pattern of rehoming, first moving from domestic to institutional settings and then, over the past fifty years, increasingly returning to family and community. Throughout much of human history, people with disability-related dependencies who survived infancy and childhood were cared for by their families. Many newborns with congenital disabilities were allowed to die to avoid the burden of their care, and many others died for lack of the kind of medical care that has become routine in the modern world. It is also worth noting that the category of disability—and the dependencies associated with it—has changed over time, along with changing definitions of work. When work consisted mostly of agricultural labor or domestic chores, a physically robust person with an intellectual disability might not have been dependent. Meanwhile, a person with mobility impairments might have been unable to do physical labor but can, with appropriate accommodations, succeed in a more modern, white-collar profession. And the majority of the "very old," a huge proportion of the world's dependent population today, would not have enjoyed such longevity in the past. This is to say that, over time, new dependencies arise while others are mitigated by medicine, technology, or changing norms. Chapter 7 will detail the emergence of an institutional culture designed to manage and/or reform a population that includes those known as idiots, the feebleminded, and the insane,[74] as well as unprecedented numbers of frail elders, particularly those with dementia. I look more closely at how institutions fail to care but also, perhaps more surprisingly, at their crucial role in supplementing or replacing family on the front lines.

The history sketched here and in the chapters that follow concentrates largely on North America, with some detours into Western Europe when relevant. I focus on those regions because they—along with China and Japan—are most immediately confronting a demographic shift in which rising numbers of dependents outpace traditional approaches to caring for them. Never before in human history have there been more people in need of care than those capable of providing for them. This is climate change of a different kind, where our built environments and social networks are becoming increasingly inhospitable to our needs. Its challenges, and any solutions we devise, will have global implications. We tend to think of care in terms of intimate, face-to-face encounters, but its transactions are embedded in larger networks that ultimately extend across the planet. The care industry has become a major economic force, driven by imperatives of growth and profit rather than the needs of dependent people.[75] Changing demographic, economic, political, and technological conditions in wealthier regions have created a rising demand for paid caregivers. Those jobs are increasingly being taken by migrants driven by precarious economies and the decline of traditional occupations like subsistence agriculture in their own countries.[76] The economies of nations like the Philippines, Tibet, Mexico, and India have become heavily dependent on foreign remittances, many from workers in caregiving professions.[77] Nannies from the Philippines and Tibet are prized by a global elite because their cultures are reputed to value superior caregiving.[78] Migrant women have created a "global care chain" that supplements the economies of their homelands but drains them of other equally vital and far less fungible resources. The absence of mothers, wives, sisters, and daughters introduces a deficit of care for those they leave behind.[79] The sociological research on migrant nurses, nannies, home health aids, and personal attendants provides a basis for the discussion of stories about paid domestic care in chapter 6.[80]

There we will see how the history of Western colonialism shadows local caregiving arrangements, meaning that representations of paid care in North America and Europe, where people (usually women) chafe under the obligations of caring for dependent family members, almost inevitably lead outward to other parts of the world, where people (usually women) need work badly enough to travel. Reading with care involves looking for evidence of those global care chains, sometimes finding it in the margins, minor characters, and peripheral narrative vision and sometimes front and center of the stories we tell about modern familial life.

Care has no inherent politics, although it is highly susceptible to politicization. What activities count as caregiving, who is responsible for doing them, who is seen as deserving of care, and what resources we are willing to give to sustain them are all political questions. Care can easily be enlisted by political conservatives to make the case for a return to "traditional" families where some women stay at home or for compelling other women to work for wages instead of getting government support to care for their children. Care is often a term for medical paternalism aimed at women, parents, the poor, or people with disabilities. The politics of care become biopolitical as they enter the domain of population management, regulating our bodies in the name of national health, safety, and well-being. Care can be given or withheld according to moral judgments about sexual practices, gender identity and embodiment, reproductive health, and education. Care also concerns the political left in arguments for a more expansive welfare state, universal health insurance, workers' rights, and affordable preschool. Its politics extend beyond the human, to causes like more sustainable food systems, animal welfare, and protecting wildlife and the environment. The notion of "self-care," which may appear apolitical, looks less so when it is marshaled to sell expensive products and services or justify turning away from the problems of others. Practices like mindfulness, exercise, and positive thinking have a different politics when applied to marginalized people—women of color, crips, or queers—who are liable to wear themselves out working on behalf of communities or causes and badly need avenues for replenishment and repair.

The notion of "radical care" has become current across a spectrum of political agendas. When coupled with "self-care" (as in "radical self-care"), it often means attending to the physical or emotional well-being of those dedicated to activism or community organizing. In the meme-ified words of Audre Lorde, "caring for myself is not self-indulgence, it is self-preservation, and that is an act of political warfare."[81] Premila Nadasen defines "radical care" as explicitly tied to leftist politics, "alternative and transformative care practices emerging from and connected to social movement organizing."[82] A 2020 special issue of the journal *Social/Text* describes radical care as "fundamental to social movements," a bridge between the individual and collective causes ranging from environmental protection to immigration policy to health care. The editors, Hiʻilei Julia Kawehipuaakahopulani Hobart and Tamara Kneese, define "radical care as a set of vital but underappreciated strategies for enduring precarious worlds."[83] I appreciate this work and the growing critical attention to "care" it has introduced across a range of disciplines and political projects. I welcome the diverse range of causes and activities that have been conceived as forms of care while hewing, in my own work, to the narrower definition of care as "the intimate and necessary labor required to sustain those who are dependent." *Why care?* I hope that this book will complement those conversations, showing the timeliness and urgency of bolstering our fragile systems of care and recognizing the exchange of care as a source of value, meaning, and creative possibility.

THE CHAPTERS AND THE SHAPE OF THE BOOK

Following this introduction, *Love, Money, Duty* consists of three parts and a coda. It is organized around the premise that the dynamics of care, while highly particular, are also structured by the social roles and spaces where it is given and received. I shape the topics of individual chapters around subject positions and environments of care, starting with the first and most intimate caring relationship between people who identify as mothers and the children who receive their care, then moving outward to the unpaid exchange of care in other familial relationships to paid care work in the home to institutions of care to caring machines. Stories about my own experiences of caring and being cared for will surface periodically in these chapters, a reminder of the standpoint that anchors my work as a scholar and writer. The book can be read sequentially, but it should also make sense to the reader who approaches it more selectively, opting to concentrate on particular chapters or read them out of order.

Part 1, "Next of Kin," focuses on care within the home and family, an umbrella term that includes biological and chosen relationships. I define "family" here as a configuration of individuals who share a private, domestic space and some sense of obligation to care for one another. Laden with assumptions of heterosexuality and other social norms, family is a crucible for forging expectations and practices of care that have radiating consequences for the world beyond home. "Familialism" is the name for the formation of unpaid care relations in a household, as well as the social logic that presumes legal and biological families to be the first responders when it comes to care.

Chapter 1 is about mothering, which I define as the essential caring activity required by all human animals, as well as the culturally constructed ideas and assumptions about the relationship between mother and child. More specifically, I address stories of "extreme mothering," about women caring for children in exceptional states of dependency. Because their experiences are so unusual, they make aspects of more ordinary mothering seem strange, opening what might seem to be natural or common sense to scrutiny and analysis. They describe worst-case scenarios but also offer strategies for survival and understanding in conditions where child care does not lead to the expected outcomes of growth, development, and independence. Chapter 2 is about the recent cohort that I call Gen S, siblings of disabled children who require extensive care and live at home. It delves into the sibling's unique standpoint as a witness and sometimes a participant in the work of care, as well as being the person who has the longest relationship with a dependent brother or sister across many life stages. Gen S narratives adopt creative forms as they testify to care otherwise concealed within domestic space. They can be unsparing in detailing the grim and isolating work, but they also describe family as an incubator for long-term, and sometimes artful, interdependencies, and they find meaning in lives spent in dependency or in caring for dependent people.

Couples and/or other chosen family configurations are the concentric circle of chapter 3, which looks at circumstances where care is suddenly thrust to the center of an adult relationship. It focuses on a historical moment when such scenarios were widespread, the early AIDS epidemic and the unexpected dependencies that made care a priority within queer families. The ubiquity of grave illness and the failure of traditional medical and political institutions forced couples and/or communities to invent caring arrangements that would have a lasting effect on health care and social services. Chapter 4 is about children and parents, gender and age-related dependency. It stages a dialogue of sorts between memoirs by women with dementia and those of the adult daughters who care for them. This is not a pleasant conversation and rarely involves anything like a neat circuit of reciprocity. Instead, the intergenerational exchange of care is fraught with misunderstanding, resentment, and expense, with occasional glimpses of harmony, and even reward. These stories experiment, at the level of form, with how to depict what Elinor Fuchs describes as "The Emergency" of impending dependency and the challenges of eroding self-awareness.

Part 2, "The Subjects of Care," is a single chapter about the memoirs of adult dependents, some with congenital disabilities that require lifelong care and others disabled in midlife. I am interested in how the onset of disability in a life course shapes attitudes toward care and how dependent people recognize and coexist with their caregivers. This is where the problem of autonomy and the sovereignty of vulnerability come front and center, as dependent people grapple with how to maintain the dignity of a self-direction that also relies so heavily on the care of others. I also consider how extreme dependency forces an interesting reckoning with genre as memoir—a literary form that seems to reflect the independence idealized by the disability and patients' rights movements—is adapted to acknowledge dependency and the work of those who maintain the body of the author. I explore the varied narrative strategies authors develop to represent autonomy-in-dependency, as well as how and why they represent the personhood and agency of their caregivers.

Part 3, "Professing Care," turns to paid care work. These chapters confront the awkward alignment of care with the temporalities of capitalism: wage labor, the time clock, hourly pay, and the shift or workday. Chapter 6 is about paid care work in the home, usually involving a direct exchange of cash for services. Where the previous chapter emphasized adult dependents with considerable autonomy, this chapter features relationships triangulated by a third party who is responsible for managing and paying the care provider. Paying attention to theory of mind—the process whereby one person makes necessary but imperfect sense of the opaque interiority of another—it looks, first, at narratives about the fraught dynamics between mothers and the nannies they hire to care for their children. Then it turns to narratives about care of adult dependents; the uncertain status of a paid caregiver whose place of work is another person's home; the meaning of work that involves such seemingly passive states as waiting, sitting, and biding time; and the coexistence of radically different perceptions of the same banal environments and events. Chapter 7 moves out of the home to institutions with a mission of care for dependent persons. As I define them, institutions are organizations where care work is distributed beyond family and home and where the mechanics of management and compensation operate at a remove from the exchange of care. It begins with the "asylum classics" of Ken Kesey, Sylvia Plath, and Susanna Kaysen, all of which criticize the impersonality and abuses of modern psychiatric hospitals. More surprisingly, Plath and Kaysen also find healing away from home and under the care of strangers, experiencing asylum in the more positive sense. The second part of the chapter looks to a newer and more diverse collection of voices and settings that represent communal care in the era of deinstitutionalization and the privatization of health care. While these works do not provide solutions to the problems of modern institutional care, they show the dire consequences of its absence, as well as glimpses of how and when caring institutions succeed.

Prompted by my disabled son's intimate and loving relationships to things, the coda, "Caring Machines," considers the care robot. A literary figure that is now increasingly a reality, care robots inspire me to reflect on those aspects of care that are unique to human beings and on those situations where caring machines might be effectively enlisted as partners in our caring activities.

I abandoned my first effort to draft this introduction in the summer of 2020, when it became clear that the global pandemic, and the care webs that it had so abruptly torn away, was not going to end anytime soon. In a passage I typed, excised, and recopied in a different context I wrote, "It is hard to understand how barely moving, accomplishing so little in a day can make me so tired. It helps me to remember that care for the self and for others is work, even if not the kind that will be recognized with money or professional acclaim." Feeling the need to make sense of my circumstances by writing *something*, I also found new forms more suited to the time and place—a short article with a very specific assignment, a personal essay, a comic—reminding me that care can be generative, although not always in the ways we expect.

The years of pandemic also burnished the form of this book. Narrative has the capacity to hide the work of care, as when it equates personal beauty with independence, erasing the many people, resources, and effort that contributed to making a single person appear beautiful. Books themselves are massive exercises in denial, shearing away not only the hours and pages of effort that went into their production but also the care work done by others that allows us to write at all. Narrative also has the capacity to make less valued forms of effort visible. I had always intended to write about my experiences as a care giver and recipient, to expose work that is typically hidden or banished to the acknowledgments, where we express gratitude for the people who sustain us, manage our homes and places of work, and watch our children while we write. But that form took on new urgency once the work of writing had to happen on the same bed where I slept, read the newspaper, held office hours over Zoom, helped my son with his home-work, and worried about expenses with my husband. The compression of my life convinced me that the *only* adequate form for this book would be a tapestry that weaves together stories of my own labors of care with more critical reflections about its representation. That is what I have done, and I hope it will be a document of otherwise invisible labor, my own and that of countless others; a tribute to the many people and resources that sustained me during the work of writing; and a resource to draw on during times of need inevitably to come.

I

NEXT OF KIN

1

THE FOLDED TIMESCAPES
OF MATERNAL CARE

I n caring, time is folded," writes Maggie Nelson. "One is attending to
the effects of past actions, attempting to mitigate present suffering,
and doing what one can to reduce or obviate future suffering, all at
once." [1] Nelson uses this lyrical image to explain how it is imaginatively
possible to mother when the future of your own particular child is
bound up with the escalating malaise of the planet. Folded time
accounts for how a mother can care, simultaneously, in the present and
in the future, for a currently living being and lives to come, about a
single, beloved person and life itself. All care requires an awareness of
past and future, often paradoxically conjoined with intense absorption
in the present moment. But maternal care is special, involving the particular interdependencies of parent and child; the sometimes-acute
clashes between a mother's experience of temporality and that of her
children; and the weight of cultural assumptions about gender, race,
biological, and social reproduction. Maternal care, and the elaborate
folds of time it requires when the future is in doubt, is the subject of this
chapter. But where Nelson becomes aware of time's folding through the
increasingly palpable signs of climate crisis, I emphasize how time is
bent out of shape when dependency intersects differences of race, gender, and ability. Long before evidence of planetary malaise universal-
ized the challenge of parenting into uncertain horizons, mothers of

people with disabilities and nonwhite mothers struggled to care in the face of grim or impossible futures. Their collective wisdom offers cautionary tales, as well as resources for caring in dire times, even as it points to the limits of taking any one caregiving narrative as an exemplary model.

"Mothering" seems like an obvious place to start this book, since it is a starting point for the experience of care. All human animals are born dependent and require mothering to survive. Because the phase of infant dependency is universal, as is the experience of being mothered, mothering is often held up as the paradigm for care ethics.[2] As feminist thinkers sought to redirect moral philosophy toward the activities and values important to women, mothering seemed like the ideal model for the virtues of nurture, generosity, and relatedness.[3] In the introduction, I described the liabilities that can come from idealizing motherhood, but they are worth reiterating here. I am interested in actual mothers, who are imperfect, compromised, and complicated as any other human animals. To equate mothering with caring virtue is to risk overlooking the oppressive burden childcare places on many of those actual mothers; it can constrain their choices about how and if they will engage in the work of caregiving, and make them targets of criticism for all the ways they fail to measure up to an imagined ideal.[4] Mothering is also easily conflated with biological reproduction and the hardwired behaviors it allegedly triggers. But we human animals have spent millennia developing social practices and institutions to distribute the care of children beyond those who have the fleshly machinery for pregnancy and birth. Janine Antoni's *Umbilical*, the artwork on the cover of this book, reflects on mothering as a relation that may begin in biology but is always mediated by artifacts and social practices. My concern is with the cultural construction of care we call mothering rather than its biological dimensions. Although this chapter focuses on the perspectives of those who identify as women, occupy the social role of mother, and care for dependent children to whom they are related by biological reproduction, the caveats I have just identified are never far from my mind. They allow me to explore what is at stake in centering mothers as an ethical prototype, the obligations this entails for actual mothers, and the extreme feats of imagination required of those whose responsibilities are far in excess of any established cultural scripts.

I also take the risk of starting with mothers because my own standpoint as a caregiver is so powerfully shaped by the experience of being one. I identify with many of the familial roles explored in this book—I am also a sibling, somebody's child, and a spouse—but my embodied knowledge of caregiving has come primarily from being a mother. It is impossible for me to write about care without recognizing how I am particularly and complexly embedded in my subject. I am a textbook "motherless mother."[5] My biological mother died when I was six, after a year and a half of illness.[6] Although my material needs were abundantly met, I have no memories of receiving the kind of care described as mothering, nor do I remember having an even remotely motherly surrogate of any kind. I was raised by a single father, family friends who came and went, and a series of underpaid caregivers. I thought very little about this aspect of my past until I became a mother myself. I now see how my self-understanding is shaped by maternal absence, as is the way I parent my two boys and share caregiving duties with my husband, their father. I have never known motherhood to be natural or effortless, a fact that makes it easier for me to scrutinize an activity many understand to be—at least in its ideal form—instinctual. It is even harder to disentangle my writing about care from my experiences of mothering because much of this book was written—or not being written, to endless frustration—amid a global pandemic that confined my family to a smallish apartment for long stretches of time. I literally could not distance my work as a writer from my work as a caregiver. Every page is marked by the often-disruptive and unwelcome demands of mothering; this also, I hope, infuses it with compassion and perspective.

Like Nelson, my experience of mothering involves "folded time." I try to imbue my children with an understanding of the historic injustice that secures their many privileges, while at the same time attending to their needs, vulnerabilities, and compelling particularities, while at the same time preparing them for an uncertain future. I am acutely aware of the contradiction between my desire to surround them with abundance and the ways our life drains the planet's already-depleted resources. As I indulge in such earnest reflection, I struggle with anger, irritation, and resentment at having to sacrifice my time for the sake of another's development. One of my sons is also intellectually disabled, meaning that the more predictable temporal folds of maternal care are often irrevocably askew. Henry made my sense of developmental time strange from the very beginning. When he was less than six weeks old, an occupational therapist described the way he gripped a rubber ring as "delayed." I wondered how an infant who had only just entered the world could already be delayed, even as—ever the literary critic, reading into things—I appreciated the term's optimistic suggestion that one day he might catch up.

With Henry, my experience of maternal time has been more unevenly folded—perhaps "wadded up" is a better description—than parenting his typically developing brother. In the strictly regimented temporalities of modernity, this wadded-up time of disability—insiders call it "crip time"—shadows certain children, marking them as deficiently slow, belated, or—worst of all—retarded, but also sometimes as unhealthily precocious.[7] Crip time pulls people with disabilities backward or sticks them in place, but it also involves narratives about the future. Getting the resources my son needed to thrive required a story about his limited potential. We justified the therapies and educational supports he has enjoyed by arguing that his opportunities for work, education, and relationships will be more restricted than those of a typical peer but that his future dependency might also be diminished with more help during childhood. For the bureaucrats, Henry's story was not about generative possibility but rather stunted growth. The price of those services was what bioethicists call my son's "right to an open future."[8]

The temporalities of my son's development are also the temporalities of maternal care. People ask me what I plan "to do" about Henry's future, a question they never ask about my typically developing son. The implication is that his need for care will be prolonged, perhaps lifelong, inevitably outlasting his parents' ability to provide it. I don't love the question, but I know that its vision of the future is likely to be accurate. I need somehow to plan for my son's potential long-term dependency without denying him opportunities to grow and have new experiences. I want him to be welcomed in a world that values speed and productivity, even while accepting that he moves at a different pace and on a more meandering path. For now, and the foreseeable future, mothering Henry is a funhouse of maternal time: everything takes longer, goes more slowly or quickly; there are unexpected roadblocks and trap doors and no apparent exit in sight. Mothering Henry has propelled my search for narratives by mothers who have found meaning in the snarled-up time of caring for a disabled child, but it has taken me far beyond a search for analogies to my own (unusual but not exceptional) experience to scenarios of "extreme mothering" that shred the cultural script of maternal care altogether.

Parents who have limned the extremes of maternal time have a lot to teach us about motherly care, and their insights are especially valuable in a world where climate change makes the future of the entire species feel more provisional and less open. This chapter looks at narratives about the limit cases of mothering. I call them "limit cases" because they represent an outer edge so intense that it forces us to define the meaning and purpose of care, distinguishing it from the many other demands and expectations of modern parenting. The child whose radically uneven development never leads to independence of any kind, the child whose development is actually a regression, and the child whose future seems so bleak that death is a better alternative: I go to these borders of extreme parenting because it is there that the most daring and innovative feats of maternal imagination are required to establish the possibilities and limits of caring for another who is interdependent but nonequivalent with the mother's own being. In each case, I am interested in how mothers describe the virtually unthinkable prospect of no future for themselves and/or their children. In finding the emotional and material resources to navigate the unimaginable, they also develop creative forms to challenge the conventions of narrative that dictate the unfolding of a life story.

TIMESCAPES OF MATERNAL CARE

Mothering, like other forms of care, is bound up with questions about time. When linked to reproduction, it begins with the potential conflict between the "biological clock" of the maternal body and the temporalities of a woman's plans for education, career aspirations, and other projects of self-development.[9] Prospective mothers are barraged with contradictory advice about timing, telling them, for example, that younger women are more likely to succeed with conception and pregnancy but that older women are more likely to provide their children with financial and emotional stability. When it comes to biology, there is simply no way to divide the time evenly. Although reproduction requires the contribution of two sets of genetic material, almost all the work is done by the body that bears and gives birth to a new life. Caring for an infant means following the temporalities of the child's body, responding to its demands for feeding, cleaning, sleeping, and socializing. The work of social reproduction—and the sacrifices of time and energy it requires of mothers—follows a similar pattern that endures long after biological reproduction is over and done with. Care pivots to the more regimented time of the clock, with the expectation that children be trained to sleep, wake, eat, learn, exercise, and play on schedule. We scrutinize and judge mothers who over- or underschedule their children. Along the way, time for care of the self is continually overshadowed by the more urgent and socially recognized demands of motherly care.

A poignant reminder of mothering time: After my father died, I found a datebook he had saved from 1974. I was five years old for most of that year. Until somewhere in August, the entries—which include play dates, doctors' appointments, chores, lessons, outings—are penciled in the script I recognize as my mother's. Several weeks are blank. This emptiness marks the period of her worsening symptoms, final hospitalization, and death. Then my father's signature black pen—larger, darker, unmistakably his—takes over. In the midst of writing this chapter, I see the datebook from 1974 as a record of his abrupt, unwanted, and necessary assumption of family care work once done by my mother. I remember him mostly as an imperfect caregiver, but I am moved by the effort to assume management of family time made by a grieving man, older than most fathers in those days, and so far out of his element.

The datebook reflects family norms that position mothers as the keepers of schedules, enforcers of bedtime and morning rituals, observers of developmental milestones, conduits to routine pediatric care. Jack Halberstam describes "family time" critically, in terms of "the normative scheduling of daily life (early to bed, early to rise) that accompanies the practice of child rearing. This timetable is governed by an imagined set of children's needs, and it relates to beliefs about children's health and healthful environments for child rearing."[10] Imagined beliefs indeed: These are the stories we make up to justify care that coexists with our own ideas about a worthwhile life. While this is an apt description of familial time, Halberstam's wording involves a telling absence of subjects. He is writing about work that requires effort, but he uses the passive voice. *Who* is responsible for all that scheduling, meeting of needs, and provision of healthful environments? The missing term is the mother, who is tasked with structuring the present around timetables that promote the child's current well-being and development into a person who can participate in the routines of adult maturity. She is held responsible for damaging her child if she is, say, too rigid during the stage that should be directed by the needs of the infant's body or too relaxed when proper care is supposed to be disciplined. I am also using the passive voice, but more deliberately. *She is tasked*: usually not by any one individual but by our collective values and expectations.

Such expectations reached a nadir in the mid-twentieth century, when the psychiatrist Leo Kanner coined the term "refrigerator mother" to describe a woman whose deficient early care was blamed for her child's autism.[11] So powerful was the impact of a cold, withholding mother that she could corrupt her child's ability to perceive and reciprocate caring feelings. And, at the other end of the spectrum, Philip Wylie's best-selling book *Generation of Vipers* labeled persistently smothering care "momism," accusing overly protective mothers of breeding men who were weak and emasculated.[12] Betty Friedan added an ironic feminist twist to this charge, blaming the feminine mystique not only for oppressing women but for producing "the homosexuality that is spreading like murky smog over the American scene." In Friedan's homophobic reasoning, the excess demanded of contemporary mothers was responsible for an epidemic of gay men, characterized by "passive, childlike immaturity."[13] From the more radical zone of the feminist spectrum, Shulamith Firestone issued an equally dire warning about intensive mothering, asserting that "'raising' a child is tantamount to retarding his development. The best way to raise a child is to LAY OFF."[14] Times change along with social norms, but the scolding admonitions against the dangers of too much or too little maternal care endure into the twenty-first century. Ironically, they have sometimes been fueled, rather than debunked, by the women's movement and the rise of subsequent feminist generations.

A well-known example of the deep entrenchment of cultural associations around maternal care is the heated responses provoked by the photographer Sally Mann's 1992 series *Immediate Family*.[15] Mann is both an artist and a mother, sometimes abandoning her post as protector and helper to get behind the camera and photograph her children. Some images deliberately call attention to motherly absence, such as a photograph of Mann's son lying on the ground with a bloody nose that stains his chin and shirt. Shot from above, it suggests that the photographer grabbed her camera instead of comforting or cleaning up her bleeding child.

In other photos, Mann's children pose nude, at once erotic and vulnerable; her tween daughter stares confrontationally at the camera, a cigarette dangling from her fingers; a young girl, topless, nestles against a man's arm, which stretches down suggestively out of the frame. Some seem to invite a pedophilic gaze; others include adults gazing at or caressing children in the frame. Where is their mother? Could she really be watching from behind the camera? Did she happen on her children in such poses, or, maybe worse, did she direct them? These images provoke us to question. Lest we write them off as examples of the more laissez-faire parenting of an earlier generation, we should remember that the photos were immediately controversial, described by critics as "manipulative," "sick," "twisted," and "vulgar." Mann responded by accusing them of conflating art with reality and of holding outdated, sentimental views on motherly care. The project and the debates it provoked attest to the power of art to make strange the qualities of dependency and care traditionally attributed to women and children and to how jarring it can be to see our expectations about the proper roles for adults and children, creators and subjects of art, unsettled.[16]

While much has been written about the scandal of *Immediate Family*, a less-remarked-upon aspect of Mann's project is the questions it raises about the conflicted timing of maternal care. Parenting is rife with potential conflict between the demands of a dependent child and the mother's own needs and desires. At the time they were photographed, Mann's children were in a transitional stage, far beyond the innate dependencies of infancy but with a debatable capacity to care for themselves or make reasoned decisions about their own safety. Would good care mean keeping these children clean and out of harm's way at all times? Or allowing them to explore and take risks? And who gets to decide? What about the mother's time? What if she wants to spend it developing her art instead of hovering over her children? *Immediate Family* takes these questions out of the realm of private, domestic life and puts them on display in galleries and art museums. It reflects powerfully on the colliding temporalities of the child's maturation and a mother's self-realization, and it asks whether a woman can inhabit, simultaneously, the roles of artist and caregiver or whether those belong to distinct times and places.[17]

Immediate Family's photographs of children who are vulnerable or in danger run afoul of cultural truisms about a child's claim on the future. Across the political spectrum, causes ranging from climate change to health care, gay marriage, education policy, race-based violence, reproductive rights, and taxation use the child as ballast to task the currently living with consideration for future generations. THE FUTURE IS OURS and LIVE AS IF OUR FUTURE MATTERS are familiar slogans that speak in the voice of a child who demands attention, accusing adults of ruining the world for their descendants. When directed at the environment, concerns about the future implicate the entire species, and the whole planet. It's not just queers who have no future, as Lee Edelman and others have influentially claimed.[18] All lives are at risk on a not-too-distant horizon.[19]

But at the scale of a human life, the child's grasp on futurity is unevenly distributed according to race and ability. While queer theory takes the child as an abstract figure, when it comes to particular children, these differences matter a great deal. The lives of children of color may be shaped by the assumption that they have a diminished future, one with fewer opportunities and grimmer outcomes. The poignancy of this social logic is captured by a political cartoon that shows a teacher asking a Black boy what he wants to be when he grows up, to which the boy replies, "alive" (figure 1.1). At the same time, Black children are subject to an accelerated future by "adultification bias," leading to a disproportionate likelihood of incarceration, sexual violence, unwanted pregnancy, and premature death.[20] The disabled child looks to similarly foreshortened horizons, their opportunities shaped by forecasts of a burdensome and unproductive future.

As the parent of a son with Down syndrome, I am often confronted with the contradictions in the disability-related version of the child's claim on the future. Many organizations and causes that support people with disabilities seek our attention with images of cute children or childlike adults (figure 1.2).[21] Aren't they lovable? Disabled children have the same claim to a bright future as other children, they tell us. Filled with potential, they merit opportunities to grow and develop. Care is an investment that will pay off in later maturity and self-sufficiency. But there is another contradictory message, suggesting we should pity these children because they will never enjoy the future open to typical peers. Faced with grim prospects, they appeal to our sympathy and our wallets. There is a reason we call them poster *children*: Disabled adults (and particularly adults with intellectual disabilities) are depressingly unproductive, stalled out, or, worst of all, in states of decline that we do not want to see. At best, images of cheery adults with Down syndrome associate disability with eternal childhood, a future

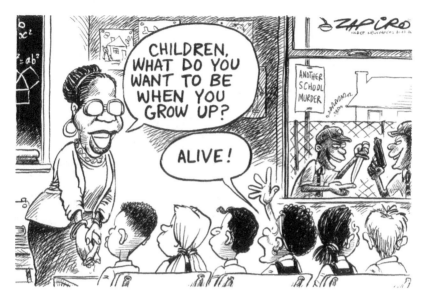

FIGURE 1.1 This cartoon illustrates the uneven distribution of opportunity and well-being according to race.

Source: Zapiro, "What Do You Want to Be When You Grow Up?"
© Zapiro, 2006. Previously published in independent newspapers.

that is limited and tediously redundant; at worst, a disabled future is expensive and painful. If the disabled child can embody hope for normalization into future independence and productivity via the right kinds of care, adults with disabilities are an unwanted reminder of a future of unending dependency, one that is not bright or hopeful or always getting better.

My disabled child's claim on the future is bound up with the weighty presumptions about motherly care that I experience on a daily basis. Mothers are expected to be the first responders when a child departs from the predictable temporalities of development, whether by maturing too soon, too late, or not at all. We assume they will shoulder the obligation to provide or manage care that extends into all foreseeable futures. When the temporalities of a child's development, maturation, and/or lifespan go off the rails, so do the temporalities of motherly care. To get at this conjunction, I turn to stories about the timescapes of

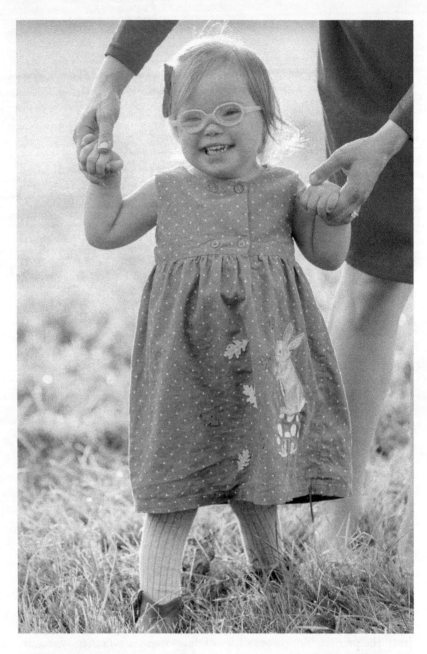

FIGURE 1.2 A publicity photo for the National Down Syndrome Society uses a winsome child to appeal to potential donors and advocates. The girl in the photo is beaming and appears to be healthy. Her clothes and grooming, as well as the adult supporting her effort to walk, suggest that she is well cared-for and worthy of care.

Source: Photo by Margot Rhondeau. © National Down Syndrome Society.

extreme mothering: when a child's physical and intellectual development are out of sync, when a child regresses instead of moving forward, and when a child is seen to have no future at all. Cases where mothering becomes permanently collapsed with a child's pervasive dependency offer exceptional opportunities to think about the possibilities and limits of a given caring relationship and the environments that sustain it. They also present interesting literary challenges. The narrative strategies of more conventional life writing are utterly inadequate to reflect on the temporalities of mothering gone awry, and its forms must be fragmented, warped, and recombined to address the extremity of their subjects.

EXTREME MOTHERING 101:
NARRATIVE TIMESCAPES

I wrote a memoir, *Raising Henry*, because I thought I had something new to say about parenting a child with Down syndrome at a moment when genetic science, education, and social attitudes toward people with disabilities were changing at lightning speed, often in contradictory ways. I also imagined my book as a tribute to precursors like Emily Perl Kingsley and Michael Bérubé, whose writing about their children with Down syndrome had been a lifeline in my early days of parenting Henry.[22] The stories of these parent-authors offered me a kind of embodied theory; their insights about interdependency and care resonated with what I would later discover in queer, disability, and critical race studies but were communicated through personal narratives that also moved and engaged. Kingsley and Bérubé taught me to challenge the normative truisms of child development. I join them in asserting, emphatically, that being slower and more dependent does not mean having no future.[23] In the face of grim doubters, we write with wonder at seeing our children develop, of realizing how much they are capable of doing, and discovering how many of their limitations are imposed by low expectations rather than lack of potential. We insist that, regardless of ability, our boys are more alike than different from any other child. And as a result, our life stories are shaped—more or less—like other life stories that follow a path from infancy toward growth and maturation.

There are good reasons, both literary and political, to follow the conventions of memoir when writing about disabled lives. But sometimes lived reality is so wildly off kilter that the conventions cannot hold. Sometimes experience itself is divergent enough that its story demands a different form. In what follows, I look to narratives about mothering children so far from the tree of normative development that the protocols of life writing must be broken and reassembled: In one example, caring for the child whose development is uneven and never leads to independence of any kind; in another, the child who has no future at all; in a third, the child whose future seems so bleak that death is a better alternative. This is my calculus: I go to the outer reaches of extreme parenting, beyond advice manuals and developmental schedules, where the future can only be conceived (if at all) through the most daring and innovative feats of maternal imagination. In each case, I am interested in how mothers find the resources to care while confronting the virtually unthinkable prospect of no future for themselves and/or their children and in what narrative strategies they use to rescript the conventions of a life story. While few parents will ever find themselves in such exceptional circumstances, we have much to learn from their trials and their creativity, especially as the future for the entire planet looks increasingly grim. We need more strategies to help us care for other humans and our environment even in the face of decline or just maintaining an imperfect now.

In addition to Bérubé and Kingsley, an essential author in my parenting library is Eva Feder Kittay, introduced earlier as a feminist moral philosopher who writes from her standpoint as a mother and a caregiver. Kittay belongs to the first generation of feminist ethicists to make care a subject of serious consideration, her contribution grounded in the experience of parenting a disabled daughter.[24] She uses this position to complicate philosophical discussions of care, autonomy, and development that had, to that point, been organized around an able-bodied norm. Like some other feminists, she conceives the interdependency of mother and child, and the webs of care that sustain them, as foundational to a more just society. But the intensity and prolongation of her daughter's need for care led her to different conclusions than any other feminist philosopher or memoirist of her time. As she rescripts the conventions of moral philosophy—typically premised on an abstracted and impersonal individual subject—she also, at the level of form, rejects the developmental assumptions embedded in more traditional autobiography—that lives unfold according to predictable milestones marked out by chronological time. The result is a generic hybrid, fusing philosophical reasoning with personal writing that both reflects and extends a theory of interdependency and care across the uneven temporalities of mother and child. While Kittay is not alone in inserting her own standpoint into her philosophy, her experience as a mother and caregiver to a multiply disabled daughter made a unique and influential contribution to the ethics of care, as well as life writing by parents.

Sesha is Kittay's protagonist, the motivation and exemplary figure for her philosophical thought. As she is memorably depicted in Kittay's 1999 book *Love's Labor: Essays on Women, Equality, and Dependency*, Sesha is a study in contrasts. At age twenty-seven, she is an attractive woman with dark brown eyes and wavy hair, a lover of music, with a powerful capacity for joy. Alongside these appealing qualities, she also "has no measurable I.Q" and is unable to speak, take herself to the bathroom, walk independently, or eat with utensils. She cannot survive without constant care and supervision. [25] On first reading this account, I was struck by its blunt list of all the things Sesha cannot do. The prevailing wisdom of disability advocacy is to avoid, whenever possible, the negative language of lack and defect in favor of "different abilities" (one could say, for example, that Sesha uses a wheelchair instead of saying that she cannot walk). Given that Kittay would be well aware of such conventions, I wondered why she favored rhetoric that emphasizes Sesha's vulnerability and extreme dependency. I think she would say, if asked, that her vocabulary is meant to support a claim about the personhood of even the most dependent people. Sesha is neither independent nor autonomous. She cannot care for herself or ask for what she needs, but she can feel and communicate pleasure. Framed in this way, Sesha can serve as a paradigmatic but also highly specific instance of Kittay's argument about the right of dependent people to thrive, while the noneuphemistic catalogue of her needs attests to the work her survival demands of others. Where the case for disability empowerment emphasizes ability and potential, the case for care rests on the justice of ensuring well-being for the most incapacitated among us, and for their care providers.

There is a temporal dimension to Kittay's ethics of care, which includes the recognition that all people develop over time, even if they do not follow the standard trajectory of human maturation. Although her daughter's abilities do not register on standard measures of intelligence, Kittay rejects the concept of "mental age," with its demeaning implication that a grown woman with decades of living and physical development is the mental equivalent of a toddler stuck in time.[26] Sesha's body and life experience are those of an adult woman; her awareness of the world, tastes in music and companions, and repertoire of nonverbal cues are the product of an embodied life history. She requires caregivers who attend to the needs of her dependent body as it grows and ages without becoming more autonomous. Kittay's vision of a just society would provide for the sustenance but also the flourishing of a community's most dependent members as they change across a lifespan.

One of Kittay's most memorable descriptions of her daughter captures the complexity of uneven development, within and between a dependent person and her caregivers. Sometimes its signs are subtle, registering as silence or innuendo. But reading with care, we can apprehend the folded time of care, an evolving web of supportive care relations that Kittay calls "distributed mothering." This is her description of a typical morning:

> Sesha, as always, is delighted to see me. Anxious to give me one of her distinctive kisses she tries to grab my hair to pull me to her mouth. Yet at the same time my kisses tickle her and make her giggle too hard to concentrate on dropping the jam-covered toast before going after my

hair. I negotiate, as best as I can, the sticky toast, the hair-pulling and
the raspberry jam–covered mouth. In this charming dance, Sesha
and I experience some of our most joyful moments—laughing, duck-
ing, grabbing, kissing.[27]

On first read, this account of an awkward, messy, loving daily
encounter captures the warm intimacy between mother and daughter
but seems to say little about care. But note, also, what is unsaid. Reading with care in mind, we might observe that Kittay arrives to find
Sesha already at the breakfast table, eating toast that someone has evi-
dently prepared for her. The extent of Sesha's delight suggests that she is
probably seeing her mother for the first time that morning. If so, it follows that someone else has helped her out of bed and readied her for
breakfast, as well as making the meal. Although that person is not
described in the passage, the work that happened between the lines of
this delightful description is central to Kittay's philosophical project.
What initially appears as a description of mother and daughter is also
an example of distributed mothering. In a just society, care of dependent people is shared in ways that also sustain their caregivers. Sometimes, the personhood of those who share the labor of care can fly
under the radar, especially when most successful. The kinds of work
that made this scene possible receive full attention elsewhere in Kittay's
philosophy.

The work that got Sesha to the breakfast table, and the workers who
perform it, are fundamental to Kittay's philosophy of care. An account
of Sesha's development must also recognize the vulnerability and aging
of those who mother her. In a more typical story of development, the
dependent child grows into an independent adult who no longer needs
the support of a caregiver. Not so for Sesha, whose caregivers will inevitably age, but without the expectation that their work will lessen or that
she will move toward autonomy or independence. Certainly she will
not reciprocate by providing for aging parents or raising children of her
own. By the time Kittay wrote Love's Labor, she had shared the work of
mothering Sesha with Peggy, a beloved caregiver, for more than two
decades. "As Peggy and Sesha age, we reach the limits of the laboring

aspect of caring," she observes. "This is a difficult and troubling state of affairs—for us as parents, for Peggy, and, if Sesha understands it, for her. Sesha's possible future without Peggy troubles me profoundly—not simply because we have come to so rely on her, but because I cannot bear the thought that such a central relationship in Sesha's life could be sundered."[28] Kittay is not sanguine about these future challenges, even as she recognizes the reality that all caring relationships change over time. Sesha may maintain her affective bonds with Peggy, but other aspects of her care will need to be distributed over multiple parties across the time and space of a life. Writing frankly about the fragile and shifting networks of care that her daughter requires, Kittay argues that a truly just society would provide for the needs of people like Sesha but also for those who sustain her over the long term, an ethic she calls *doulia*.[29]

Imagining the temporalities of motherly care is not just a theoretical exercise, because it affects how we act in the present and plan for the future. An extreme and notorious example is the case of Ashley X, a girl with a genetic condition that rendered her intellectually disabled and completely dependent on the care of others. Her parents nicknamed her a "pillow angel . . . because she always remains where she is placed, which is usually on a pillow."[30] Calling their daughter an angel implies innocence and virtue.[31] This image was threatened when Ashley began to show signs of precocious puberty at age six. Her parents worried that a mature body would be harder to care for and more vulnerable to sexual abuse. Advised by doctors and bioethicists, they decided on a solution that became known as the "Ashley Treatment," a series of surgeries and medications to block their daughter's growth and physical development. In the years since it became publicly known, the case has been the subject of ongoing controversy. As the mother of an adult woman with a similar level of dependency, Kittay weighed in to criticize the decisions of Ashley's family. All people will mature and develop regardless of ability, she argued, and no child's growth should be determined by the conveniences of her caregivers, no matter how well intentioned. She also cautioned that the family could not know, when Ashley was just six, how their own feelings and beliefs would evolve over time.

There is no way to predict what it would be like to care for Ashley when she became a woman, work that might bring joy and satisfaction, as well as new burdens.

I'll admit to finding Kittay's side of the story utterly persuasive, as do most scholars I know in the field of disability studies. But in the years since Ashley's story broke, I've also befriended M, a colleague who speaks openly about opting for the same treatment for her multiply disabled son. She is a single mother of twins who has a demanding job and lives in a New York City–sized apartment. I have no doubt of her love for her children. M's story was an important stop on my listening tour through the zone of extreme parenting. Hearing her reminds me that life is complicated and that any particular caregiving scenario is bound up with the needs and desires of multiple other parties. I'm not arguing for the suspension of all ethical judgments, even as I acknowledge that there are no easy answers to our caregiving dilemmas. Invariably, care involves asymmetries, the sacrifices of some to ensure the sustenance of others.

Another way to describe these cases, in line with the themes of this chapter, would be to say that these parents tell competing stories about the future. Where my friend M and Ashley's parents believe they can foresee the future accurately enough to justify an irreversible medical intervention, Kittay accuses them of prematurely foreclosing the future for themselves and their children. Care always takes time and takes place in time, in ways that may be inconvenient, costly, or unpredictable. There is no treatment that can suspend Ashley, or her parents, in time. That we know for certain. And the stories we tell about a child's development—as well as the development of their caregivers—have real consequences for the care they receive and those who provide it.

My son, Henry, is very different from Sesha or Ashley or M's son, but Kittay's insights about developmental futurity resonate with my experiences as a parent. Our family has always engaged in distributed mothering. Supported by a network of teachers, therapists, sitters, camp counselors, health care providers, and others, I share Henry's care with his father and Angela, a paid caregiver who has known Henry since he was an infant. Angela is an absolutely vital resource whose work allows me to parent, earn an income to support my family, and continue my career as a professor and writer. I love her dearly and also sometimes resent needing her. I pay for her time, even as I acknowledge that her work is priceless. She accepts payment, while expressing a devotion to my son far beyond any monetary compensation. She acts as a composite of nanny, doting and permissive grandmother, friend, and playmate. She makes up excuses to give him snacks, shares inside jokes with him, and takes him home to visit with her family. As Henry entered his teen years, he continued to see Angela as his best friend but also to need different kinds of care. His body matured; he started to shave, use foul language, and had a crush on a girl at school. I also recognize that Angela is growing older, along with my son. She is now in her mid-sixties, with grandchildren of her own, as well as the kinds of impairments that are common in advancing middle age. I hope and expect that she and Henry will continue to be dear friends, even as I confront the fact that their interdependency will need to evolve. Guided by thinkers like Kittay, I am trying to manage dependencies that are dynamic, unpredictable, but also inevitable as long as life persists.

Where Kittay considers dependency over a span of decades, different questions about maternal care arise when the future of the dependent child is gravely attenuated. The author Emily Rapp confronted this devastating scenario when her fourteen-month-old son, Ronan, was diagnosed with Tay-Sachs disease, a fatal genetic condition that would lead to his death before the age of three. Where the dependencies of Sesha and Ashley X promise to be prolonged, requiring extensive planning for the future, Ronan's dependency meant that his life would end all too soon. How is a mother to care for a child with no future? But how can she not? How to value a life with no potential for growth, and how to do so without losing herself entirely? In her memoir *Still Point of the Turning World*, Rapp writes of mothering for the present.[32] Struggling to live in the now, she looks for value in the time she shares with her son, rather than his future promise. This is a radical departure from the culture of modern parenting, where care often takes the form of prodding and withholding, boundary setting, nagging, cajoling, and enforcing. The goal of this unpleasant cycle—aptly captured in the title of Jennifer Senior's book on parenthood, *All Joy and No Fun*—is to make our children the best possible version of a future self.[33] Rapp's terrible situation makes all of that seem trite. "There would be no vocab jars for Ronan," she writes. "There was nothing he needed to prove or do or become. He could stay a beautiful acorn; he didn't need to grow into a tree or realize his potential. He disproved Aristotle's teleological theory that potential is the key to life."[34] Free of the weighty obligation to the future, Rapp finds beauty in the image of her son as dormant and enclosed in a protective shell. Read closer, the limits of this metaphor point to the horrifying reality of her situation. Ronan cannot persist, nutlike, in an embryonic stasis. He will progress, but tragically so, toward decline and certain death. The script of childhood development torn away, Rapp has to figure out how to mother a child who can neither stay where he is nor grow to maturity.

There are multiple folds in the timescape of Rapp's memoir. She writes about a past self contemplating an inevitable and unthinkable future, one that she already occupies by the time of her writing. She is doing exactly what she found so unimaginable, living on after her son's death. The deviant temporalities of mothering Ronan give her work a form. Where Kittay breaks with memoir by using fragments and glimpses of a life to illustrate a set of ethical principles, Rapp's memoir captures how care's time pools and eddies, even as it flows forward.[35] Its narrative movement is strikingly different from the brisk pace of her previous memoir, the readable coming-of-age story *Poster Child*. It also differs from more conventional illness narratives, which tend to measure out time by the emergence or abatement of symptoms. *Still Point* gives surprisingly few details about the course of Ronan's disease, or the daily work of caring for him as it progresses. Each chapter represents a month in Ronan's life, but there is no play-by-play account of his decline and little discussion of bodily changes of any kind. Instead, consistent with its title, *Still Point* is a record of pauses where Rapp thinks, perceives, and sometimes just *is* in interdependency with her son. The form is ruminative but not pathologically so. Care leaves its imprint in a shape that is recursive, lyrical, and pensive.

Caring for Ronan is one theme of Rapp's memoir, but it is always coupled with accounts of *being cared for*. The advice of other mothers who have gone through the same experience emphasizes duty to the dying child, with some version of: "*He needs you. You are his mother. This is your task, hellish as it might be. You have no choice.*"[36] Where they dwell on obligations, Rapp attends to the resources a caregiver needs to sustain her difficult task. Rejecting the image of the mother as a selfless and infinitely available fount of care, she represents herself as someone who also needs to be cared for. She is lucky to have many offers of help, and she accepts them. A deep and extensive web of distributed mothering includes caring parents and relatives; a strong circle of friends and neighbors that provides food and companionship; a network of families that have faced similar tragedies; her flexible and rewarding job as a writer and teacher of writing; opportunities for regular exercise; inspiring natural settings; access to medical specialists, caregivers, and therapists (with insurance coverage good enough to go unmentioned); a spinning-yoga class to raise funds in Ronan's honor; travel to conferences for families and caregivers; participation in a Reiki healing group, treatment for mother and son by a Japanese sensei/acupuncture expert; a therapeutic visit to the Kindred Spirits Animal Sanctuary; a swim therapy class; vacations to a hot springs mineral spa; a writers' retreat in southern Spain; a palliative care training weekend at a Zen center; and, eventually, Rapp's discovery of new and enduring love along with the demise of her marriage to Ronan's father. Where Ronan's illness is terminal, *Still Point* emphasizes sustenance, a principle that guides the shape, as well as the content, of the story it tells. When the other mothers tell Rapp, "*you'll survive*," her memoir unpacks the tools needed for survival. Its catalog of restorative activities attests to the amount of labor and resources required to uphold caregivers and the importance of allowing oneself to be helped.

Emily and Ronan are the first of many examples of an interdependency involving terminal care to be introduced in this book. Their story captures the tedium, redundancy, muteness, and occasional small-scale satisfactions of tending to a dependent with no future except death. When the dependent is a child, the scripts of motherly care are shredded as attention zooms in on comfort and subsistence in the present. The laser-like focus of needs and resources is time-bound. The webs of care that form in such circumstances can, and usually must, eventually be unraveled. In Rapp's story, this means that, impossible as it may have seemed during Ronan's lifetime, his caregivers have a future beyond the terminal horizon of his illness. A new web of care develops to sustain those who must live on. If Rapp is to follow her own wisdom, the best way to honor her child and to mark their continued interdependency is to survive to tell their story. In doing so, she insists that survival is not—like the many accomplishments recounted in her earlier memoir—a feat of individual will but the collaborative product of buoyant networks of care. Nor is human mothering a self-obliterating symbiosis; in some form or another, interdependency evolves into paradependency, with mother and child having increasingly distinct needs and timescapes. Rapp's situation is exceptional, but it can also be exemplary, a caution against parenting that is so future oriented it loses sight of what is precious in the present, a call for mothers to recognize their own needs for sustenance and take help that is offered, and a reminder that the life spans of mother and child overlap but are not coterminal.

It might seem that one memoir is enough to document the life of a child who lived less than three years. But Rapp went on to write a second book that covered the same period and its aftermath. *Sanctuary*, the successor to *Still Point*, is worth mentioning for the way it details the reservoirs of bad feeling that had been pushed to the sidelines of the earlier memoir. Where that account dwells on the survival strategies of a mother surrounded by abundant webs of care, *Sanctuary* details the extreme physical and emotional toll of fulfilling her care obligations. The less salutary consequences of mothering a dying child include relentless grief, anger, resentment, and exhaustion. The strain of caring for Ronan destroyed Rapp's marriage and led her to compulsive sexual encounters and flirtation with suicide before the tenuous repair recounted later in the book. It is one thing to advise mothers to cherish the present and care for themselves and quite another actually to follow your own advice as your child is dying and afterward. The timescape of *Sanctuary* extends into the wrenching, unimaginable future where a parent lives on, continuing to be part of the turning world, after a child's death. It is a valuable companion to *Still Point* for its unsparing account of the costs of care work when there is no other choice, its happy ending (There is a marriage! There is new life!) feeling more like a literary device because-you-have-to-stop-somewhere than a real conclusion.

In a final example of extreme parenting, these two temporal dimensions—struggling to care for a child that has no future (interdependency) and attempting to live on after that child is gone (paradependency)—are folded together into one narrative. We have seen how mothers like Rapp and Kittay confront the particularly intense or prolonged dependency of a child sustained by webs of care that help distribute their labor. Toni Morrison's *Beloved* is also about mothering a child under the most difficult circumstances, but with important differences.[37] It is a work of fiction, and it is set in the past. And it centers on a child whose exceptional dependency is not caused by illness or disability but by an environment that makes it impossible to mother effectively. Morrison's protagonist, Sethe, is a former slave who has risked everything to gain freedom for herself and her children, committing infanticide to save her daughter from approaching slave catchers. Regardless of individual health or ability, a slave, by definition, does not possess bodily autonomy or ownership of their labor. Slavery presents an additionally devastating impasse to women who are forced to bear and nurture children they cannot mother and whose future is gravely foreclosed. Confronting such a horrific future, Sethe decides the greatest act of care she can provide for her child is to kill her. But even in death her daughter is not liberated; instead she is doomed to endure as a restless, resentful ghost. Haunting is the literary form Morrison gives to the lingering interdependencies of mother and daughter, a symbol for the persistence of mothering even in the absence of a child. Beloved, first as an impish spirit and then as an embodied woman, represents the devastating consequences of a depleted network of care that fails mother and child, family, and the surrounding community.

Although fiction, *Beloved* is based on the true story of Margaret Garner, a fugitive who killed her own child rather than see her returned to slavery.[38] The affordances of fiction allow Morrison to give a voice to Beloved, a nonlinguistic dependent child. Her character offers an alternative perspective on the tensions that flare up when the interests and needs of mother and child collide irreconcilably. The mothers of actual children who have little or no capacity for language—like Sesha, Ashley, or Ronan—are required to speak *for* a dependent, voiceless Other. Each adopts a singular narrative voice to represent the entanglement of their needs and desires with those of a dependent self.[39] Fiction allows Morrison to portray the subjectivity of the dependent, nonverbal child in language, casting it as sometimes continuous but often in conflict with that of her mother. Whether a disembodied ghost or a robustly corporeal stranger, Beloved is fully capable of self-expression. Her gestures and words express what a toddler (and later a mature, but equally dependent, woman, perhaps something like Kittay's Sesha) might say if she could convey the intense love and aggression evoked by a maternal presence, doing her best to care and (inevitably, from the frustrated child's point of view) falling short. At the level of form and content, *Beloved* exposes interdependency not as a state of being but as a process that must be continually renegotiated, sometimes in the presence of conflict, resistance, and incompatible needs.

In *Beloved*, the interdependency of mother and child is perverted by slavery. Like all humans, enslaved people are, in Kittay's words, "some mother's child," but the care they give and receive is gravely compromised by the mother's unfreedom in the present and the difficulty of imagining a future that is bright or open. Sethe mothers her children in the shadow of past maternal abandonment. She remembers her own mother as brusque and neglectful, seemingly unable to form a caring attachment to a child destined to be a slave. She is left behind when her mother runs for freedom, an attempt that ends in capture and punishment by death. Sethe last sees her mother's mutilated corpse hanging from a tree as a warning to other slaves contemplating escape. Living on in the aftermath of slavery and infanticide, Sethe endures by tending to the immediate material needs of her family, while beating back thoughts of the past. The effort of maintaining this deliberate amnesia leaves her no means of imagining another future or of meeting her living daughter's emotional needs in the present.

The unexpected arrival of two visitors—her old friend and soon-to-be romantic partner Paul D and the mysterious, needy stranger Beloved—challenges her determination to live narrowly in the present, offering new and ultimately irreconcilable affiliations and versions of interdependency. Beloved and Paul D differ starkly in the kinds of care they need and offer to provide. Paul D promises the more mutually sustaining, companionate relationship of two autonomous adults, while Beloved, although a grown woman, occupies the position of an utterly dependent child. Putting Sethe in the position of mother, she makes burdensome demands but also offers the rewards of thriving under good care. Sethe finds caring for Beloved enriching and depleting, anxiety producing, and deeply satisfying. While not disabled in any straightforward way, Beloved is a dependent family member whose precarious health and challenging behaviors require extra time, resources, and attention. With her childlike mentality and mature physical form, Beloved embodies the temporal paradoxes of the permanently dependent child. We have seen how the mothers of Sesha and Ashley X confronted worrying questions about a dependent daughter's transition from childhood into physical adulthood, how to care for and protect their daughters as their bodies and desires matured, and how to provide for a long-term dependent, all as they contend with the aging and frailty of their own bodies. While actual mothers get only one chance to parent a particular child—each making dramatically different, if similarly irrevocable, choices—in fiction, the daughter Sethe killed as a toddler can return, equally dependent, as a full-grown woman with verbal speech, bodily autonomy, and sexual desires. Her manifestation forces Sethe to confront the consequences of her choices but also seems like an opportunity to compensate for her past actions.

The interdependency of mother and a particular child endures even after the death of that child, whose absence makes it impossible to complete the care of mothering. But where a mother like Emily Rapp experiences that loss as an individual, Morrison writes of a more collective experience of trauma. *Beloved* reads like an allegory for a community confronting the impact of a generations-long deficit of care. Any hope for repair must also be collective. This hard-earned understanding comes only at a point of crisis. Initially the trouble seems confined to an individual family, increasingly isolated from neighbors and community. Sethe tries to break the cycle of loss without understanding that no one individual can go it alone. Their household turns inward, shutting itself off from the world. But the needs of Beloved, Sethe, and Denver become irreconcilable without a broader web of care to sustain them. Beloved needs too much; Sethe and Denver reach the limit of their ability to care for her. Beloved's body swells, and her demands escalate; her caregivers become weak and frail.

Sometimes those most in need of care are so exhausted they can't even recognize their own depletion. As Sethe's resources dwindle, she can neither seek care nor imagine living otherwise. It is Denver who realizes that she must venture out of their isolated domestic unit. Asking for help, in this novel as in life, is an act of courage, a scary acknowledgment that you have needs, with the even scarier risk of relying on someone's else's capacity to give. Her neighbors respond with generosity, as people often do in desperate times. They recognize that Sethe, on the front lines of prolonged and intensive caregiving, is also in need of care. And Sethe, after alienating her neighbors by flaunting her self-sufficiency, is finally compelled to accept their help. This mutual recognition enables the exorcism of the greedy, demanding, embodied Beloved, in this reading a figure for exingency without reciprocity or the possibility of completion. She leaves behind the painful memory of a child whose future was foreclosed and the formation of a fragile community of care surrounding Sethe and Denver.

Beloved explores the fissures of care that endanger Sethe, her family, and a community unable to put the past to rest or contemplate a better future. Its story of neglectful and murderous parenting might be explained in terms of the failures or madness of a particular mother.[40] We live in a society that is particularly quick to condemn Black mothers when their children come to harm.[41] The novel complicates such easy answers by embedding its protagonists in a community whose resources of care for those in need have been drained, leaving a mother unable to imagine the future as anything other than the repetition of an unbearable past. It does not exonerate Sethe for infanticide, but it does distribute responsibility by embedding her crime in a web of inter-dependencies. "This is not a story to pass on," Morrison cautions at the novel's end, memorably gesturing to the contradictory necessity of for-getting and transmitting the past. The shifting meanings of "pass on" include strategies that acknowledge trauma and loss while preserving the ability to care about and for the future.

By setting *Beloved* in the nineteenth century, Morrison is not sug-gesting that the problems of care it introduces are behind us. Care is an aspect of particular relationships that are always embedded in net-works, meaning that its absence has effects that radiate through popu-lations and over time. Just as good care is an investment in the future, a care deficit can be transmitted from one generation to the next. At the time of the novel's publication in 1987, many Black women still strug-gled to mother in the absence of material resources and robust webs of care. The workfarist policies that compelled poor women to take jobs in exchange for benefits reflected an ongoing failure to recognize mother-ing as work and the lack of social commitment to care for those in need. Morrison's warning against abandoning families exhausted by genera-tions of care's absence was as relevant then as it was one hundred years before. But *Beloved*'s story about parenting in the face of an impossible future also speaks to readers in the twenty-first century in ways Mor-rison might not have imagined when she wrote the novel.

This chapter began with the increasingly evident signs of climate change, which make the future tenuous for the entire species. I pointed out that, at a moment when it is hard to know how to mother any child, the parents of children with disabilities can offer alternative ways to think about the temporalities of motherhood. So can the parents of BIPOC children (sometimes also disabled), since the ravages of climate change are not evenly distributed. People of color disproportionately bear the brunt of environmental collapse, since they disproportion-ately live in environments vulnerable to pollution and natural disaster. These burdens are vividly illustrated in the recent work of the artist

Titus Kaphar, whose 2019 series *From a Tropical Space* is about Black motherhood and care in an atmosphere of unfolding emergencies, fast and slow.[42] Although Kaphar works in a static medium; his paintings have much to say about the passage of time. He is best known for reproductions that insert a Black presence into classic works of art, drawing the viewer's attention to a history of its erasure from the Western canon. The paintings in *Tropical Space* are different in that they do not reference canonical artworks, either in content or style. It is as if their subject required the artist to search for a new form, more oriented toward future than past. In these images, Black mothers care for children that have vanished, but so recently that the precise shape of their bodies remains as a silhouette that seems to be cut out of the canvas, leaving white space behind. Interdependent with their absent children, these mothers are sometimes also under erasure, with the extremities of their bodies abstracted or gone altogether. Sometimes they appear in ordinary-looking contexts—waiting for a Greyhound bus, pushing children in strollers, braiding hair on a stoop, standing in a kitchen—while other paintings depict an atmosphere of crisis, the aftermath of a storm or the signs of a medical emergency. Usually the women are alone, although occasionally they appear in pairs, with each looking off in a different direction. They do not comfort each other or find solidarity in shared circumstances. Even when the settings are mundane, they are colored in lurid hues of pink, purple, and teal that suggest a toxic environment and portend future ill health. Against this sickly palette, the white spaces left by eerily absent children in Kaphar's paintings make a powerful statement about the limits of mother-child interdependency. Even as women engage in the intimate gestures of caregiving, their children vanish, leaving the mother's body suspended in rocking, cuddling, pushing, braiding, hugging, cradling. This is a future that no mother wants to imagine but that some are forced to live. Paradependent, they continue to exist, to have needs, and live in bodies, while bearing indelible memories of the children who depended on them.

What would these mothers say if they could talk? A short story cowritten by Kaphar and Tochi Onyebuchi gives voice to one of them. She connects her child's erasure to an unknowable future. "She doesn't know what's waiting for her," the mother reflects, "even as the vanishing happens." In the face of this ominous but unspecified disappearance, the mother longs to arrest time. "I want to wrap this moment in my arms," she says, even as she is helpless to stop the process of loss.[43] All mothering is about separation. This speaker could be describing the ordinary experience of watching a child grow and mature, but the accompanying painting says otherwise. Kaphar describes his subject more specifically as "a haunting narrative of black motherhood wherein fear and collective trauma crescendo to the disappearance of their children."[44] The ominous vacancy left by the child's disappearance and the wash of flat, confrontational color suggest this is not a natural process. These mothers do not look like they are celebrating a child's passage into a bright, open future, but rather cradling absences whose small size and childish outlines suggest they are premature or tragic. Even when there is more than one woman in the frame, they do not support, look at, or otherwise acknowledge each other, their isolation as devastating as the vacant spaces where children should be. All mothering relationships exist as part of networks in a social fabric, and the aloneness of Kaphar's subjects shows theirs to be fragile and inadequate.

Much as they speak to the particularity of Black motherhood, these paintings are also about mothering as such. The relationship between mother and child is, by definition, asymmetrical, its interdependencies necessarily temporary and shifting. It is possible for a child to care for a mother, but *to mother* means to be a giver, not a receiver, of care. Even as the child is depicted as an absence—their location and fate unknown—the mother's body retains its memory in her pose and the direction of her attention. The work communicated by these bodies is uneven. The silhouettes left by the children's bodies recline while the mothers engage actively. They care by doing work, as they push, hold, cradle, stroke, braid. Their postures and expressions appear mournful but resigned, attesting to the obligatory nature of their labor. Even for those who most eagerly chose it, mother*ing* is grueling, sacrificing, and sometimes oppressive work. It is marked by a generational divide since a mother is, by definition, significantly older than her child, shaped by decades of accumulated experience before its arrival. She knows the dependent child's life story from the beginning, while it enters hers midstream. There will be separation, interdependencies broken and rearranged. Motherly care is time-bound. In the best-case scenario, the child she nurtured will live into an unknown future after she is gone. All childhood is ephemeral, and all children are vanishing, whether they are maturing or their lives are shortened tragically by death. This dynamic process is inevitable to mothering. Its particular impact on relations of care will be further clarified by looking at the very different timescapes of siblinghood and how the more elongated lateral relationship of brothers and sisters shapes the way they imagine and engage in acts of caring for one another.

2

THE ELONGATED TIMESCAPES
OF SIBLING CARE

F or many people, our longest relationship to another person will be with a sibling. Unlike *mother* or *parent*, *sibling* is a noun but not a verb. And although siblings sometimes do care for one another—emotionally or physically—unlike mothers, they have no prescribed obligation to care. In the smaller and more generationally compact modern family, there is little protocol for assigning caregiving tasks to one sibling or another, although there may be a period when an older child is charged with tending to a younger. As children grow into adults, there is no agreement about the extent and nature of any sibling's caregiving duties, or even that they will provide one another with care of any kind. This means that siblings have unique and underappreciated experiential knowledge about care within the family. And all the more so when one sibling is exceptionally dependent, requiring care that is more intense or prolonged than a typically developing child.

Toni Morrison recognizes this in *Beloved*, giving Denver, the younger sister, an equal voice in the dialogue that emerges among a mother and her daughters. Embedded in the household she shares with her mother and needy older sister, Denver has a distinct perspective on the dynamics of care within the family. Barring untimely death, she will live with that special knowledge for longer than her parents, her outlook changing and enriching with time. Sibling perspectives on care over the long term are the subject of this chapter, which focuses on the asymmetries of need that arise when one brother or sister experiences pervasive, long-term dependency, profoundly shaping domestic life in ways that may be undetectable to outsiders.[1]

When we consider care over a lifetime rather than during just the years of childhood, the shifting dynamics of siblinghood come into focus. Just how unpredictable its long-term trajectory may be, and how unexpected the onset of dependency, is powerfully illustrated in Christina Crosby's 2016 memoir, *A Body Undone: Living on After Great Pain*.[2] Crosby's primary subject is the aftermath of a bike accident that left her quadriplegic, but the book also follows the changing circuits of care in a sibling relationship. As a child, Christina's sense of self was defined by siblinghood. She was less than two years younger than her brother Jeff, whom she strongly resembled in looks, interests, and abilities. Brother and sister were fiercely competitive and the best of friends. When they fought, Christina, who was taller and bigger, was often the winner. Then came the bodily changes of puberty, along with gendered expectations about how boys and girls are supposed to behave. Held back by biology and society, the teenaged Christina no longer felt like her brother's equal. A much more divisive twist of fate intervened in early adulthood, when Jeff was diagnosed with multiple sclerosis, which would eventually end his life. Over several decades, Jeff's health and physical abilities declined, while Christina thrived. They remained close, and sometimes Christina helped care for Jeff.

Everything changed again when Christina had a near-fatal accident at age fifty. She writes about waking up in the hospital and seeing Jeff's wheelchair at the foot of her bed. "I vaguely knew the word 'quadriplegic' now applied to me, too," she writes, "though my mind revolted from that likeness as a coincidence entirely too improbable to be true."[3] For a brief period, Christina and her brother entered an unwelcome new form of twinship, as wheelchair users dependent on others for help with many aspects of daily life. But soon after Christina learned to use her own wheelchair, Jeff became too weak to operate his, and it was Christina who hovered at the edge of Jeff's hospital bed. By the time of her brother's death, Christina had known him longer than she had known either her parents or her beloved partner, Janet. From childhood to middle age, they had seen each other through dramatic life changes that put each in the role of providing for, and receiving care from, the other. While Crosby's story is remarkable, it also attests to the unforeseeable course of any sibling relationship that unfolds over many decades and stages of life.

Siblinghood gets a chapter of its own because it is a ubiquitous and deeply meaningful relation embedded in practices of care that are far less scripted (and less well recognized) than those associated with mothering, or most other forms of kinship examined in this book. While individual parents or families may have strong beliefs about how siblings should relate to one another, there are few standardized cultural narratives about siblinghood, and it remains understudied compared to other kinship roles.[4] For at least a century, Freudian theory held sway over psychosocial understandings of family life, which centered on hierarchical relationships between parents and individual children.[5] Freud saw mothers and fathers as the predominant factor in shaping a child's development, with siblings registering primarily as competitors for parental attention.[6] Such heavy emphasis on parent-child dynamics overlooks the fact that siblings often provide our most influential and enduring family relationships, whether hostile or amicable.

Many people cannot remember a time before their siblings were born, and, like Christina and Jeff, they often retain that connection through many stages of life, long after the death of parents or other adult authority figures.[7] In childhood, siblings are our most constant and immediately accessible role models. They may school us in the virtues of cooperation, fairness, and responsibility. Often an older sibling will care for or protect (and/or torment) a younger, whereas later in life, those roles may be complicated or reversed. Siblings also provide early lessons about inequality, competition, and conflict.[8] Maybe, like my boys, they share a room where each becomes an unavoidable (and often unwelcome) companion and witness to the other's private life. As members of the same family, siblings have no choice but to share food, clothing, chores, toys, and the affection of their parents. As members of the same generation, they may share values and beliefs that are different from those of their parents. In this, they provide our earliest introduction to interdependence, forming a basis for care relations with peers in the wider world. Arguably, siblinghood defines even the selfhood of single children, who may identify as an "only child" or "singleton." This identity, which many carry over a lifetime, emerges from the absence of a relationship presumed to be the norm.

While inequality is baked in to all siblinghood,[9] I am interested in the asymmetries that arise when one brother or sister is unusually dependent and in how more typical siblings write about the dynamics of care within the family. As in the previous chapter, I take these situations of extreme dependency as special cases that highlight, with particular intensity, the limits and gaps in our current systems of care but that also offer insights about care among more typical siblings and other lateral relationships beyond the family. Across a varied range of stories, I identify a set of features particular to the sibling's-eye view of dependency and care. First, the sibling's role as a witness, a partisan observer of the care required by a vulnerable family member, and an actor within those exchanges. Siblings may recognize the rewards of intimacy with a dependent person while also testifying—often with anxiety, resentment, or anger—to the staggering amount of maintenance work that person requires, much of it invisible to outsiders, much disproportionately heaped on mothers. They see, and may be directly affected by, the wearing away of mothers and others who do the uncompensated work of sustaining vulnerable people. Second, the sibling's lateral relationship to the dependent person. Unlike the inherently hierarchical dynamics of mothers and children, siblings are generational peers whose stories attest to the selfhood of dependent brothers and sisters, providing an intimate view of their capacity for growth, development, and reciprocity. A brother or sister who is exceptionally dependent can also serve as a model—for better or worse—for engaging with peers in a world where ability, good fortune, and success are unevenly distributed. The family becomes a crucible where siblings practice survival, coexistence, and even collaboration in the context of inequality.[10] Third, the long term of siblinghood. Sibling narratives introduce a new perspective on the temporalities of care. Questions about development and futurity taken up in the last chapter look different when considered from the prolonged, lateral, and evolving position of siblinghood. When siblings know one another over a lifetime, they acquire firsthand knowledge of the instability of care giving and receiving roles and how to maintain (or sever, or restore) a relationship as they move across a spectrum of dependencies.

The sibling dynamics that interest me are the product of relatively recent historical circumstances that made it more likely for exceptionally dependent children to be raised as part of a household and cared for by their families. These include the closure of institutions that once would have housed chronically ill or disabled children and the innovation of portable medical devices that are relatively easy to operate. Once more medically fragile and/or disabled children began to live at home, a new generation of siblings would grow up as embedded observers and participants in the care work transferred to their families. For our purposes, "siblinghood" is less about a biological relation than a social role within a family unit. A "sibling" is a peer who shares a household and at least one parent with other children, and who maintains relationships to brothers and sisters that continue into adulthood. As they come of age, the brothers and sisters of dependent siblings began to write. Let's call them Gen S. Within that cohort, I am especially interested in the challenges of storytelling when a brother or sister is not only physically dependent but intellectually disabled in ways that impede their access to self-narration. As we will see, Gen S siblings often arrive at magnificently intuitive understandings of neurodiversity that put them in the forefront of disability inclusion, but they also understand the costs of inclusion for those caregivers who do the hard and wearing maintenance work it requires.

FIRST GENERATION, INCLUSIVE

Sibling inequality is as old as humanity itself, but the forms it takes and its implications for care are historical. Since the 1970s, the intersection of medical innovation and the closure of residential institutions shaped experiences of growing up with a severely disabled brother or sister in ways distinct enough to produce a cohort.[11] The group I'm calling Gen S comprises the first children in many generations to grow up in a household with a disabled sibling. And for the first time, children with injuries and illnesses that would have once been fatal were living longer, fuller lives than ever before. Those with intellectual disabilities, many of whom, in past generations, would have spent their lives in residential schools or hospitals, increasingly lived at home. Gen S narratives show that the new atmosphere of inclusion that has prevailed for the past half-century has profoundly reshaped sibling attitudes toward care. *How* they have been shaped is less clear. The insights to be gleaned from sibling narratives are inconsistent and sometimes contradictory. As such, they capture a spectrum of experience particular to its time and to the lateral intimacy of a sibling relationship.

Only in the last fifty years has it become the norm for children with intellectual disabilities in the United States and Western Europe to be raised in a household along with typical siblings. A hundred years ago, an intellectually disabled family member would have been a shameful secret. In the era of eugenics, a person classified as "feebleminded" cast doubt on the fitness of their relatives and, if allowed to reproduce, was forecast to perpetuate inferior bloodlines for future generations. When a child was diagnosed with feeblemindedness or idiocy, experts advised that institutionalization was in the best interests of the entire family.[12] We see this logic at work in William Faulkner's 1929 novel, *The Sound and the Fury*, where the intellectually disabled Benjy Compson is a source of worry and embarrassment to his family. Although he grows up at home, household servants are tasked with keeping him quiet and out of sight. His younger brother Jason sees Benjy's care as a burden and, as soon as their mother dies, "was able to free himself . . . from his idiot brother" by committing him to the state asylum.[13] Across the Atlantic, Virginia Woolf wrote resentfully of sharing a household with her half-sister Laura, "a vacant-eyed girl whose idiocy was becoming daily more obvious, who could hardly read, who would throw scissors into the fire, who was tongue-tied and stammered and yet had to appear at table with the rest of us."[14] Like Benjy Compson, Laura was removed from the household to an asylum after her father and stepmother found it too hard to care for her.[15] The 1988 film *Rain Man* tells a more recent version of this story, about Raymond, a man with autism who has been so effectively erased by institutionalization that his brother, Charlie, doesn't know he exists. Charlie learns that he has a brother only when their father dies, leaving Raymond a vast inheritance.[16] Hijinks ensue as Charlie schemes to get the money for himself, leading to a series of adventures that teach him to appreciate his brother. These were the early stages of Gen S consciousness, reflected in Charlie's dawning awareness that his brother has abilities and even talents, as well as needs.

In this chapter, I consider narratives by and about Gen S brothers and sisters, who came of age during and after the movement to shutter residential facilities for people with disabilities. For the first time since the rise of the nuclear family, there was a widespread commitment to raise disabled children at home, include them in their communities, and educate them at local schools. As a result, for the first time in modern history, it would be common for children with exceptional dependencies to grow up alongside typical brothers and sisters. This shift was deeply consequential both for dependent people themselves and their siblings. Sibling narratives affirm the value of including dependent and neurodiverse people in a household without avoiding the associated difficulties. They tell us that deinstitutionalization has enriched family life, but also that it has been scandalously incomplete. There is little good in closing residential facilities without providing adequate support for the households and communities charged with caring for former residents.[17] When a disabled sibling is also medically fragile, Gen S narratives introduce another modern dimension of care, the redistribution of work once done by paid medical professionals to unpaid family members.

The troubled process of deinstitutionalization and the demands it makes on siblings who outlive parents or other guardians are not just things I've read about. My parents' closest family friends adopted a son in 1965. From the beginning Diane asked doctors about her baby's delayed development and medical issues, but they dismissed her concerns, as did her husband. It took four years for Josh to be diagnosed with an intellectual disability. Diane adored her son, adopted a second child two years later, and raised them together, even after she and her husband divorced and he cut Josh out of his life. Only when I started to learn the history of disability many years later did I realize that Diane's commitment to keeping her son at home after his diagnosis was still somewhat remarkable for the time. When Josh was eight, she published a personal essay with the revealing title "The Lonely Search for Help," about the frustrating lack of advice on how to meet Josh's behavioral and medical needs.[18] She writes bluntly of the struggle to care for her son, while never suggesting that he doesn't belong with his family. Eventually Josh would go to boarding school because there was no other appropriate option for him. The closest residential school was a two-hour drive from home. Still, he remained a valued family member who received regular visits and was welcomed home on vacations and holidays. Now that I, too, am raising a disabled son—supported by more abundant, if still insufficient, social and government resources—I realize how alone Diane must have felt as an early and unwitting pioneer at inclusion. It is easy for me to see what she could have done better, but I also now have more understanding of what it must have been like to invent the—now well-oiled—wheel of "special needs parenting."

What I remember about growing up alongside Josh is his goofy sense of humor and knack for imitations. If he heard a funny sound once, he would repeat it hundreds of times, sometimes adding it to the eclectic playlist of quotes and noises he would utter for decades after. (A perennial favorite among us kids riffed on overhearing his parents at an intimate moment). He loved rock music, playing his drum set and singing along in a loud, joyful, and tuneless voice. He wore coke-bottle-thick glasses that were often askew. He was also prone to violent tantrums that sometimes ended in property damage (a dented car fender, a hole in the wall, broken records and drums). Sometimes he hurt his sister, Naomi. I remember the time he slapped her while she was having her temperature taken, shattering the glass thermometer in her mouth. Another time he jumped on her in a fit of frustration while we were standing on a dock, everybody rattled by how easily they could have rolled into the icy water surrounding it. Naomi remembers that Diane would force Josh to apologize after these incidents and then assume the matter was closed, telling her daughter to forget about them. She never did.

Diane's primary tactic for managing Josh's behavior was to take him shopping or ply him with food. By the time she wrote her essay she was castigating herself for having "mistakenly indulged almost every whim." She continues, "I have painfully realized my mistakes, and I have started to set a variety of limits on him. I was doing Josh a disservice by expecting nothing of him."[19] As a younger person, I felt free to blame Diane for the coddling that reinforced her son's misbehavior. I was sure their conflicts could have been managed differently by setting clear boundaries and asking more of him. But reading the essay now, I am most struck by her isolation. She was a working mother, trying to get by. As she carted her child from one expert to another, I wonder why nobody gave better advice about his care and development. Maybe there was none to be had. There were few, if any, support groups or established advocacy organizations. Even as she accepts responsibility for her mistakes, I'm aware of how oppressive it must have felt that they were hers alone. I can understand why many families thought it was safer and healthier to commit a disabled child to care outside the home. And I can also see the challenges Josh's family confronted. They were the first generation to try inclusion, enabled by the preliminary impetus to return people with intellectual disabilities to their communities but hamstrung by the absence of local care networks for people with disabilities and their supporters.

Diane was the mother of two children. But even as she confesses her worries about Josh, she says nothing about Naomi, who was four at the time. She does not write about parenting her daughter; she doesn't seek advice or try to imagine what it was like to grow up as Josh's sister. Maybe she didn't think these questions would interest her readers, or maybe they never occurred to her. Like all siblings raised in the same family, Naomi's identity formed as she grew up alongside her brother. Because she is a younger sister, there was no life before Josh. They shared a room, each witnessing the other away from the eyes of parents and other adults. By the time Josh went to boarding school, Naomi's sense of self had been firmly shaped by the space and experiences of living with Josh for over a decade and the family they continued to share. Now that Diane and her second husband are dead, Naomi has inherited guardianship of Josh. Sometimes he says to Naomi, "You're my mom now." His words express awareness of his own dependency and the heavy responsibility she now bears. "No I'm not, I'm still your sister," she answers. She has not rejected the role of managing Josh's care, but her words express the unchosen and laterally imposed nature of her obligation. This is the trajectory of many dependent adult siblings, given that children in a modern family are likely to be generational peers who will outlive their parents.

More families of my generation understand the importance of preparing siblings who are expected to inherit guardianship of a dependent brother or sister. But because they were first and dealing with their own frailties, Naomi's aging mother and stepfather did not do anything to ease this transition. They did not include her in discussions about Josh's future care, passing down a bureaucratic morass she is still trying to navigate. In many states, parents are legally required to support adult children with disabilities, but there is no such requirement for siblings.[20] At the same time, it is inconceivable that Naomi would abandon Josh to care of the state. He is her brother and she loves him. He is also a dependent adult in declining health. They live in different cities, and she spends hours trying to arrange for his care. She takes time off work to attend meetings and deal with the bureaucracy of guardianship. The staff at his group home calls her to report his infractions. He breaks his own things when he gets angry. Sometimes his glasses or hearing aids are lost, leaving him blind and deaf. He had to be assigned a different room after shouting racial slurs at the neighbors outside his window. Periodically he is hospitalized for cellulitis and other mounting medical complaints. He seeks the attention of nurses by using foul language and insults.

When I talk to Naomi, I am aware of the uncompensated burdens she shoulders, the drain on her personal days, the unpaid hours she spends on paperwork, talking to staff and social workers, gathering information from lawyers and counselors. Some brothers and sisters care for each other at different points. It goes without saying that Josh will not, and never could have, reciprocated by caring for Naomi in her own phases of dependency. Her work is mostly invisible, and I probably wouldn't recognize it if I weren't writing this book. She would face the same obligations if she were Josh's brother, but I also know her sense of duty is shaped by being a woman in a culture that expects women to do more than their share of the care work in their families. In addition to inheriting legal responsibility for Josh, Naomi has inherited the felt sense of responsibility expressed by her mother in the essay written half a century before.

Naomi and other siblings of her generation are pioneers who grew up without role models, expert advice, or a community of peers. By the time Josh was a child, a body of knowledge was starting to emerge about raising and educating children with intellectual disabilities. But their siblings were an afterthought. Nobody saw them as a special cohort, and siblings did not recognize themselves as having an identity or a shared set of experiences. Only in the 1990s, as Gen S came of age, was there an acknowledgment of their unique standpoint. They had needs of their own, as well as a wealth of experiential knowledge about navigating families where the distribution of ability, health, intelligence, and opportunity is radically uneven. A genre of sibling advice literature has defined a new identity, the "special needs sibling." A whole industry of self-help books, support groups, and online forums has emerged to support these siblings, addressing their emotional needs and providing resources to advocate for their disabled brothers and sisters. Care is central to this genre, since it starts with the premise that family dynamics, and the identities of those involved, are shaped by the exceptional dependency of one child. Sometimes the "special needs sibling" genre frames sibling experience in a more negative light, exploring the resentment of typical brothers and sisters who felt silenced, neglected, or burdened with unrealistic expectations. Sometimes it focuses on the unexpected joys and benefits of having a disabled sibling.[21] Sometimes it addresses the caregiving concerns of adults who inherit guardianship of a dependent brother or sister or want to become advocates.

Sibling self-help literature now offers something for almost any constituency, with different advice depending on whether the target audience is children, adolescents, or older adults. There are even different flavors for the more common disabilities, most notably autism and Down syndrome. Although varied in content, these works share the presumption that the identities of typical and disabled siblings are relatively fixed and, almost always, that a sibling's "special needs" are congenital. They are always oriented toward an imagined audience of typical siblings, who are also the informants. Their voices appear in quotations and anecdotes, and there is no such thing as an unreliable narrator, nobody to invoke the indelible law of nature that there are always at least two sides to every sibling story. Disabled siblings do not get to speak at all. They are spoken for by their siblings and sometimes by experts, as evidence of one position or another. We do not get the full story of any one family but rather a chorus of sibling voices attesting to similar feelings and situations. This is to say that advice literature is a genre, meaning it has conventions that presume a certain audience and a given set of expectations for its content. It tells you your experiences have been shared by others and gives you strategies others have used to manage it successfully.

Literary narratives about siblinghood can do something different. Absent the imperative to be helpful or offer a coherent message, literature can explore the variability of a lifespan and the tangled life networks that intersect it. Crosby's *Body Undone* does not provide a neat package of wisdom about caring for a disabled sibling. Identities like abled/disabled are unsettlingly fluid, suddenly changing course and intensity. Given a situation "too improbable to be true," she makes no claim to be representative of anything other than the unpredictable reversals of fortune that can happen. In what follows, I look at Gen S memoir and autofiction—novelizations based on a sibling's lived experience—with the recognition that narrative can be opaque, contradictory, frustrated, redundant, or inconclusive. There are multiple sides to a sibling story, which literature can bring out. This might make it feel less reliable but points to a foundational truth, that siblinghood is relational, an identity always interdependent with at least one other person. Literature stays with the trouble. It disrupts the production of coherent advice or actionable outcomes, but in doing so it adds another layer to the varied meanings of care that this book seeks to understand.

Time is of essence to siblings, as it is to all caring relationships. In this case I am interested in the long-term nature of siblinghood and also how the timing of disability onset shapes attitudes and interpersonal dynamics. The majority of literature and advocacy around the "special needs sibling" assumes that disability is congenital or early onset. I found no such advice literature for siblings whose brothers or sisters become ill or disabled after a relationship is already established, as was the case for Christina and her brother, Jeff. But the timing of when, in a life course, a sibling becomes dependent has a significant impact on how brothers and sisters think about their care. I get at this dynamic by comparison. First, I look at Paul and Judy Karasik's collaboratively written 2003 *The Ride Together: A Sibling Memoir of Autism in the Family*, where a brother's disability is baked in to his identity and that of the family. I then turn to two works—Jon Pineda's 2009 memoir, *Sleep in Me*, and Akhil Sharma's 2014 autofictional novel, *Family Life*— about siblings who are suddenly disabled in adolescence, their newfound dependencies forcing a rearrangement of identities, plans, and relationships.[22] For the former, I use the phenomenological concept of "always already" to capture a sibling's experience of a brother or sister whose dependency is a normalized and constant feature of family identity, while the latter examples concern the acquisition of dependencies that are abrupt, unexpected, and transformational.

ALWAYS ALREADY: THE TEMPORALITIES OF A CONGENITALLY DISABLED SIBLING

Near the beginning of the collaboratively written sibling memoir *The Ride Together*, the cartoonist Paul Karasik draws a single neuron, a star-shaped blotch against a black background, before drawing his brother, David. Sometimes, he explains, the instructions driving neural development get "scrambled," producing the symptoms of autism that David began to exhibit as a toddler. By anchoring David's disability in biology, Paul rejects the theory, popular at the time, that it was caused by a failure of maternal care.[23] There would be no David without his autism. And as the book's subtitle, *A Memoir of Autism in the Family*, suggests, David's younger siblings had no life before him, nor did they ever belong to a family without disability in its midst. Autism is *in the family*; their knowledge of disability is intimate and unselfconscious, at least initially, a kind of organic understanding that is a special feature of early sibling experiences. The always-already temporality of sibling-hood is the context for a story that begins prenatally and extends over some decades into the unresolved present.

In a household with multiple siblings, there are also multiple per-spectives on family life. *Ride Together* creates dialogue among different points of view, each sibling-author adopting the form best suited to the story they want to tell: Paul, a cartoonist, working with comics, and Judy, a writer, using prose memoir. Juxtaposed in a single chapter, some-times the voices of brother and sister relate different events, and sometimes each describes the same event from their own perspective. Gender shapes how each sibling bears witness to the caregiving activi-ties performed by adults in their household and, later, how they approach the responsibility of their brother's care. We see how their views on dependency work are directly tied to the gendered divisions of labor within the family, established by their parents and transmitted to the next generation. Paul speaks primarily as an observer of the care work done by women, while Judy is increasingly enlisted as a partici-pant. Paul's comic follows the evolution of a sibling relationship from neuronal growth to growing up in a shared family home to adulthood. Comics are an ideal medium for illustrating a sibling's-eye view, fil-tered through the lens of adult understanding. Paul the boy has no caregiving responsibilities and engages busily with friends, hobbies, and imaginative play. But Paul the adult artist draws the care work that sustained him and others in the household into the background. These activities appear to Paul the boy as an uninteresting blur, but Paul the adult shows their importance to maintaining family life.

In the comic book world devoured by boyhood Paul and David, the heroes are Superman and his cohort, but the unquestionable hero of *The Ride Together* is Joan, the Karasik family matriarch. Joan is the antithesis of a refrigerator mother, a reliable source of warmth and encouragement to her four children. In an episode depicting a chaotic family dinner, Joan is a constant, steadying presence in almost every frame. Sometimes she is visible only as a comforting arm, a hand holding out a plate of food, or from behind as a silhouette directing family activities. When David and his father get into a fight that ends with a broken chair, Joan fixes everything emotional and physical: She manages to soothe David's agitation, send her husband away to calm down, and then—when the human care work is done—to repair the damaged furniture.[24]

In another episode, boyhood Paul, who has an active fantasy life as a comic book Secret Agent, dashes out the door carrying his briefcase (figure 2.1). In the background of the frame—and of Paul's boyish awareness—we see his mother pushing his grandfather in a wheelchair. At the end of the episode, Paul returns to the house, running into the family's paid African American housekeeper, Dorothy, who is leaving after a long day of work. Together, these images tell a story about how care is experienced differently by different members of the household. In the background and at the margins of Paul's sequences is a story about the racialized women's labor that allows his boyish body and imagination free rein. In this way, Paul's comics depict the development of a long-term relationship from mutual dependency to a present where David's care is managed by his adult siblings. It is a detail too perfect to banish to a footnote that I took a weeklong Zoom seminar with Paul Karasik in the summer of 2020. He began by telling us he might occasionally need to get up because he was caring for his mother, at the time aged one hundred, who was lying in bed in the next room. This incident adds many layers of meaning to a story of care work, gender, and generation.

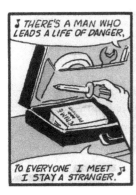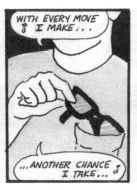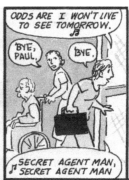

FIGURE 2.1 In Paul Karasik's comic in *The Ride Together*, Paul takes up his secret agent tools and persona while caring labor is visible in the background.

Source: From *The Ride Together: A Brother and Sister's Memoir of Autism in the Family*,
by Paul Karasik and Judy Karasik. © 2003 by Paul Karasik and Judy Karasik.
Reprinted with the permission of Washington Square Press,
an imprint of Simon & Schuster LLC. All rights reserved.

The last chapter of *Ride Together* gives David an opportunity to participate in his own story. In Paul's final comic, he and Judy show David a draft of the book and invite him to contribute. David seems uninterested. "Listen," Paul asks, "at least tell me what we should say you're up to now?" David demurs, walking away with the words, "oh . . . this and that."[25] It is time for his favorite TV show. Although David leaves Paul and Judy behind, Paul's art follows him out of the room. The ensuing frames show David his own. He begins to speak as an imaginary superhero, one of the many TV and radio personalities that populate his vivid inner life. He is a person who thrives on routine and repetition, returning to familiar narratives at predictable times. Ending the book on this note, Paul and Judy allow David to speak on his own terms, in a form representative of his own storytelling preferences. This sequence also reflects on the deep knowledge siblings have of one another: Paul doesn't have to follow David because he knows exactly what his brother will do when he leaves the room. Here disability is a shared experience of family, rather than that of a lone individual and his problems. David

may be the person with an autism diagnosis, but he is a son and a sibling, meaning that autism becomes a relationship, an interdependency
involving, among other things, the give and take of caring activity.

The same story looks very different from Judy's point of view. As her
prose sections alternate with Paul's comic, they fill out the picture of
family life. Because she is a sister, Judy is a far more implicated, if often
reluctant, witness of adult caregiving. Her side of the story does not
begin in childhood but in her thirties, as she witnesses the frailty of her
aging mother with alarm that is not shared by her two nondisabled
brothers. Judy is angry at their reluctance to plan for the inevitable, and
fears she will be compelled to replace her mother as David's caregiver.
"I saw myself holding my brother David's hand, leading him through
his days, big emptiness all around me," she writes.[26] This is not the welcome emptiness of an open future but the bleak foreshortening of a
sister's options. She can imagine what that future might hold because,
since childhood, she has witnessed her mother perform the work of
caregiving for the entire family. Judy appreciates that Joan did it with
joy and efficiency—while having no desire to follow in her footsteps.
She resents being positioned as the designated caregiver simply because
of her gender. Her narrative affirms the work of women who are expert
caregivers, without suggesting that they are good caregivers because
they are women or that familial care responsibilities are the natural
obligation of wives, mothers, daughters, or sisters.

A crucial chapter in Judy's story is called "Independence," which at first
seems ironic, given that it is largely about caring for dependent people. In
addition to David, the household includes Joan's elderly father and her
sister-in-law (known as Sister), who is intellectually disabled, nonverbal,
and uses a wheelchair. Although the teenaged Judy removed herself from
caregiving obligations, her memories of that time reveal that she was a perceptive witness to the work performed by her mother, aided by their hired
housekeeper, Dorothy. "During the period when Grandpa and Sister lived
on Lenox Street," she writes, "caretaking was the main event in the house."
In considerable detail, Judy describes the repetitive labors of caring for
the household, which involve washing clothes, washing bodies, washing dishes, cooking, entertaining, watching David, dispensing medicine,

and starting all over again. She suggests that dependency work need not be tedious and unsatisfying, nor does the presence of adult dependents need to be burdensome or depressing. This is because Dorothy and Joan are gifted caregivers who create an environment where "everyone was treated equally; the presiding spirit calmly asserted that this whole scene—wheelchairs, bedpans, and the constant static of unconnected language—was just another way people lived."[27] Although Dorothy and Joan are collaborators, it is worth noting that the Karasiks enjoy a household of dignity and calm because they can afford the help of a paid caregiver, a Black woman with dependents of her own to support. We will return to Dorothy, and the experience of professional care workers, in chapter 6.

Judy identifies the paradox of good caregiving, which is best when most invisible, when the hard and necessary labor of nurturing and sustaining seems pleasant, effortless, and natural. It is easy to forget that such activities are work, or to overlook them entirely. That is, until something goes wrong. Judy fully appreciates Joan and Dorothy only in their absence. When her parents go on vacation, they hire a night nurse to care for her grandfather. Judy hears him calling for help and realizes the nurse is ignoring him, but also that she doesn't know what to do. "The house was cluttered with the accessories of healing—wheelchairs, a walker, a tray for false teeth, bedpans, a potty chair, cotton wool, rubbing alcohol, a shower stall with a flexible stainless steel hose instead of a regular shower head," she writes, "but still I was ignorant, the classic educated fool. I was afraid." Judy's desire to help is toothless in the absence of knowledge or experience to tell her how to act. Having witnessed the failure of care, eventually she does act by calling Dorothy, who leaves her own family in the middle of the night to come to their rescue. The chapter ends with Judy's more complicated understanding of the "independence" in its title: "It wouldn't be until years later that I would learn how to lift someone, how to change a bed underneath someone, how to feed a grown person who ate only soft food. But that night I learned that a person needs to know these things, to be independent."[28] In Judy's revised understanding, care of the self is only a narrow aspect of being "strong and independent"; the feeling of independence is often more like *interdependence*, which includes the acknowledgment of one's own vulnerability, as well the ability and will to care for loved ones in need. Yet even as she comes to appreciate talented caregivers and to learn some caregiving skills of her own, Judy resists the idea that women are naturally inclined to care. She writes frankly of her distaste, finding the work of tending to someone else's needs as a diminution of her own horizons, rather than an activity that is mutually sustaining. There will be no seamless transfer of David's care from one generation of female kin to another.

A sibling perspective on adult dependents like David—who has no inclination or capacity to tell his own story—can be especially valuable at a stage of life when parents and other older guardians are aging or dead. By the time David was placed in residential care in the 1980s, the process of deinstitutionalization was well underway, and his experience is evidence of its many failures. As large facilities closed, clients with more manageable behaviors and medical needs were relocated to community housing. David belongs to a class of people whose complex dependencies continue to make them eligible for an institutional placement.[29] In the book's most devastating chapter, Judy learns that David has been physically (and perhaps sexually) abused in the facility where he lived.[30] The news prompts a shift in perspective from seeing David as a burden on her freedom to the recognition of his point of view. He is vulnerable and, in an unsafe environment, becomes a victim. "I imagined David frightened," she writes. "He calls out in his words that we understand but other people don't. My tall elegant awkward brother, crying, as he falls."[31] Like Paul, Judy has a sibling's capacity to imagine her brother's feelings and actions, as well as being one of the only people who can understand his efforts to communicate. The scenario she describes is wrenching, as is her realization that, in the absence of parents, she is the person who can best translate David's desires and needs for care. As with so many caregiving situations, this is not a role she chose or built into her plans, but she is willing to take it on. Judy assumes her place in a web of care required by her vulnerable brother, acknowledging the extra emotional labor demanded of her as a sister surrounded by male siblings.

Judy's narrative closes with a livable resolution. David has been relocated to a facility where he seems stable and content, and she is happily settled in Italy with a child of her own to care for. From this distance she remains attuned to a care economy that could easily be overlooked precisely because it is functioning effectively. David's new home is staffed by migrant care workers whose salaries sustain the families they left behind.[32] One nurse tells Judy he can afford to visit his children only once a year. Judy, who is briefly separated from her own husband and child while visiting David, feels the gulf that divides her from this Black man who supports his family from afar. Her story ends with the uncomfortable awareness that her choices—to live in Europe, to care for her child but pay others to care for her adult brother—are enabled by workers whose circumstances are far more constrained. Their stories will receive more attention in chapter 6.

The Ride Together is an unfinished story of care, a bifocal siblings' perspective on dependency through many life stages that includes the differing viewpoints of brother and sister. Always already, Paul and Judy know David as an older brother, a source of competition, jealousy, companionship, and amusement who is more than his diagnosis. As adults, they tell stories about their childhood that testify to their parents' caregiving, commemorating activities so ordinary, and so cloaked in domestic privacy, that they would otherwise be lost to time. They also speak as adults who have inherited responsibility for, if not physical provision of, their brother's care. They draw attention to the people who do the work that allows them to have lives apart from David. Unlike the evenhanded advice of sibling self-help literature, *The Ride Together* speaks with a messier polyvocality that testifies to the more ambiguous, and sometimes contradictory, raw (or rawer) materials of remembered sibling experience over the long term.

BEFORE AND AFTER: SUDDEN TEMPORALITIES OF SIBLING ACCIDENT AND INJURY

Nearly all the current sibling advice literature is about brothers and sisters with congenital or early-onset illness or disability, meaning that dependency is inherent to a child's developing identity, experience of

siblinghood, and the dynamics of family. A very different perspective
on care emerges when a sibling becomes dependent later in life. A cata-
strophic event like illness or accident throws familiar patterns of
caregiving into crisis, disrupting established sibling identities and relations, especially when it results in a more long-term dependency. Where
once a brother or sister was known through more mundane dynamics
of sibling rivalry and companionship, everything changes with the
abrupt and irreversible onset of dependency. Whatever coming-of-age
story was being written is violently shredded. For perspective on how
siblings have navigated such wreckage, I turn to two works—Jon Pineda's
Sleep in Me, and Akhil Sharma's *Family Life*—each narrated by a brother
whose admired older sibling is transformed by a severely disabling
accident. In each case, a sudden reversal of fortune renders a once-
vibrant teen vulnerable and dependent, and the long-term dynamics of
sibling relatedness are scrambled.

A new plot emerges. Parents who nagged their kids about homework
and chores redirect their energy toward keeping a badly injured child
alive. The space of home, with its ordinary messes, becomes cluttered
with equipment of care. Routines are disrupted, a healthy child or children pushed to the sidelines. The body of a teen on the cusp of sexual
maturity—and its attendant concerns with privacy, attractiveness, and
erotic discovery—suddenly recenters on the primal functions of moving, breathing, eating, and excreting. In each case, a younger sibling
bears witness. He sees the gendering of care as the lion's share of work
falls to his mother, only sometimes with the support of professional
caregivers, who are also female. He sees the mountains of paperwork,
the meetings and phone calls, and bureaucratic negotiations required
of families of long-term dependents. But he is also a reluctant participant, enlisted to help with care work, household maintenance, and
other unwelcome responsibilities. The expected division of care is
upended as he is asked to give more while receiving less. This pair of
narratives shares another key feature in that both Pineda and Sharma
(and his semiautobiographical protagonist) belong to immigrant families. This vantage makes them aware of how ethnicity and culture shape
attitudes toward dependency and dependency work, as well as the role

of the state in determining how and if it will subsidize the care otherwise performed by family.

At the center of *Sleep in Me*, Jon Pineda's coming-of-age memoir, is the story of his older sister Rica, who, as a teen, was gravely injured in a car crash that left her permanently dependent, with brain damage, seizures, and paralysis on one side of her body. Rica has only minimal capacity for language and no chance to tell her story before her death a few years later. But her brother Jon is a witness to, as well as a participant in, her transformation and the new care routines it demands. He attests to the worry, expense, and sacrifices required to sustain his sister, the burdens that fall disproportionately to his mother, and the impact of Rica's debilitation on his relationships outside the family. But youth and proximity also allow him to assimilate his sister's condition, incorporating it into a new normal that includes more ordinary sibling rivalry and companionship. In the end, Jon's most tragic childhood experience is not Rica's disabling accident, but the failures of care that end her life.

The story of an acquired disability is always divided into before and after, each stage, in Pineda's memoir, associated with different forms of care. Instead of the belated or atypical always-already trajectory associated with congenital disability, an accident violently interrupts development. The immediate physical injury may be localized in a particular body, but the disruption radiates throughout the household and social network. As Rica's sibling, Jon is implicated in the accident, which marks the course of his development as well as hers. Pineda characterizes the teenaged Rica of the before-time as preoccupied with relatively ordinary adolescent self-care: A high school cheerleader, she diets and tries to minimize the appearance of the broad nose and dark skin inherited from her Filipino father. The Rica of the after-time is utterly dependent on the care of others. Pineda describes his sudden awareness of her vulnerability when he finds a strange teenaged boy staring at her naked, comatose body in the hospital. The boy runs away; the encounter is fleeting, but the traumatic "evil of that moment" lingers.[33] Jon feels chagrin at his delayed reaction and fear at what could have happened, recognizing a new duty to protect his sister from violence.

The abruptly grown-up Jon is also charged with mundane responsibilities. Where the Rica of Before had struggled to manage her weight, her injured body becomes a weight to be borne by others. One memorable passage represents the weight of Rica's body as a burden that requires the unwelcome interdependency of brother and sister.

> The idea of weight.
> Whatever it wants it gets. My sister on me now. I'm thirteen again. I'm fourteen. Fifteen. My loose arms slipping under hers. Move forward and then adjust, inevitably counter. For these moments, we appear to be dancing.
> No, not dancing. There is nothing graceful in what I attempt, nor in what her body allows.[34]

The appearance of dancing, but not really, not in ways that are rhythmic and vital. Jon's embrace of his sister is clumsy and resentful. He makes a greedy, demanding "weight" the agent, emphasizing the absence of a human culprit: Neither Rica nor her family members can be blamed for the unwanted situation that has befallen them. This passage also captures the conflicted temporalities of care: The work is redundant and cyclical, but the worker develops, his age advancing with each sentence. The essential nature of this work becomes tragically clear with Rica's death, which results from the failures of those she depends on to bear her weight. While staying in a rehab center, she slumps in her chair and suffocates before anyone notices. Her family's worst fears—that she would be harmed if left in the care of strangers—are realized. Having carried his sister's weight for years, Jon carries the most awful burden of all when he serves as a pallbearer at her funeral. He recalls the unwieldy weight of her coffin: "She was heavy, surprisingly so, and there was some minor struggle placing her into the back of the hearse." This is the last of his many struggles with Rica's passive body, although her memory will have a weight of its own. "There was still the weight of her absence to figure," Pineda writes. "None of us would be prepared."[35] Caring for Rica was a burden, but not an entirely negative one. It also structured family life, particularly for her mother.

Care takes up time and space, and its absence can bring emptiness and loss of purpose instead of (or even along with) freedom. Rica's loss is a further weight to be negotiated by those left behind.

Pineda earns the tragedy of Rica's loss by showing how, amid the suffering and difficulty associated with her injuries, her life continued to be a source of meaning, companionship, and, sometimes, pleasure for her siblings. In the shared environment of home and family, Jon is especially well positioned to observe the subtle ways Rica's personhood endures—her tenderness, foul language, cheesy sense of humor—even as many of her capacities are impaired. His anecdotes attest to the endurance of self in her cursing and pranks. Rica's younger brothers provide another view of her life as a disabled person. Unlike Jon, they have few memories of a time before, and fewer responsibilities for Rica's physical care. This standpoint means that they do not see her primarily in terms of deficits. Pineda tries to imagine how his brothers might tell a story in which disability is always already an aspect of Rica's identity, rather than the product of grievous injury, pain, and loss. "They have known her mostly as this person who must rely on them," he observes.

She is not broken.
We are the ones who are broken.[36]

Brokenness registers in relation to a feeling of lost wholeness. The younger brothers can see Rica as intact without ignoring her disability. Where the rest of the family is "broken" by their melancholic attachment to the person she was before, the younger children see her dependency as a feature, not a bug.

In a family where the narrator is one among multiple siblings, brothers and sisters provide context. They show how any one account is shaped by the standpoint and experience of its teller, and suggest (or, in the Karasiks' case, include) alternative versions of the same story. These show how perspectives on care are informed by gender and family role but also by age, birth order, and temperament. *Sleep in Me* is Jon's story, so his experiences dominate, but he is also part of a family, a participant-observer in its webs of care. As a sibling, he attests to the unwelcome experience of caring for a dependent older sister, while also being a witness to the uneven impact of her care on different members of the household.

There is no such perspective available in a nuclear family where there are just two siblings. When one child is incapable of self-representation, the other's voice provides the sole testimony to sibling experience. This is the situation in Akhil Sharma's autofictional novel, *Family Life*. As the only sibling of a suddenly disabled brother, Ajay, the narrator, has no peer to share his experiences or modulate his perceptions and feelings. His isolation is compounded by the fact that he is a recent immigrant to the United States. His aspiring, middle-class family has only recently relocated from India, leaving them far away from a community that might otherwise share the burdens of care work.[37] *Family Life* begins as a conventional immigration narrative, but the plot detours sharply when the Mishras' cherished eldest son, Birju, is gravely injured in a swimming pool accident. Sophisticated medical interventions allow him to survive a coma but leave him in a persistent vegetative state. The novel offers an immigrant's perspective on a health care system that takes extraordinary measures to save lives without providing adequate care for the severely disabled who live on. The expectation that family, especially female relatives, will serve as care managers, nurses, and cheerleaders for their medically fragile son destabilizes the Mishras' tenuous foothold in the United States. The majority of Sharma's novel is about how a sibling experiences the dramatic reorganization of family life around care for his dependent brother. Narrating in first person, Ajay describes the initial upheaval in his family with the unsentimental, self-absorbed, and often darkly comic voice of a child, his understanding changing as he matures.

Family Life is particularly good at capturing the full spectrum of emotions a child may experience when a sibling is gravely injured or sick. Ajay is used to being cared for by doting parents and his elder brother, with minimal expectations of reciprocity. After the accident, he sometimes expresses pity and concern for his brother, but he is also resentful, lonely, and selfish, particularly as a new normal sets in, with adult attention focused on Birju's care. There is a doubleness to his narrative perspective, which reports on his parents' distraction with the unsentimental self-absorption of a child, but comes from an adult author, writing decades later, with a more sympathetic understanding of adult responsibilities and worries. With Ajay as a guide, the novel peels back the Mishras' outward-facing restraint to reveal the more ignoble aspects of family life; he is witness to the rage, frustration, and despair of his parents' most unguarded moments. Predictably, most of the care work falls to his mother, who gives up her paying job to tend to Birju. Unlike the cheerful, patient mothers in previous narratives, Shuba expresses her worry and exhaustion as anger, shouting at the doctors, hospital staff, and care workers, as well as her husband and younger son. Ajay's father, Rajinder, provides the family's only source of income, and he strains to meet the mounting costs of Birju's long-term care. He responds to stress by binge drinking, making him unable to help with Birju and causing him to soil the house with vomit and urine that his wife has to clean up.

The child Ajay alternates between compassion and judgment of his parents' weaknesses. But by far his greatest condemnation is reserved for the public and private institutions that promise (often brokenly) to help dependents and their families. As a child and an immigrant, he has an especially damning view of the victims' compensation received by his family. The financial settlement provided by the owners of the pool is grossly inadequate to the expense of Birju's ongoing need for care. In one darkly comic passage, Ajay attempts to sum up the time his parents expend on caring for his brother in monetary terms. Doing the math from the standpoint of a bright but naïve child, he exposes the unseen and undercompensated care work expected of the family and the hypothetical financial losses it sustains as a result.

My father had said that financial settlements were based on how much the person injured could earn. As I walked, I thought of how much the money meant in terms of hourly pay. I reasoned that my mother went to the nursing home every day. She was there from eight thirty to seven. This meant she worked about ten hours a day, seven days a week. I was there from three to seven every weekday and both days on the weekend. I was not working all the time, though, when I was home. My father was also there on weeknights and weekends. If I were to undercount, my father and I each spent twenty hours a week at the nursing home. Birju was damaged all the time, and so this could count as a hundred hours of work a week. Two hundred and ten hours a week times fifty weeks was about ten thousand hours a year. If Birju remained alive for ten years, there was a hundred thousand hours of work. Six hundred and eighteen divided by a hundred was six dollars and eighteen cents.[38]

Ajay's childish calculations draw attention to the unpaid family labor, the care work outsourced to friends and relatives that helps minimize costs to hospitals, nursing homes, and insurance companies.[39] His account of care work includes more passive states like sitting, waiting, exerting a presence. Birju's family does work when they visit, reminding staff that he is loved and protecting him from harms that befall unattended residents. Priceless, nonspecific, and time-consuming, such preventative contributions only exacerbate the difficulty of accounting for the monetary value of Birju's care.

In addition to the hours of watching and tending, Birju's care also involves bureaucratic labor. Unlike the cyclical, slow, and intimate time of physical caregiving, the time of care management is stupid, boring, and repetitive. Ajay describes the long hours his parents spend researching, filling out paperwork, paying bills, and making phone calls to argue with the insurance company over medical supplies and nursing care. After Rajinder earns his salary outside the home, he devotes his weekends to the unpaid labor of securing care for his son. The table that should be a place to gather for a family meal is instead covered with objects related to the managerial care of a medically fragile dependent, "insurance forms . . . rubber-banded stacks of letters, a stapler, his checkbook, and a yellow legal pad on which he wrote letters to the insurance company."[40] Ajay doesn't do the work himself, but he experiences it in the absence of his father's attention, the clutter, and the subdued atmosphere of the household.

While *Family Life* focuses most intently on the aftermath of Birju's accident, it follows the long term of severe disability by looking several decades into the future. We know the Mishra family will come through the immediate crisis because the novel begins with a middle-aged Ajay gently teasing his seventy-two-year-old father about being a "sad baby."[41] There is no mention of Birju. Ajay's silence resists the kind of prurient curiosity about the future displayed by outsiders throughout the novel. But it is also evidence that this is a sibling's story. Birju's accident is a major event, but not the sole defining feature of Ajay's selfhood. His deliberate silence signals that it is less important for the reader to know how and if Birju lives or dies than how his accident shapes his brother's life. A key aspect of Ajay's maturation is his understanding that, unlike his parents, his fate is not bound to caring for Birju. While siblings sometimes do grow up to become guardians of disabled adult brothers and sisters, they don't have to. We don't know whether Ajay avoids this future because his brother died too soon or because of choices made by his family. We do know that he is successful enough to support his parents financially. His story is a reminder that there is no predetermined legal or social script for sibling relationships, especially as they age into adulthood. Unlike his parents, who are obligated to care for their son whether they want to or not, Ajay can choose a life apart from their burdens. Together with the Karasiks', his story—told over the long term—shows that sibling care can take a variety of forms, sometimes involving management and financial support to distribute the work, if not doing the hands-on support directly.

The members of Gen S are now well into middle age, and their stories about distinctly modern experiences of siblinghood, dependency, and care are circulating. They break new ground, but without leaving a straightforward path for those coming behind. Their diversity is evidence that there is no one-size-fits-all model to care for long-term dependents; nor is there one for the relatively unscripted status of siblinghood obligations and bonds, even when a brother or sister lives with intense and prolonged dependency. Siblinghood is an utterly ubiquitous social role, but it has no particular narrative arc. Nonetheless, I have tried to show commonalities among the perspectives of those who share a household and a set of parents with an exceptionally dependent brother or sister and belong to the same generational cohort. Sibling-hood is a relation of profound, intimate, and unchosen interdependency, although its responsibilities and long-term commitments are less clear-cut than those of parents and children. That lack of clarity can be disorienting and scary, especially when it involves the well-being of a vulnerable person. But it also forces an important reckoning with the meanings of care, work, and family.

This chapter focuses on literary narratives because they allow for the ambiguity and emotional nuance that are essential ingredients of all prolonged caring relationships but especially pronounced in sibling-hood. Narrated from the viewpoint of a sibling who is both witness and participant, these stories emphasize care work that is at the margins of most life writing. With the irreverence of familiarity, sibling narrators are willing to say when it absolutely sucks; what aspects of care are dis-gusting and undignified; what makes them sad or resentful; and how and why they love a particular, imperfect, and dependent fellow human. They also show us how and why the temporal arc of sibling dependency matters. It matters whether a condition is congenital or early onset—meaning that it is always already an inherent part of a brother or sister's selfhood and perhaps more fully assimilated into the dynamics of fam-ily life—or a result of later illness or disability that causes an upheaval in a household.

The absence of a robust critical conversation should not be taken as a sign that siblings are marginal to care in a family. Their importance cannot be overstated, and the insights they offer are socially relevant far beyond particular situations where a child is exceptionally ill or dis-abled. Siblinghood is a lateral relationship that often models how we will interact with peers in the world beyond the family. Inevitably those horizontal relationships will be asymmetrical, characterized by imbal-ances in resources, needs, and abilities. The relationship I formed with my younger sister must have anticipated and shaped, in myriad and infinitely complicated ways, my relationships with coworkers, neigh-bors, and friends. While mothering is often held up as a paradigm for care, siblinghood is a less hierarchical model for imagining our interdependency with others and our responsibility to care for those who are dependent. And sibling narratives can get at the rewards of interdependency, but also at the deep-seated antipathy, resentment, and resistance that entanglement with dependency may occasion.

I write this chapter surrounded by the unfolding drama of sibling development. My boys remind me of Walter and Gary, the brothers in the 2011 movie *The Muppets*. Gary (a human played by Jason Segel) is tall, clean-cut, and handsome, while Walter (a Muppet) is short, cute, and hapless (figure 2.2). They are kindred spirits who wear the same

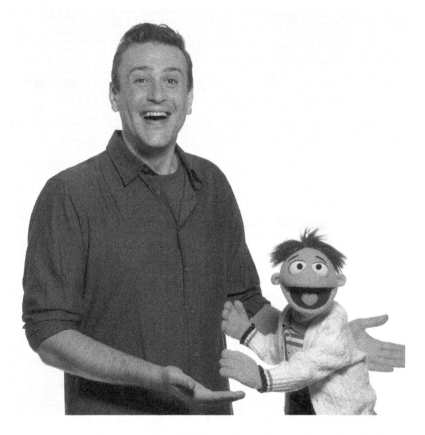

FIGURE 2.2 A publicity photo from *The Muppet Movie* showing Gary (played by Jason Segel) and his Muppet brother, Walter.

Source: © Disney.

clothes, enjoy the same activities, and are the best of friends. That is, until they become aware that man and Muppet are fundamentally different, their individual desires and needs seemingly irreconcilable. When Walter's newfound kinship with a community of Muppets throws Gary into an identity crisis, he sings, soulfully, about his doubts. "Am I a man, or am I a Muppet?" he asks as he confronts an unwelcome choice between his brother's new friends and his human fiancée. In the film's Hollywood-happy ending, Gary doesn't really have to choose. Man and Muppet occupy a spectrum that can be negotiated. The brothers maintain their friendship while each also finds belonging in a group of his own kind. Each will have the opportunity for independent growth without sacrificing his brother's love and support.

My sons—ages fourteen and sixteen at the time of this writing—are also the best of friends, although they never wear matching clothes, brush their teeth in sync, or sing tuneful duets. Like Gary and Walter, one is tall and the other short; one enjoys easy success at sports, friendship, and academics, while the other has little interest in these measures of accomplishment. One of my sons is also multiply disabled, and the other is typical. Sometimes their differences matter hardly at all as they pummel each other, exchange rude text messages, and play on the Xbox. But sometimes they seem as profound as the species divide between man and Muppet.

My typically developing son, Noah, is a witness to my work as his younger brother's caregiver. He hears me cursing Henry's slowness in the bathroom, our elaborate negotiations over bed and screen time, my sharp response to reports that he was disruptive at school. Noah sees me worn out by the physical labor of scheduling and maintaining his brother's life, even as he conveniently forgets that I do similar chores for him. Noah may no longer need help in the bathroom, but he too makes messes that he doesn't clean up, requires someone to fill out endless forms for school and camp, and expects someone else to prepare dinner. But because his brother's dependencies are more atypical— prolonged, unpredictable, time consuming—it is easier to see caring for him as work and to forget about the many other tasks of maintenance our family requires.

Noah also witnesses the necessity of distributed care, although he usually notices only when it fails. I am his brother's primary caregiver, but I share those responsibilities with his father and a complicated network of nonfamilial caregivers that includes friends, teachers, therapists, camp counselors, and volunteers. Noah also witnesses my work as an employer of paid caregivers. There is no employee handbook for Henry's care, and he is not yet capable of representing (or tending to) his own needs. What Noah sees in his peripheral vision is the obscure labor I perform to archive the details of his brother's needs and habits for use in training other people to provide him with care, most of it mental, but sometimes recorded in lists, instruction manuals, and guidebooks. He witnesses my efforts to treat Henry's caregivers with respect, learn from them, and compensate them financially for the valued work that they do. I think Noah benefits from being my sometime-witness, but I also want him to enjoy the self-absorption of adolescence, the feeling expressed by Judy Karasik that one is "strong and independent," however illusory that may be. And when the care network I've organized works as it should, it is almost invisible, allowing Noah, like Paul Karasik, to be rushing out the door while his mother stays a minor character in the background. Only when one or more of the nodes malfunction does care work come sharply to the forefront, as it did in the months of pandemic seclusion our family recently experienced.

Noah is no silent onlooker. Increasingly, he too provides care for his brother, infusing it with his own adolescent style. He decides they will eat the takeout food directly from the container with their bare hands or play baseball indoors or gaze into their respective screens without talking. He also reminds me that he is a witness, with regular editorializing on my abilities as a parent and on the limitations of Henry's other caregivers. Sometimes he commiserates. More often, he is a critic. To his ears, my voice is overly condescending, manipulative, or kinder than his brother deserves. He is quick to tell me when I have breached his brother's privacy and instructs me to be more patient or stricter, more lenient or gentle, angrier or more compassionate. Sometimes he enlists his brother in rebellion against parental authority. Together they bang their utensils on the dinner table, drive parents from the room with screeches and howls, jump on the furniture, or hog the TV to play video games. They laugh when we plead with them to go to bed or sit still, and they accuse us of being old, boring, and tired. Sometimes they cuddle, with Henry nestling against Noah's chest, while Noah rests his cheek against the top of his brother's head. These alliances can be touching or annoying; they are also evidence of a relationship separate from and only partially visible to my parental gaze. They remind me that neither son remembers a world without his brother and that, hopefully, this present is an opening chapter in a lifelong relationship. There is some chance each may end up knowing his brother longer than any other person.

I'm not sure what Henry understands of the future. He doesn't talk about much beyond our plans for a summer vacation and return to school in the fall. Having seen Noah learning to drive, he tells me, vaguely, that he too wants to drive a car. Noah is more likely to think ahead, sometimes including his brother in his plans and concerns. When he was younger he talked of buying a house with a wing for Henry or an apartment they would share as roommates. Sometimes he asks questions about where his brother will live, whether he will go to college, and what jobs he might have. Even as I want Noah to think of Henry as an individual with an open future, I also want him to consider how disability shapes Henry's opportunities and aspirations. I introduce him to adults with Down syndrome, who I hope will help him imagine a range of possible outcomes for Henry. I want Noah to be prepared for his brother's future dependency, even as I hope he will try to reshape the world to maximize Henry's opportunities. I want Noah to feel he has abundant choices about where his own life will go, but I also hope he will want an ongoing relationship with his brother. I realize the burden of the many ambitions and desires I have for my older son.

Ironically, in some respects Noah is the brother with the less open future since it is hard to imagine an outcome where he avoids the burdens of aging parents, as well as a disabled brother. Christina Crosby's story reminds me that our family's future could be rearranged by accident, illness, or other misfortune at any time. And Noah could throw up his hands, cut all ties with his immediate family, and move to a distant part of the world. He could also be like Ajay Mishra, in *Family Matters*, withdrawing to a sustainable distance without severing relationships. But in the most likely case, Noah ends up caring for someone more dependent and outlives the rest of our nuclear family. This is not necessarily a grim future, since caring can be one, often meaningful, aspect of a lengthy and evolving life trajectory. Burdens can be more or less onerous, unwanted or welcome. A sense of responsibility toward others doesn't have to compromise a life filled with varied and worthwhile experiences, nor should care be the exclusive responsibility of immediate, biological family. I hope that I am giving both of my sons tools to develop a supportive circle of nonbiological family and friends, and that their care networks will be robust and wide ranging. Siblings, like families more broadly, can be an essential resource for care, but they aren't always, and they have limits. Later in this book I'll consider the possibilities and shortcomings of alternatives or supplements to the unpaid care work of siblings and other familyish people.

My boys are a part of something new, no longer Gen S, because the groundwork of inclusion has been laid. But what that means for the future and how it will affect care relations is an unwritten story. As I close this chapter, perhaps more than any other in this book, I am aware that I write myself off the page. In the absence of more tragic outcomes, my sons, like so many other siblings, will have a relationship that endures long after I'm gone. Each will see more of how his brother's life develops, and, as adults, they will likely know each other more intimately than I will know either of them. I will be a character in stories they tell to other people. An understanding of family focused only on parents and children misses how the prolonged relationships among siblings and with other lateral peers inform attitudes about care giving and receiving. So too, renewed attention to siblings might prompt a reconsideration of mothering as the primal referent for caring relationships. There are few, if any, experiences that replicate the bond between mother and child. Perhaps the rivalrous, complicated, and unscripted relations among siblings are a more fitting model for how family dynamics get perpetuated in caring relations in the world beyond. And if that is the case, then we need to look beyond the neat, transparent-seeming accounts of advice literature to the variety, ambiguities, and contradictions of sibling narrative.

3

LATERAL KINSHIP AND THE
BORROWED TIME OF HIV/AIDS

n Tony Kushner's epic *Angels in America* there are some artful care-givers and some who fail miserably when needed most. In one of the play's more devastating scenes, Louis abandons his longtime partner, Prior Walter, while he is hospitalized with an AIDS-related ill-ness. When Prior accuses Louis of acting like a "criminal," Louis responds, sardonically, "There oughta be a law."[1] There oughta be, but there isn't. There are no legal regulations on his behavior, however cow-ardly and unethical. There are no lawful options to cement the rela-tionship between these men, nor is Louis required to care for his sick partner in a time of mass death. When Louis moves out of their shared apartment, Prior has no biological family to look out for him, a vacancy emphasized by his hallucinations of ghostly Walter ancestors who heckle rather than comfort. Into the vacuum steps Belize, a queer nurse and longtime friend who takes up the slack, as Black and Brown people are so often required to do.[2] A more surprising source of comfort is Hannah, a visiting Mormon drawn to Prior's sublime visions of angels. She keeps him company in the hospital, even as she is not very good at caring for her own adult son. The end of the play brings neither closure through death (tragedy) nor renewal of romantic ties (comedy). Instead Prior lives on, having forgiven Louis but unwilling to take him back. In the last scene, Prior, Louis, Hannah, and Belize assemble at Central

Park's Bethesda Fountain—named for a biblical site of healing—a diverse and improvised group unevenly committed to caring for Prior and for one another.

Angels was among the most celebrated of many HIV/AIDS narratives that began to appear in the early-mid 1990s in the United States and Britain, as the epidemic swept through the arts world. Varied in form and tenor, these works belong to a moment when questions about dependency, care, and family became an urgent priority for the ill and their supporters. They landed with particular irony for gay men who were estranged from their biological families. As Louis's biting comment implies, gay couples' commitments were not sanctioned by law—no matter how closely they resembled heterosexual marriages— nor were they legally bound to care, as are parents or wedded spouses. In Kushner's play these circumstances lead to a devastating betrayal. More typically, gay men and their support networks took extraordinary measures to care for one another in the face of abandonment by their families of origin, government, and established health care institutions. Often their devotion went unrecognized, and many faced devastating exclusions from their partners' medical decisions, hospital rooms, and funerals. But the epidemic also saw the creation of new and more inclusive narratives about kinship that would have a lasting effect on health care policy and collective social understandings of family.[3]

Narratives about the transformative impact of HIV/AIDS on care and chosen family are the subject of this chapter. Continuing the discussion of horizontal relationships from the previous chapter on siblings, I turn to the kinship assemblages of LGBTQ people, which may or may not include couples at the center. I argue that, at a moment of widespread death and debility, their care arrangements operate on "borrowed time," a phrase I adopt from Paul Monette's 1988 memoir about caring for his gravely ill partner, Roger, while confronting his own seropositive future.[4] "Borrowed time" aptly describes the temporal consciousness of the first generation of people with HIV/AIDS, who experience each moment as a precious and agonizing postponement of a dreaded inevitability. Borrowed time is not yours to own, and its sweet pleasures come at a steep price. Living on borrowed time means caring for one another in the face of imminent and certain death, a known future that informs how one lives in the present and reassesses the past. To appreciate its value without lapsing into despair at its impermanence requires constant and exhausting vigilance. In what follows, I consider representations of care on borrowed time from the first stage of the epidemic and its aftermath, paying attention to how different narrative forms—fiction, memoir, photography, drama— respond to the particular temporalities of terminal illness. I am interested in how these stories commemorate the care work of those lost to AIDS and their supporters but also in how they reshape understandings of kinship and care outside of heteronormative family institutions. My conclusion turns to Matthew Lopez's 2018 play, *The Inheritance*, to consider the legacy of the AIDS crisis on subsequent generations of gay men caring for one another. I started this book with the observation that exchanges of care are particular to a time and place. This may be the chapter where I am most aware of care's specificity. At the time most of these stories were written, an AIDS diagnosis was almost always fatal. Today, it is a treatable condition for some populations, while continuing to devastate others.

HISTORY, TEMPORALITY, KINSHIP

"THERE ARE NO GAY MEN MY AGE," cries Henry Wilcox in *The Inheritance*, "not nearly enough."[5] Now in his sixties, he is referring to the wages of AIDS on a generation for whom a diagnosis meant almost certain death. That time, when widespread illness forced care work into the foreground, reconfiguring kinship arrangements and priorities, is the historical impetus for this chapter. The emergence of HIV/AIDS—an illness initially associated with gay men and IV drug users—is an ignoble episode in the history of government and institutionalized health care, and historians have documented the impact of delays and inaction. The physical suffering of the sick was compounded by failures of care, rejection by biological family, social ostracism, and compromised treatment by medical providers. Firsthand accounts from San Francisco General Hospital's AIDS clinic in the early 1980s describe janitors dressed in hazmat suits, doctors and nurses who avoided their patients, sheets going unchanged, and food service staff who refused to enter the rooms of infected patients.[6] The shortcomings in professional care placed a tremendous burden on supporters of the ill, shaping their loss and its aftermath.

Sometimes those debilitated by AIDS had legal and biological relatives to care for them. But what happens when family, the institution positioned as the default resource of care, turns away from those in need? Many of the LGBTQ people who came out during the sexual revolution of the 1960s and 1970s had been shunned by their families of origin. Estrangement and rejection by biological family is a common theme in LGBTQ literature of the period, an absence brought into the foreground by the dependencies of grave illness. "The most common link between all gay people," the protagonist of Sarah Schulman's 1985 novel, *Rat Bohemia*, laments, "is that at some time in our lives, often extended, our families have treated us shabbily because of our homosexuality. They punish us, but we did not do anything wrong." Another character calls his fellow ACT UP members his "family," which to him means "we are so intimate that we can act out all of our pain in front of each other. We can tell each other the truth."[7] Here, family is defined not by law or religion but as the group that offers absolute acceptance and mutual understanding in a time of crisis. "For gay people, our friends form our nuclear families," writes the LGBTQ activist Urvashi Vaid. "While our communities take on the role of an extended family system. . . . Our family commitment to each other is not forced, but desired."[8] Without throwing out the concept of family altogether, these voices attest to the urgent task of reconfiguring it to meet the needs of a vulnerable population.

"Chosen family" is the term often used to describe such voluntary social networks, which may span generations but typically consist of generational peers drawn together by dedication to care for one another. Kath Weston's foundational 1991 ethnography, *Families We Choose*, explored the kinship arrangements of gay men and lesbians in Northern

California's Bay Area in the decades following the sexual revolution. Weston's research also coincided with the first decade of the AIDS epidemic. Her study emphasizes how illness brought care to the forefront of LGBTQ family values and tested the commitment to be present in times of need. "When people told relatives and friends that they had AIDS," writes Weston, "kin ties were reevaluated, constituted, or alienated in the act, defined by who (if anyone) stepped forward to offer love, care, and financial assistance for the protracted and expensive battles with opportunistic infections that accompany this disease."[9] Sometimes chosen family centered on long-term partnerships unrecognized by law but otherwise similar to those of married couples. Paul Monette describes his relationship with Roger as "the 'group of two' that Freud calls a marriage."[10] But sometimes kinship arrangements were more situational, as the requirements of caring for a gravely ill person transformed loose social networks into something more binding. In these cases, caregiving patterns and activities were often vague and piecemeal. Like siblinghood, there is no dominant social script to determine obligations for giving and receiving care in a makeshift familyish assemblage, especially one that springs up at a moment of crisis. Narratives about caring for people with AIDS attest to the creativity and tenacity of such transient communities but also to the rivalries, conflicts, and undercurrents of resentment that arise in an emergency where everyone is exhausted and overtaxed and roles are constantly being improvised and reinvented.

I use the term "chosen family" to describe the kinship of LGBTQ people caring for one another, while being mindful of its limitations. Despite its name, chosen family is often formed under conditions of constraint, particularly in the time of AIDS. Acting as family to a gravely ill person is stressful and exhausting. "I wanted to run away, I wanted it to be over," confesses Amy Hoffman in *Hospital Time*, a memoir about caring for a friend dying of AIDS.[11] The social network assembled around Hoffman's friend, Mike, is loose and improvised, formed out of necessity rather than choice. Although Hoffman calls Mike's circle a "family," I am aware that some queer people reject the term altogether, believing that the odor of heteronormativity is baked into the word itself.[12] Elizabeth Freeman draws on Pierre Bourdieu's concept of "practical kinship" to describe the intimacies of queer people as an alternative to family. As she summarizes, "kinship is a set of *acts* that may or may not follow the official recognized lines of alliance and descent, and that in any case take precedence over the latter in everyday life."[13] This emphasis on practice is an apt way to describe the care assemblages of people with AIDS and their supporters, and it is one that allows me to include narratives about care for people debilitated by illness who have no families, chosen or otherwise. Still, I will also refer to "chosen family" when appropriate because that is the descriptor most often used in the narratives themselves and in the new health care policies and customs that emerged in the wake of AIDS.[14] I use this language with awareness of its imperfections, as well as its potential. An affiliation "chosen" under evident constraint can draw attention to the gaps between legal and biological definitions of family and the practical social arrangements people develop to care for one another.

The "borrowed time" in the title of this chapter refers to care in that indeterminate and uncertain period of postponement before death, as it is experienced by the ill person as well as those who care for and about them. Fatal illness shapes the temporality of care in AIDS narratives of the 1980s and 1990s. Dying has its own clock, as does the work associated with it. Its timing is unpredictable and makes no exceptions for the needs and desires of the living. Caring for someone with a terminal illness promises none of the rewards of recovery or reciprocity, a difficult situation we have already encountered in Emily Rapp's account of mothering a dying son in chapter 1. Care is given because it is necessary, racking up endless social debt with no hope of repayment or even recognition. Borrowed time is paradoxical: It may seem to pause but also to speed up, to be both structured and formless, empty and impossibly full. So much of the time of grave illness is spent waiting, in bed or at bedsides, in medical appointments, enduring treatments or respite from treatments. The time of waiting may feel painfully slow and elongated by suffering, confusion, and the redundant chores of caregiving and receiving. It may seem boring and pointless and empty. But borrowed time is contradictory because it is also infused with a sense of urgency and preciousness, of the need to experience and be mindful of each hard-won moment. What if this is our last chance? Will tomorrow be the day everything changes?

On borrowed time it is both essential and impossible to live only in the present. Time is colored by an acute awareness of an impending future that is delayed but inevitable. Writing of queer ecology in an age of climate change, Sarah Ensor argues for an "ethics of temporariness" that involves accepting, rather than attempting to stave off, an antici-pated loss. She argues that aspiring to "save" the environment is doomed to failure because it is a nostalgic project that can only succeed by restoring wholeness. Instead she proposes that dwelling with inevi-table impermanence and frailty could prompt more sustainable action in a world blighted by climate change.[15] Informed by queer theory, Ensor extends this ethic to social relationships, where vulnerability can be the basis for caring with tenderness and determination to make the time we have matter. In the readings to come, I am interested in the effects of terminality on narratives about care in the first-generation experi-ence of AIDS. I consider what it means to care when there is no long term, in stories about how the borrowed time of fatal illness shapes kin-ship practices. And I look at how care on borrowed time may inspire formal choices, including the flamboyant style of Kushner's *Angels in America*, the gossipy voices of Monette's *Borrowed Time* and Susan Sontag's "The Way We Live Now," the collaborative process made visi-ble in Tom Joslin and Peter Freedman's documentary film *Silverlake Life*, and the visual tropes in Terese Frare's photojournalism.

My understanding of borrowed time is shaped by my own childhood experience of improvised care networks in a time of terminal illness. My parents were married heterosexuals: he the breadwinner, she a musician who cut back on career to be the primary caregiver for two biological children. Our conventional household was upended when my mother was diagnosed with terminal cancer that led to her death eighteen months later. I was six; my sister was four. We were all living on borrowed time, although I was too young to know that. I was not the ill person or her caregiver, but I was a witness and a casualty. What memories I have of my mother involve her being cared for rather than providing me with care. As our domestic life imploded, a loose network of friends and neighbors stepped in to care for us, and I remember mother-adjacent people, usually but not always women, doing motherly things for me. This was practical kinship, involving generous people attending to work that needed to be done rather than fulfilling the obligations attached to a particular social role. The care was haphazard and unpredictable, with one person taking me for a haircut, another buying me pajamas, an occasional play date or sleepover. This chapter is underwritten by my experience of the networks of care that can form in a sudden crisis; the ambience of tenderness, devotion, resentment, and grief they generate; and the difficulty of preserving them in the aftermath of tragedy. Formed in haste, those webs unspool and reconfigure; I'm sure I have forgotten many acts of kindness and comfort. I like to think they were extended without expectation of a response. Toward the end of the chapter, I consider what it would mean to repay the debt on borrowed time. In the version I explore, those who benefited from or witnessed the provision of care reciprocate by offering care to others in need. Writing this chapter has caused me to think a lot about the asymmetrical circulation of debts and indebtedness, and whether I have or will ever give as much as I once received.

A "GROUP OF TWO": QUEER COUPLES ON BORROWED TIME

By the mid-1980s, AIDS had already assumed a recognizable narrative form, and it was not pretty. "Only four thousand had died by March '85," writes Paul Monette, "but already we all knew stories of men left incoherent in their own excrement, abandoned overnight by friends, shipped back to a fundamentalist family to pay the wages of sin. They were chained to their beds with dementia in New York. They lost their houses and all their insurance. The most horrible death in modern medicine, people said."[16] As the decade continued and these stories proliferated, the narrative tropes of misery and abandonment endured, becoming more emphatic with each repetition—the inadequacy of medical institutions, loss of belongings, neglect by government, rejection by biological relatives, destruction of social networks—all culminating in an awful death. In these stories, "family" is not a bedrock of support and unconditional love but a wellspring of moral condemnation that hypocritically abandons the ill and dying in their time of greatest need.

The horrific failures Monette describes are a backdrop to a story of care at its best. *Borrowed Time* is a memoir about the tenacious love he shared with his long-term companion, Roger, who died of AIDS, not alone but in the company of his parents and life partner. Monette returns repeatedly to the jarring contrast between his life and the broader crisis to emphasize their good fortune and suggest how easily things could have been otherwise. His story is a testament to exceptional care amid a population-wide crisis in which many more died alone and uncared for. Beginning with his title, the narrative is suffused with a sense that time at the end of life is "borrowed," precious, unpredictable, unearned, and finite. Borrowed time coincides with other temporalities, including the couple's long relationship, the distorted and frenetic time of crisis, and an unthinkable future paradependency, in which a seropositive partner lives on, bereft and likely to face an equally awful and untimely death.

The plot of *Borrowed Time* tracks the arc of fatal illness. It begins with the appearance of Roger's symptoms, follows his cycles of debilitation and recovery, and eventually his passing. The chronological movement of the present detours to recount the relationship he enjoyed with Paul for over a decade before. The story of a devoted partner nursing a beloved to untimely death is a recipe for sentimentality, and Monette often leans into the emotional undercurrents of his material. Embracing sentiment, his narrative is an antidote to the toxic image, circulating widely at the time, of the lone gay man as an uncaring vector of contagion. By the mid 1980s, the epidemic had already assumed a familiar moral cast, blaming individuals for irresponsible behavior, underwritten by the thoughtless hedonism of an entire subculture.[17]

The most enduring symbolic figure in this myth is Patient Zero, an antihero made famous by Randy Shilts's bestselling documentary, *And the Band Played On* (1987), which was published a year before *Borrowed Time*. According to that narrative, AIDS was introduced to the United States by a Canadian flight attendant, Gaetan Dugas, who used his lay-overs as opportunities for orgiastic tours through the nation's gay urban nightlife. Shilts depicts Dugas as a textbook villain who knowingly infects his victims before telling them, "I've got gay cancer. I'm going to die and so are you."[18] It is hard to think of a more succinct statement of uncaring. But did it actually happen? In the last decade, genetic sequencing technology has exonerated Dugas from this notorious post-humous legacy, proving that neither he, nor any other identifiable indi-vidual, could be held responsible for infecting an entire population.[19] The insights of science have been buttressed by more nuanced portraits of Dugas's character and relationships that complicate his image as a cartoonish bad guy.[20] These were not available at the time of Monette's writing, but sentimentality offered a counter to the panicky stereotype of the selfish, sex-crazed gay man.

In Monette's memoir, the borrowed time of Roger's illness is given meaning by looking back at the time before. Paul and Roger under-stand themselves as a married couple. Although unrecognized by law, their commitment is strengthened by the experience of grave illness and the limited horizon it introduced. Monette rewrites the homopho-bic narrative of Patient Zero with a more salutary alternative, "the story of a kind of bond that the growing oral history of AIDS records again and again. Whatever happened to Roger happened to me, and my numb strength was a crutch for his frailty."[21] Roger's medical crisis brings them closer together, deepening bonds that are already in place. Each small-scale act of comfort in the present loops into the fabric of a long-term, committed relationship. Caring acts fold the present of grave illness into the shared past accrued by the two men. The intimate knowledge of each other acquired over time is stored as muscle mem-ory that allows Paul to care for Roger, and Roger to complete his care.

The performance of sickbed care in the present also draws the couple together in new ways, equally laden with sentiment. Repeatedly,

Monette describes a seamless interdependence: He grips Roger's shoulders "as if I would fuse us into a unit." In their final days "I couldn't think at all anymore without thinking first about Rog," and Rog says to Paul, "with a mixture of astonishment and tenderness, 'But we're the same person. When did that happen?'"[22] Paul's care for Roger can sound a lot like sex, involving skin-to-skin contact, the exchange of fluids, exposure of vulnerable areas of the body, and a quasi-mystical sense of union. Indeed, in the time of grave illness spanned by Monette's memoir, the exchange of care between a sick person and a beloved partner takes the place of sex in serving as the physical enactment of their utter interdependency. The borrowed time of grave illness makes the acts of intimacy Monette describes both precious and dreadful. Care on borrowed time involves a set of actions, but it is also about navigating an almost unbearable emotional paradox. Borrowed time requires the couple to maintain enough awareness of the awful future to experience each moment with gratitude. But they also have to manage that awareness enough to avoid ruining the time that they have, as it narrows from weeks to days to moments.

The concept of time "borrowed" also suggests a temporary transfer of resources, since any gain made by Paul and Roger must involve an expenditure by someone else. When the sociologist Georg Simmel identified the dyad as the fundamental unit of social life in 1955, he also recognized that no pair exists in isolation; couples contain "the scheme, germ, and material of innumerable more complex forms."[23] Monette constantly alludes to those more complex forms, describing a network of caring people that allows him to make the most of his time with Roger. At their best, these friends, acquaintances, and professional associates understand that Paul and Roger need not face-to-face care but a scaffold—sometimes distant and unseen—that allows them high-quality time together. Given Monette's account of hostility between men with AIDS and their families, Roger's parents are an unusual node in their network. Monette describes them with loving appreciation, one of the notable ways his memoir rewrites the script of AIDS as a domestic drama rather than a morality play or horror story.

Another source of support comes from hired care workers and housekeepers, who are exceedingly hard to find at a time of uncertainty about sources of contagion and prejudice against the ill. In the end stages of Roger's illness, Monette gives particular credit to a paid caregiver named Dennis (who is, unsurprisingly, a nonwhite person). In cataloging Dennis's routine, he shows the repetitive, ongoing nature of the work. "He'd help Rog get up and dressed in the morning, serve him breakfast, massage his legs, sit with him by the phone dialing Roger's business calls."[24] These tasks are mundane, but their effects are invaluable. Having good care means that Roger can expend energy on activities he finds meaningful and that Paul and Roger can make good use of the limited time they have left together. When time is measured out in moments, preserving a dying man's "liveliest hours" is a treasured contribution. Monette ensures that Dennis's work—the kind that is so often forgotten and undercompensated—will be remembered by recording it in print.

Although print is his chosen medium, Monette repeatedly describes writing—even records as basic as a calendar notation or a diary entry—as inimical to the utterly absorbing, present-oriented work of end-of-life care. He makes this contradiction a feature of the narrative, which can only be produced retrospectively. Other media do a better job with immediacy, capturing care at its most intense extremes. Film was the chosen medium for another couple, Tom Joslin and Mark Massi, when they told a similar story of caring for a beloved partner on borrowed time. Unlike writing, film can more directly record present realities, no matter how debilitated its creator may be. A subject can just *be* in front of a camera without any extra expenditure of thought or energy. In this case, it allowed Joslin, who was dying of AIDS-related illness, to be the author of his own story, with those who cared for him as a supporting cast. With the push of a button, the camera frames him in an environment and relationships with others, who sometimes appear onscreen, sometimes partially visible in the background, or present as ambient sound.

Joslin conceived the 1993 documentary, *Silverlake Life: The View from Here*, as a "diary" about his experience of AIDS. While a print diary is traditionally a private, individually authored form, Joslin's project is collective, including his longtime partner, Mark, and, later, his friend and former student Peter Friedman, who edited and produced the film after both men had died. Film is an inherently collaborative art, but *Silverlake Life* embeds interdependency into its form, as well as its narrative content. Framing and camera position document Joslin's growing debilitation. Sometimes the camera is mounted on a tripod, allowing Joslin to record himself alone during moments of particular vulnerability and physical weakness, late at night or resting in bed. At other times, Massi holds the camera, his disembodied voice heard over the soundtrack as the picture is trained on Joslin. Sometimes the camera follows the two men more voyeuristically into medical appointments, massages, and therapy sessions. Although Friedman is largely invisible through most of the film, his role as an organizing presence becomes clear in a voiceover near the end. He is there to document Massi's decline after Joslin's death and describes the posthumous work of assembling the film. In revealing the process of its construction, *Silverlake Life* presents filmmaking itself as a collaborative act of care. Joslin's devoted partner and friends care for him by continuing the work he started, which also becomes a gesture of care for Massi as he mourns Tom's loss and confronts his own illness.

As with *Borrowed Time*, much of the "view from here" provided by *Silverlake Life* consists of the small-scale, redundant daily work of care giving and receiving. Care is a focus of nearly every scene in the film, and almost all of the work is done by Massi. We see him doing housework and chores, making food, measuring out and administering medications, and taking Tom to the therapists, alternative healers, and medical experts who surround the couple. Neither man inhabits his role seamlessly, and the film doesn't try to hide their mistakes and shortcomings. They are in a bleak and unenviable situation. In one scene, Tom films himself waiting in the car, weak and exasperated, while Mark completes a series of errands. Tom is cross and uncomfortable, Mark is impatient and dismissive, and the atmosphere of tension attests to the affective demands of care work for both givers and receivers. In another scene Mark angrily tells their therapist about Tom's refusal to take his full dose of medication. Mark is concerned that Tom is hastening his own death, while Tom weakly asserts that he is doing the best he can. Later in the film, Mark feeds Tom some food that upsets his stomach, then confesses fear that his bungled caregiving has only made Tom worse. The scene reinforces the depth of Mark's devotion, as well as the difficulty of knowing how to care for someone at the edge of death. We are also reminded that although Mark is healthier than Tom, he also has AIDS and fears being left alone, sick, and uncared for. The scenes of his decline soon after Tom's death underscore the extent of his own illness throughout the time that he was a devoted caregiver to his partner.

Film is an apt medium for depicting the long term because of its capacity to cut between past and present. A committed partner or other members of a chosen family can show care by acknowledging that the dying person had a self before their illness and the narrowing horizons it inevitably occasions. In this sense, nostalgia, and its coupling with sentimentality—feelings often associated with pathological attachment to the past—can be a healthy resource for enduring a difficult present. The "ethics of temporariness" requires being in the present while also being aware of how it is shaped by a better past. Joslin conserves the past by incorporating footage that documents his long and happy relationship with Mark into *Silverlake Life*. Film and photos of the couple in better times attest to Tom's prior self, as well as the history that informs Mark's gentle ministrations to his dying partner. We see what the frail man in the film's grim present represents to him, and we anticipate what he will lose with Tom's death. Surveying the long term of their relationship also allows these men to aerate the present with moments of levity, and even joy. But they also share spots of meaningful borrowed time even in a present that is shadowed by grave illness. Their personhood is not confined to the roles of sick person or caregiver; we see them dancing, shopping, strolling through the Huntington Library's botanical gardens, watching the LA Marathon. They make jokes, relax in a swimming pool on vacation, and cuddle on the couch. These reciprocities attest to the persistence of a long-term partnership even against a backdrop of suffering and loss.

Old footage also documents unhappier long-term relationships, providing a sometimes brutal record of the disappointments of Tom's biological family. Genetic kinship is decidedly not the grounds for unquestioning acceptance. Unlike the loving parents that support Paul and Roger in *Borrowed Time,* Tom and Mark endure the all-too-common experience of rejection and condemnation by their families of origin. Using scenes from an earlier autobiographical film about coming out, Joslin shows his parents openly expressing their homophobia, making it obvious why Tom would not turn to them in his time of need. In one scene, Tom's mother negates his commitment to Mark by expressing disappointment that her son would not have a "family," a term she equates with having a wife and children. Tom's father is much worse, describing his son's sexuality as "awful" and "embarrassing" and Mark as ugly and abnormal (although "pleasant"). Tom's brother and sister-in-law are more sympathetic, but distant.

It is hard to think of a more potent symbolic crucible of family estrangement than the awkward Christmas Tom and Mark spend with the Joslins during Tom's last months of life, all captured in the film. They debrief on the return flight, expressing relief on landing at LAX. Clearly, home is their shared house in Los Angeles, not the house where Tom was raised. In what was rapidly becoming a sad trope of AIDS narrative, we see Tom's biological family arrive in LA as he is dying. Tom's mother belatedly expresses appreciation for the care Mark provided her son. A more official acknowledgment of Mark's role comes from the coroner, who lists him—in the presence of Tom's family of origin—as "next of kin" on Tom's death certificate. Some rituals of care are local and site specific. In 1985, such a gesture might have been possible only in an artsy, socially progressive community like Silverlake, where "kin" is identified in terms of caring actions rather than biology or legal recognition.

In the households of Mark and Tom, Paul and Roger, caregiving duties are assigned according to need and ability rather than gender. Like siblinghood, these relationships are lateral and relatively unscripted, compared to that of a married couple or parent and child. But at a time when AIDS was a fatal illness, there was one consistent component to that script: It forced care to the center of kinship arrangements and domestic life. In these narratives, each partner makes good on a long-term commitment to be the primary caregiver for the other, often with exacting tenderness and, occasionally, blunders and grudging exhaustion. The recipient completes his care, sometimes with gratitude, sometimes resistance, and sometimes simply by living for another day. On borrowed time, they know that care, no matter how loving and attentive, will ultimately fail to sustain life. Under such extreme duress, some relationships broke or floundered, while others stood up to the brutal test of terminal illness, where care cannot be rewarded by recovery. At a time when gay men were often painted as sex crazed, shallow, and pathologically self-absorbed, narratives like *Borrowed Time* and *Silverlake Life* documented the unseen labor of care, but they also did other important political work in giving couples' deep and enduring commitments a recognizable narrative arc.

QUEER SINGLES

Sometimes people die alone and uncared for, especially in an epidemic, when caregivers and institutions are overwhelmed. Many more die after being cared for inadequately, especially when illness is conjoined with an epidemic of prejudice and fear. Not all of those with AIDS-related illness were lucky enough to be nursed by a beloved partner; many others found themselves in Mark's situation, dying of AIDS after losing the partner who was best equipped to care for him. Care for a sick person in the absence of biological family or a committed life partner became the subject of a second set of narratives, about the ad hoc networks formed by friends and neighbors at a time of crisis. Sometimes these improvised familyish communities were a source of creativity and strength, but they also floundered. In theory, building a web of care might sound utopian, but when someone is dying and nobody is obviously in charge, there is plenty of room for confusion, resentment, and failure. I am especially interested in narrative treatments of those vulnerable places where care networks fray or collapse altogether because it is in these spots that we see most clearly the value and difficulty of care work—both giving and receiving—as well as opportunities for the world to be otherwise. "Oh why couldn't I simply love Mike and be generous!" laments Amy Hoffman after her friend dies of AIDS and she is haunted by memories of the bad feelings that compromised her gestures of care. Failure erupts into her narrative with an exclamation point that punctuates the temporal divide between the past ("I wanted to run away, I wanted it to be over") and the present, when she regrets not her actions but the attitude behind them.[25] Where we have seen narratives about long-term partners employ sentimental tropes to describe an arc of love and loss, this section turns to the more varied forms used to represent impromptu circuits of distributed care, the ambient feelings they generate, and the more lurching qualities of borrowed time experienced by a social network.

The improvisational care networks that spring up around a single person who is gravely ill are the subject of Susan Sontag's 1986 short story, "The Way We Live Now."[26] In the background are notable absences and failures that have, by now, become familiar tropes in narratives about gay men with AIDS: The family of origin lives somewhere that is not the Chicago, Los Angeles, San Francisco, New York, or other urban center where the sick man makes his home; they are distant or estranged, having earlier rejected his identity/social choices; they appear only at the very end stages of his illness; and they are mostly an unwanted nuisance. In Sontag's story, the man's mother (referred to as "the mother" rather than with a possessive or a proper name) is described by his chosen family as a threatened imposition, so much so that one friend is assigned the task of "keeping the mother in Mississippi informed, well, mainly keeping her from flying to New York and heaping her grief on her son and confusing the household routine with her oppressive ministrations." Later, after she insists on coming, it is a sign of the man's recovery that "the mother was persuaded to fly back to Mississippi." Like the sick man himself, "the mother" has no voice of her own, nor does anyone consider her actions to be gestures of care in intent or consequence. Into the vacuum left by biological family, a loosely configured web of care radiates from the dying man, described by one speaker as "the family he's founded, without meaning to, without official titles and ranks."

Distributed care inspires the form, as well as the content, of Sontag's story, which is structured as an extended stream of gossip and confession. It consists entirely of fragments spoken by people variously attached to the sick man, one voice washing into another. The subject of concern never gets to speak for himself. His voice emerges only through citation by others, the collective "we" of the title (which one friend calls a "utopia of friendship" and another calls "pathetic") functioning as the story's protagonist. It is as if the lack of embodied characters or a consistent narrative voice signals, at the level of form, the absence of a partner or biological family. There is no designated point person to manage the sick man's care or provide a coherent report on the course of his illness, although the dialogue is often dominated by Quentin, who, we learn in a parenthetical aside, "was proud of their friendship" and clearly thrives on being at the center of the action. But there is no collective agreement about Quentin's authority. Instead the story is an echo chamber where rumors spread and conversations flow loosely from one topic to another, moving from firsthand description to hearsay to emoting. Sentences may begin in the voice of one character and end with the voice of another. Where narrative convention identifies individual speakers by setting their words off with quotation marks and paragraphing, Sontag runs their words together to capture the way information travels from person to person, exuding an ambient cloud of feeling that mixes sadness and worry with less noble impulses like self-importance, curiosity, or reticence.

Another way to describe the story's content is to say that it voices the collective unconscious of care in a loose-knit community. Most speakers do not talk directly about care, speaking around it by discussing the health and emotional well-being of the sick friend. But as they do so, some jockey for position, overreaching to insert themselves into the thick of care management and delegation, while others voice concern without action, only later to express their feelings of guilt or to be the subject of recriminatory gossip among their friends. Surprisingly little of the conversation concerns the sick man's actual needs or expressed wishes. Instead, his friends discuss who is doing what and how they feel about it; they evaluate the quality of other people's actions, interactions, and motivations, as well as their own, and measure who seems most appreciated by the sick man and who is simply a bother. "We're rivals for a sign from him of special pleasure over a visit," a friend named Betsy remarks, "each stretching for the brass ring of his favor, wanting to feel the most wanted, the true nearest and dearest, which is inevitable with someone who doesn't have a spouse and children or an official in-house lover, hierarchies no one would dare contest." Betsy's words capture the competition and self-interest that may be an undercurrent when an illness requiring attention and care emerges within an unstructured network of friends. In place of hierarchy there is lateral spread, a makeshift collective instead of centralized care management. Sontag takes advantage of fiction to voice feelings that might otherwise be unspoken or spoken and then forgotten. The negativity surrounding care given in a spirit of selfishness or competition tends to evaporate when the crisis resolves, grievances quickly replaced with more sanitized memories. Sontag's story attempts to capture the feeling of being in the midst of a care crisis, where the expected sentiments of compassion and generosity can coexist with self-interest, pettiness, and rivalry.

As its title suggests, "The Way We Live Now" is also concerned with the time of care, specifically how to represent the time of the present. In stories about couples, we have seen how time together is borrowed—a loan guaranteed by investment in their shared past—against the moment when death will force them apart. The "now" of Sontag's story is also borrowed in that it signals a transitory and unowned present. "Now" is undeniable as it is experienced but impossible to represent because it is gone even as it happens. The voices of the dying man's friends sometimes ring shallow or self-absorbed, but they also strike a more earnest chord in their efforts to remain in the present and to infuse their dwindling time together with meaning. They pay tribute to a personhood that illness threatens to eviscerate by restoring the details of a complex self—their friend's taste for licorice, the one-night stands who poached from his collection of *maki-e* lacquer boxes, his favorite books and plants and photos—they knew from a time before illness. This too is care.

The story ends on a note of self-reflection, as the dying man's friends consider how best to preserve the now where he is still alive. "I was thinking, Ursula said to Quentin," in the last lines of the story, "that the difference between a story and a painting or photograph is that in a story you can write, He's still alive. But in a painting or a photo you can't show 'still.' You can just show him being alive. He's still alive, Stephen said." These characters are speaking in the language of borrowed time. Caring for and about a friend who will soon be gone, his intimates struggle to preserve a present that is always slipping away. For these fictional characters, much like Sontag herself, representing the now is a question of form, as well as performance: Not only are they concerned with *acting like* their friend is still alive but also with the preferred medium *for depicting* the continuity of a life. They conclude, self-reflectively, that narrative is superior to visual images. The adverb "still" represents temporal persistence—caring, rather than *cared*—a bridge between past and present that unfolds anew with each rereading. By contrast, a painting or photograph captures only a static moment that is already gone. This story was published almost a decade after Sontag's influential essay collection *On Photography*, and she would continue to reflect on the properties of visual images over the course of her career. "The Way We Live Now" ends by affirming the literary over the photographic as a medium for communicating the temporal consciousness of end-of-life care.

Given her interest in AIDS and photography, it seems like Susan Sontag would have written about the most famous deathbed image of the time, Therese Frare's 1990 photograph of thirty-two-year-old David Kirby surrounded by his grieving family, but I have never found it mentioned in her work. Often called "The Photo That Changed the Face of HIV/AIDS," this is perhaps the epidemic's most iconic image, often credited with turning the tide of public sympathy toward the ill and their families.[27] I suspect Sontag recognized the photograph's historic importance, but she might also have argued, more critically, that its power came from mobilizing sentimentality, earning compassion for a dying man only by returning him to the arms of a heteronormative nuclear family. In *On Photography*, Sontag was explicit about the historical connection between the nuclear family, which she described as "that claustrophobic unit," and the nostalgic properties of photography that seek to conserve "the imperiled continuity and vanishing extendedness of family life."[28] With this in mind, she might have accused Frare's portrait of obscuring the personhood of its subject. Where the chosen family in Sontag's story seeks to protect the dying man from his biological family, Frare's photo seemingly infantilizes her subject by putting him back into the arms of his parents. It effectively erases Kirby's history as an activist who left the small town in Ohio where he grew up to work on behalf of gay rights in California.[29] Sontag might also have observed the photograph's unsubtle religious connotations, the dying man's striking resemblance to traditional depictions of Jesus Christ, an analogy reinforced by the image of outstretched hands on the wall behind his head. And she might have noted the unseen but controlling presence of the photographer, who positions the camera as a voyeuristic onlooker to this private moment of tragedy.

Sontag never made this argument, and—given her concern with how metaphors stigmatize the ill—there is an equally plausible case to be made that she would have appreciated the photograph's success at changing public sentiment for those affected by AIDS. Despite what her character Ursula says at the end of "The Way We Live Now," visual images do not always rob their subjects of vitality and continuity. Sometimes photographs tell stories, make connections, engage in dialogue, and preserve the life of their subjects.[30] I can think of no better way to describe this image than as a scene of care for someone "still alive" but poised on the edge of death. It captures an instant of borrowed time running out and preserves it for those who live on in its wake. Its still-ness is not static, since the image feels mobile, its subjects deeply, and actively, engrossed in one another. The positioning of bodies, particularly the placement of hands, communicates embrace, enfolding, encircling. But even as it captures this family absorbed in caring activity, the photograph does not erase the cruel shortsightedness of their homophobia or the inadequacy of their far-too-belated regret. If the composition is laden with religious connotations, they are hardly comforting. This is surely a family in hell, well aware of their complicity in their son's suffering.

When the characters in Sontag's story talk about "the difference between a story and a painting or photograph," they suggest an either-or relationship. But more often than not, photographs and stories come to us together, each medium lending meaning to the other. Published in *Life* magazine, Frare's photograph and the article that accompanied it had an immediate impact. The iconic image, shorn of the surrounding story and photos, also continued to circulate beyond that initial publication, mostly to public acclaim, although widely criticized when included (in a colorized version) in a Benetton ad campaign.[31] Instead of detaching from its context over time, which Sontag saw as the fate of documentary photography, the Kirby photograph has taken on significance as the story of its origins and afterlife have been uncovered and the history of the HIV/AIDS epidemic recorded. If this is an image of borrowed time, its story is also about efforts to repay debts incurred, adding a chapter absent from other narratives of care and chosen family we have considered. There is more to be learned about care from widening the temporal frame of our discussion to follow the afterlives of those who cared for a dying man.

When the photograph first appeared in *Life*'s November 1990 issue, it was accompanied by a short article that set the scene. Frare was a journalism student and volunteer at Pater Noster House, an AIDS hospice in Columbus, Ohio, where Kirby was a patient. The broad outlines of his story sound a lot like the nightmarish scenario described by Paul Monette, in which sick men were "shipped back to a fundamentalist family to pay the wages of sin."[32] Kirby had been living in Los Angeles, estranged from his family. When he became ill, he decided to return home to Ohio. But he was not "shipped back," nor was he a passive victim. He continued to work as an activist for the remainder of his life and was eager to be photographed by Frare, seeing it as a way to promote awareness about HIV/AIDS by making his illness publicly visible.[33] By the time of the famous deathbed scene, Frare had been photographing Kirby for about a month.

Looking at the well-known photograph with care, another detail becomes apparent. On the left side of the frame, an arm reaches in to touch Kirby's emaciated wrist. Its presence indicates other people in the room, at least one more caregiver, as well as the photographer who chose to crop them out of the frame. The *Life* article identifies the owner of the arm as a volunteer named Peta. Although he is outside the frame of the most famous image, other photographs show him caring for Kirby, his demeanor gentle and attentive. Later, Frare would tell the story of how her famed photograph came to be. On that day, she and Peta were with another client when they received news of Kirby's impending death. She followed Peta to Kirby's room, watching him tend to the dying man by holding his hands and addressing him softly. Frare kept a respectful distance until the family asked her to photograph them saying their goodbyes.[34] Knowing that Frare was not a voyeuristic intruder but an invited participant in the deathbed scene changes the meaning of the photograph's composition. Now the person holding the camera seems more like a connective link in the circle of care gathered around the dying man. Her decision to crop most of Peta's body out of the frame accords this family their private moment of grief, without erasing his presence altogether.

The power, as well as the limitation, of Frare's iconic photo, is its emphasis on Kirby's biological relatives to the exclusion of others who cared by and for him. It attests to the shrinking world of a dying person, while granting perhaps unwarranted recognition to the nuclear family unit.[35] As we have seen, by 1990, the story of biological family that rushed to the bedside of a dying man they had previously scorned and rejected was already well known and extensively criticized by AIDS activists. "Who among us has not sat through the memorial service in which the traditional family arrives—tearful, entitled, sometimes penitent—to claim a place at the end of a life which they earlier abdicated?" asks the activist Urvashi Vaid, with evident bitterness.[36] Frare's photograph appears to commemorate, if not to affirm, this pattern. But this is another case where an expanded temporal frame changes the meaning of the moment suspended in the image itself.

In the three decades since its first appearance, "The Photo That Changed the Face of HIV/AIDS" has become part of a more complicated story about kinship, dependency, and care. It suggests that even if the debts incurred by borrowed time can never be repaid, they can be redistributed. That process begins by shifting attention to Peta, barely visible in the iconic photo but pictured—in the original magazine piece—in a wider-angle shot of Kirby's bedside, his expression and body language a study in compassionate attunement. The story of these photographs needs to expand back into the past, as well as the future. And it could use more protagonists. Peta, an active if not always visible participant in the deathbed scene, was of Native American (Oglala Lakota) and white ancestry and nonbinary gender, although using the pronoun "he." It was through her friendship with Peta that Frare became a volunteer at the hospice, where he was already working. After Kirby's death, Frare continued to photograph Peta until his death of AIDS-related illness two years later. Unlike the Kirby photographs, which cover only the final stages of decline, Frare had time to create a thicker portrait of Peta that includes images of him swimming and riding a motorcycle. In one especially arresting photo, he smokes in bed, wearing lingerie and a wistful expression, long hair tumbling luxuriously over one shoulder.[37] The photos of Peta in healthier times attest to the ravages of AIDS but also emphasize the extent of a life beyond the status of patient. Taken together, these images show the fuller personhood of a caregiver and document Peta's transition from provider to recipient of care as he became increasingly debilitated by illness. They also illustrate the surprising emergence of a chosen family devoted to Peta's needs and determined to recognize his contribution to the precious time borrowed at the end of David's life.

Having witnessed the expert care Peta provided to their dying son, the Kirbys resolved to do the same for him as his illness advanced. This was a remarkable turn of events, given that they had presumably rejected their own son when he came out to them. But their struggle to care for David had been a transformative experience. They witnessed the devastating impact of homophobia firsthand when their son was shunned at the small-town hospital where he was treated for his illness.

"Even the person who handed out menus refused to let David hold one [for fear of infection]," Kay Kirby recalled. "She would read out the meals to him from the doorway. We told ourselves that we would help other people with AIDS avoid all that, and we tried to make sure that Peta never went through it."[38] She praised Peta as a fearless and intuitive caregiver who offered their son intimacy where others tried to avoid him. Putting Frare's most famous photograph in the context of a longer documentary project, its story evolves from one about the failure and belated regrets of nuclear family to a familyish network of care in which beliefs, acts, and relationships evolve in response to changing circumstances (figure 3.1).

Frare's photographs capture the afterstory of David's death, which is also the ongoing story of those who survive him, and their attempt to make good on the debts they had incurred. Kay and Bill Kirby kept their promise to remain a part of Peta's life, caring for him as he became increasingly ill and dependent. While they could not undo mistakes

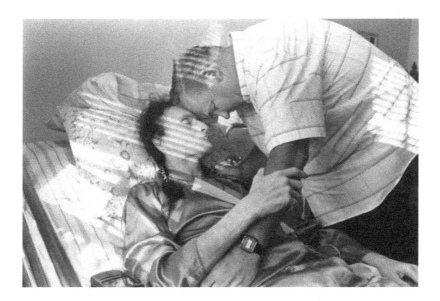

FIGURE 3.1 Bill Kirby touches foreheads with Peta, his body language suggesting attunement to Peta's suffering while Peta appears to draw solace from Bill's touch.

they had made as biological parents, they could behave differently by affirmatively choosing kinship with Peta. They facilitated his transition from caregiver to recipient, protecting him from the slights their biological son had endured in the hospital. Frare's photographs document their changing relationship as roles shifted and values were reconfigured.

The image of a parent who has not succeeded in caring for their biological son caring instead for another man in the absence of his own family, chosen or otherwise, brings us back to the beginning of this chapter, which opened with Tony Kushner's *Angels in America*. So very different in genre and medium, Kushner's play and Frare's photography tell similar stories about care in the time of AIDS, the limitations of biological and legal family, and the networks generated by a felt sense of kinship. They show how webs of care emerge, thrive, or falter on the borrowed time of terminal illness, and sometimes how care is redistributed in its aftermath. They matter not just as historical artifacts but because their subject—the diversified care configurations and resources that emerged out of the epidemic at its crisis point—would endure long after AIDS became a manageable chronic condition. While historians have written of these shifts, art does a better job of rendering the transitory and highly specific textures of end-of-life care particular to their time and place.

The legacy of that era is the subject of Matthew Lopez's 2018 play, *The Inheritance*. The play centers on Toby Darling and Eric Glass, a thirtysomething couple, and the events that occur as they cross paths with members of a younger and older generation. The youthful include Adam, a talented and aspiring actor, and Leo, a seropositive sex worker. For Adam and Leo, as well as the slightly older friends in Toby and Eric's circle, an AIDS diagnosis no longer means living on borrowed time. Its conversion from a death sentence to a treatable infection changes the way gay men think about sex and relationships, as well as their attitudes toward the past and the future. Having sex no longer carries the risk of an irreversible deadly illness. In the play's present it is even possible to repair past actions that once would have had lethal consequences. After an orgiastic night in a Czech bathhouse, Adam finds that he is HIV positive. Thanks to his good connections, he can quickly access PEP therapy that reduces the virus to undetectable levels. His peers also think differently about the future, regardless of infection status. Some plan to get married and have children, making choices that would have been unthinkable to their predecessors in the 1980s.

The remnants of that decimated older generation are represented by Walter and Henry, a long-term couple that survived the epidemic. As the story unfolds—rewriting *Howard's End* by E. M. Forster, who appears at various points in the play—we learn about the country house they bought to retreat from the infectious environment of New York in the 1980s. Their plans go awry when a chance encounter with a dying acquaintance prompts Walter to convert their home into a makeshift hospice for men in the end stages of AIDS. Decades later, Walter recalls caring for his first patient: "I cleaned him when he fouled himself. I held him as he wept in grief. I comforted him as he screamed in pain. I had no idea I had such strength."[39] As borrowed time ran out, care centered on such small and incredibly meaningful acts. The recipient, no matter how appreciative, is long gone. There is no witness to record them, and they would be lost without Walter's recollection, which he transmits across generations by sharing it with Eric. There are no do-overs in life, but this is art. By including their conversation, the play preserves a memory of this fleeting past that can be recaptured each time it is performed.

The house is the eponymous "inheritance," the play's most concrete symbol of the legacy of that period. In the end stages of cancer, Walter asks that the house be left to Eric. Although Henry and Walter's sons disregard the dying man's request, his wish is unexpectedly fulfilled when Eric (ignorant of the bequest denied) *does* inherit the house by marrying Henry. He also takes up Walter's commitment to care for men in need, past and present folding unevenly together. In the 1980s, a younger Henry had shunned the house where Walter harbored dying men. He has a second chance with Eric, who insists that they take Leo in and care for him as he suffers from AIDS-related illness and drug withdrawal. Unlike the men Walter cared for, Leo also has another chance and improves markedly under their care.

Like Frare's photographs, *The Inheritance* provides a more long-term view of borrowed time. In one way, its debt can never be repaid. Eric laments that his cohort has been "robbed of a generation of mentors, of poets, of friends and, perhaps, even lovers."[40] True enough. Individual lives lost cannot be recovered. But in another, that beleaguered generation secured the future for those who come after. The good health and varied choices enjoyed by Eric and his peers are also an inheritance. Its riches are evident in the present where Lopez's play is performed. While that legacy is visible, the play also preserves an uninheritable but equally valuable past: the gestures of comfort and succor between a dying person and their intimate circle in those days narrowing to moments, poised between life and death.

4

SLOW EMERGENCIES AND THE CARE-TO-COME

Dementia in the Family

When the sixty-four-year-old feminist psychologist Sandy Bem created a file called "memoir" on her computer, she believed it was already too late. Earlier that month she had been diagnosed with amnesiac mild cognitive impairment, a prelude to Alzheimer's. Her doctor urged her to write, telling her that others could benefit from Bem's efforts to make sense of her experiences of cognitive change. In her journal, she wrote bleakly of "a mind that could be so alive one moment with thought and feeling building toward a next step and then someone erases the blackboard. It's all gone and I can't even reconstruct what the topic was. It's just gone. And I sit with the dark, the blank."[1] To Bem, who had always equated her sense of personhood with intellect, reason, and drive, the diagnosis was a death sentence. She was determined to end life on her own terms, when her cognitive changes amounted to a loss of the self she once had been. As her condition progressed, Bem made adjustments that allowed her to participate in, and continue to enjoy, many activities with considerable independence. When her daughter Emily had a baby, Bem became an unexpectedly doting grandmother. She discovered that her "new brain" was content with the mundane activities of caring for a small child, finding herself much more patient and forgiving than she had been as a mother. Bem also had a devoted caregiver in her husband, although they had separated fifteen years before. Nonetheless, she was determined to take her own life while she still had agency, and, five years after receiving her diagnosis, she did.[2]

The continued potential to enjoy some activities, and even discover new pleasures, did not strike Bem as sufficient reason to keep living. Her judgment was consistent with the particular brand of feminism she endorsed in her life and writing, one that prized autonomy and self-expression above all else. She had challenged the patriarchal narrative in which women are predisposed to be passive and dependent but not an equally powerful narrative that sees dependency as a tragic erasure of personhood. She did not seem to value such classically feminine virtues as nurture, empathy, and relatedness, qualities that were heightened rather than dimmed by her dementia. Nor did she recognize that there could be meaning in allowing others to care for her. Much as she cherished life, Bem valued independence of thought and action more. To her, the diagnosis meant only a slow but inevitable and costly loss of reason and sovereignty.

Next to infancy and childhood, old age is the stage of life most likely to involve pervasive dependency, making it a necessary chapter in my account of care. It takes a distinctly modern form with the collective aging of the world's population. We are no longer talking about the rare individual who lives into oldest old age (defined by the NIH as 85+), but a demographic shift that entails growing numbers of vulnerable, elderly people and their caregivers. Enamored of productivity, independence, and rationality, we moderns prefer not to imagine future vulnerability and need. Age-related dependency is a situation nobody wants to think about until it is upon us, in the form of our own frailty or that of someone we love. Our world is saturated with images of vigorous aging and a host of products, spaces, and services designed to enhance its quality. Many are determined to age in place, caring for themselves in environments designed for younger bodies. In the United States, we live in homes accessible only by car, with stairs that must be climbed, slippery showers, and kitchens with high cabinets. Yet the truth is that those of us who live into old age (and certainly oldest old age) will inevitably have to contend with the need for more care, combined with a diminished capacity to provide for ourselves.

While Alzheimer's affects a far narrower population, age-related dementia (and other adjacent conditions) is an important test case for care because it involves large numbers of people with cognitive and physical dependencies, the needs of an increasingly frail body intersecting with an altered capacity to make reasoned, autonomous decisions. For my father-in-law this meant a body strong enough to crash around his property wielding agricultural tools but unsteady enough to fall, start a fire, or lose a limb. There was an argument for allowing him to take those risks, given the pleasure he got from working outdoors. But we are interdependent beings. His right to autonomy impinged on the well-being of his wife, who cared deeply about the safety of his body and their home. Aging in place became unsustainable sooner than anybody could have imagined. As with other forms of dependency, when it comes to age-related frailty, family members are our frontline providers, working without compensation to give or manage care for those in need. And as with other interdependencies, the lion's share of the work falls to wives and daughters, an arrangement rarely welcomed by anybody.[3] We must find better ways to *imagine* the care-to-come as a step toward designing more habitable environments for vulnerable elderly populations, as well as the resources to sustain those charged with their care.

This chapter looks at narratives by authors living with dementia and those who have cared for a parent with dementia. It emphasizes mothers and daughters because these are the social positions most associated with caring instincts and activities, and most likely to be strained by conflicting expectations, desires, and needs. In many ways, their stories reinforce the known outlines of a problem, putting a human face on a diagnosis that portends a protracted loss of self and the stress and expense of caring for a dependent elder. There cannot be enough of these stories. We need more, and we need to read them more attentively, to understand the scope and import of a mounting crisis of care. But my interest in these narratives goes beyond their status as evidence of a social problem, to the way they detail the timescapes of care that I will call "slow emergency." This term is inspired by Elinor Fuchs, who describes the ten-year period of her mother's Alzheimer's as "the Emergency."[4] A "slow emergency" is a seeming paradox, a situation of extreme magnitude and urgency whose full extent unfolds at a pace that makes it only gradually apparent.

Emergency is more commonly used to denote a sudden catastrophe (the car crash, the explosion, the gunshot, the fall). It may involve a paradoxical experience of acceleration and the sensation of time moving in slow motion. It may also induce temporary amnesia, an absence of recall surrounded by memories of the time directly before and after that quickly sediment into a story. By contrast, the pace of a slow emergency is so incremental that it may not be perceived until there is a sufficient accumulation of change. In this way, it is akin to Rob Nixon's concept of "slow violence," which describes the problem of environmental devastation that occurs over many generations.[5] Nixon identifies a mismatch between the temporalities of the planetary environment and those of human consciousness, which makes it difficult to reconcile the massive and cataclysmic implications of climate change with the horizons of a lifespan (an imaginative gap that has unfortunately narrowed considerably, even in the time since his book's publication). These differing scales of perception at least partially explain why it is so hard to know how to act responsibly on an individual level. Which actions count and which are just sustainability performance? Literary and visual arts play a key role in his account because they can illuminate temporalities otherwise inaccessible to human understanding. While dementia extends over months and years, not generations, it follows a similar trajectory of becoming apparent via gradual revelations rather than through a single dramatic catastrophe, while ultimately being no less calamitous. And like climate change, any data-driven knowledge about age-related dependency—in its full, all-encompassing urgency—is enhanced, at the level of feeling and conviction, by the imaginative lens of the arts.

This chapter explores the unfolding of slow emergency in narratives by those with dementia and their caregivers. I begin with women authors who took up the prompt offered by Sandy Bem's doctor, writing memoir in an effort to hold on to a self that seems to be unspooling from—or perhaps retreating irrecoverably into—its own past. Gerda Saunders's *Memory's Last Breath* (2017) and Wendy Mitchell's *Somebody I Used to Know* (2018) are first-person accounts of cognitive change that knocks the temporal arc of a life history askew, each also aspiring, through the act of telling, to create a more sustainable world for other people with dementia and their caregivers. Even as they feel the urgency of writing while they still can, these authors experience slowness on many different registers, from the pacing of everyday cognition to the rate of moving through the world to the progression of the disease. Slowness also gives time to reflect on dependency and care, as women who found purpose in providing for others reluctantly confront their own impending need. Both reach their imaginative limit at the prospect of a dependency that renders them unable to reciprocate, demanding care that has no completion other than death. It is there that someone else needs to take ownership of the story. For that perspective, I turn to memoirs of daughters who cared for mothers with dementia, Elinor Fuchs's *Making an Exit* (2005) and Roz Chast's *Can't We Talk About Something More Pleasant?* (2014). Unlike the maternal memoirs, which are written in anticipation of future dependency, these filial memoirs are written retrospectively, in an attempt to make sense of an imperfect response to slow-moving crisis. From the caregiver's perspective, slowness is more firmly associated with the at-first-almost-imperceptible advance of debility, the delayed response of those summoned to intervene, and the costly and stressful prolongation of life-in-dependency. Slowness makes the emergency of dementia care difficult to perceive and all the more expensive, demanding, and tragic to address.

Occasionally, these narratives find opportunity in slowness. Dementia's gradual, uneven progression allows life writers time to account for themselves. It conserves some unexpected resources of selfhood while opening others that have been buried or dormant. Sometimes the effort to communicate this experience prompts experimentation with narrative forms, lending variety to the more predictable rhythms of memoir. Lest this sound too celebratory, slowness does not always yield good reading. It can lead to redundancy and cliché, as life writing echoes the tedium of life experience or shifts in cognitive capacity. Still, slowing down allows these authors to apprehend the networks of care that already sustain them and requires them to build new nodes, even as they become aware of the inequities on which those networks subsist. For daughters who have shouldered responsibility for dependent elders, only on looking back is it possible to recognize the arrival of slow and unwanted parental dependency. Only in retrospect can they identify the reserves of effort and ingenuity demanded of them, as well as the many others—often less economically advantaged women of color— who help distribute the burdens of care. And only when the care is successfully distributed are they able to identify moments when slowing down facilitated an artful attunement between a daughter and a parent who has come to be associated with burden, toil, and conflict. Those moments when time seems to eddy or suspend are fleeting but also precious because they show us how and why it is worth caring in the absence of hope for improvement or recovery. In the work of each author, I find efforts to practice and capture the arts of interdependency.

NARRATIVE FORMS OF THE GRAY TSUNAMI

Once upon a time it was relatively rare to live to advanced age, and the condition referred to as "senility" was accepted as a normal aspect of the aging process. Twenty-five years before Alois Alzheimer would identify dementia as a disease, Ralph Waldo Emerson greeted his cognitive changes with complacency. When a friend wrote to ask about his health, Emerson replied, "Quite well; I have lost my mental faculties but am perfectly well."[6] Today it is hard to imagine equating the loss of "mental faculties" with good health, but Emerson wrote at a time when the onset of what we now know to be dementia was neither tragic nor pathological. Those days are long gone. In the decades after Emerson's death, the changes he experienced would be identified as the symptoms of a degenerative disease. And in the ensuing century, a dramatic increase in the number of people living with the inevitable frailties of advanced old age meant that it would become much harder to provide them with the care they required. Some of them would also have dementia that made them unable to manage the circumstances of their own care. While not all elderly people get Alzheimer's, the likelihood of developing some form of dementia increases greatly with age.[7] In short, more people living longer means more people with dementia and the dependencies it entails.

People aged sixty and older are the world's fastest growing population. At the start of the millennium, the U.S. Census identified a 38 percent increase in the number of Americans over age eighty-five and the highest-ever median age of 35.3 years.[8] Since then, predictions of a gray century have become more extreme. In 2010 there were 16 people over age 65 for every adult between ages 25 and 64; by 2035 the United Nations estimates the number will be 26.[9] A 2015 report predicted that the elderly population of the United States would double by 2050 and that the number of "oldest old" (age 80 and up) would more than triple.[10] While the AARP hailed this data as evidence of improved health care, rising standards of living, and better nutrition,[11] other commentators describe it as a "gray tsunami," a looming crisis that threatens to wash over the world's population.[12] They portend a dramatic shift in the "dependency ratio," the proportion of dependents to wage earners. Even those with the good fortune to remain vigorous and healthy will inevitably become more dependent. Medical science has had undeniable success at prolonging life, but strategies to care for those who live on have lagged far behind. Until the moment it affects us directly, few of us value the work of those who care for the elderly or the environments in which our dependents and their supporters are sustained. Energy is a limited resource, our commitment to continued economic growth and productivity increasingly at odds with the imperative to care for those who are vulnerable and the work it entails. The crisis is thus not with aging itself but with the burdens of care in societies that have not adequately prepared for population-wide, age-related dependency.[13]

As with other dilemmas of care, the problem of age-related dementia is also a problem of gender. Women are far more likely to be diagnosed with Alzheimer's than men, a statistic only partially explained by their greater longevity. In addition to genetics, being a caregiver for someone with dementia is itself a strong risk factor for developing Alzheimer's. An estimated 60 percent of Alzheimer's caregivers are women, many of them already charged with caring for children or other dependents.[14] When women are not able to care for themselves or their kin, it is usually other women—usually low-paid immigrants of color—who take their place. In becoming dependent, women-identified people face another barrier. If you are conditioned by gender to be a giver rather than a recipient of care, you are likely to experience particular dread at a diagnosis that promises future neediness, rendering you dependent on the care of others.

Sometimes dread forces a reckoning that generates usable strategies to prolong autonomy and make dependency less burdensome. But more often it leads to denial. Life writing about Alzheimer's draws attention to a pervasive social problem that most of us prefer to ignore. Sometimes other people's stories offer creative resources for getting by, giving order and meaning to chaotic experience; sometimes they offer insights about how people avoid and deflect, defense mechanisms that are easier to see in others than in ourselves. Writing by and about Alzheimer's speaks to unavoidable asymmetries of caregiving; the differences between caring for an elderly person and caring for a child; the politics of "aging in place"; and the race, gender, class, and regional determinants of elder care. Equally important, and far less remarked upon, are the aesthetic dimensions of Alzheimer's narratives. In his study of Alzheimer's, *The Forgetting*, David Shenk writes: "While medical science gives us many tools for staying alive, it cannot help us with the art of living—or dying."[15] Shenk's characterization of living and dying as "art" gestures to a key role for literature in apprehending those aspects of felt experience that get overlooked when care is approached as a problem of individual maintenance (how to keep a body alive or safe or docile) or population management (how to keep a large number of bodies alive or safe or docile). The most interesting works adopt literary forms that illuminate the temporalities of slow emergency, enhancing our understanding of what it means to give or require care under such conditions, and creating possibilities for imagining more just and sustainable ways of caring.

WRITING THE SELF WITH DEMENTIA

The concept of an Alzheimer's memoir is something of a paradox because a memoir is, by definition, a work of reminiscence. How can a condition diagnosed by loss of memory produce stories that require it? The author with Alzheimer's seeks to narrate the self at the very moment the self threatens to dissolve. She uses words to confront a situation in which language becomes elusive. She is an unreliable narrator whose fractured story speaks with absolute accuracy to the reality of a mind in transition. I am interested in how writers with Alzheimer's and other forms of dementia adapt the conventions of life writing to represent the unspooling of past from present selves and make sense of their new-found dependencies. As some connections are frayed and broken, others are revealed or forced into being. Those who identify as women and mothers—important identities for both the authors I consider—wrestle with the reversals involved in becoming recipients, rather than providers, of care. It is also worth noting the particular qualities of early-onset dementia that make writing a viable outlet. These authors' relative youth and vigor shape the experience of disease, increasing the likelihood of living with dementia-related dependencies for an extended period of time. As they contemplate dependencies to come, they seek images and modes of expression to represent an interdependent self in flux. For each woman, death is not the endpoint of their efforts to imagine the future, but rather a state of dependency so pervasive that they require care in the absence of self-awareness.

Wendy Mitchell, a single mother and successful management-level employee of Britain's National Health Service, wrote her 2018 book, *Somebody I Used to Know*, about living with early-onset dementia.[16]

Forced to retire from a job she loved—one ironically dedicated to care for others—Mitchell describes the incredible difficulty of transitioning from care giver to recipient, looking with dread to a future in which she is reduced to bare need, a body requiring care without the capacity to reciprocate. As someone who thrived on supervising and supporting others, she recognizes the work involved in accepting help. She also insists on the personhood of dependent people, even those with cognitive dependencies that require assistance with reason and self-direction. As she strives to retain personhood in the presence of a debilitating diagnosis, she develops strategies to cope with her newfound dependency and uses writing to translate her experience into usable advice for others. While her memoir is the most straightforward—in literary terms—of those I consider, its very conventionality is radical, a statement of persistent self-awareness amid a condition associated with its erasure.

Mitchell's excellent title speaks volumes, announcing estrangement from her subject, a "somebody" whose competencies and lived experience are no longer familiar. The "you" she addresses is not just somebody but *a somebody*, belonging to a class of contemporary women who define themselves through their professional accomplishments. That past self was tirelessly independent and absolutely capable; it was gratifying to be her and painful to let her go. She found purpose in caring for and protecting her children, as well as being a professional who managed others with order and competence. Mitchell acknowledges her distance from that self by addressing her in second person. The author is somebody but not *a somebody*, and part of her narrative is a prolonged and regretful goodbye to that sense of her own professional importance. But *you* is also limited, despite believing herself omnipotent. She lacks the self-reflection to write memoir and has no capacity to envision a future where she will become slower, needier, and less able. Even while mourning her departure, Mitchell chides the past "you" for its failures of imagination and details the abilities of an "I" writing in the present.

Writing memoir is part of a process of learning how to be a self that is more interdependent, transitional, and humble. Mitchell finds that she has to work just as hard to accept care as she did to give it. She wrestles with a profound resistance to relying on others. Like most disability accommodations, her condition requires some relatively minor changes in habit and environment, and others that are time consuming and cumbersome. Dependency resets the pace of life from the forward rush of the workplace to the slower, more unpredictable registers of crip time. Dependency also eventually means asking for help. The activation energy required by this step is steep, but the results are gratifying. Mitchell learns that when she identifies, rather than tries to hide, her diagnosis, strangers respond with generosity. When she asks for care and others provide it readily, this is an expression of autonomy that extends her capacities even within a heightened state of dependency. Recounting her successes gives Mitchell a sense of purpose. She may not be the same somebody she once knew, but she is a somebody, a writing self whose encroaching dependency can be turned into a resource for others.

The same cannot be said of Mitchell's identity as a mother, a role she finds incompatible with dependency. We have already seen how "mother" is so defined by caregiving as to be both a noun and a verb to describe the most tender, attentive forms of relation. What does it mean, then, to be a mother who is no longer capable of providing care for her daughters, and who will also soon need care herself? If care could function as a neat circuit of reciprocity, that would be one thing. Parents care for children in their dependency and, in turn, are cared for when they become dependent. That happens exactly never. As a single parent, Mitchell thrived on doing double duty for her daughters, but in a time of illness her unattached status means that her daughters are first in line as care providers. She denies the cultural platitude that women have a natural or intuitive desire to care for their own mothers. Where she actively chose to become a mother, willingly assuming the obligations of care that might entail, her daughters did not choose their association with a dependent elder. While they might love her dearly, Mitchell believes it is unethical to use affective bonds as a justification for unpaid labor. In another time and place, the injustice Mitchell uncovers might be the grounds for a revolution. In this context, she is one frail woman writing a memoir that she hopes will be useful to her readers. In this context, while she is still capable of making autonomous decisions about her future, Mitchell insists that she will opt, unenthusiastically, for institutionalized care rather than depending on her daughters.

Mitchell knows the modes of self-care and advocacy she describes are strategies for the present. Her symptoms are relatively mild, and she maintains considerable autonomy, supported by a small network of caring others. Although not the same somebody she once knew, Mitchell can remember that person. She retains the self-awareness to help herself, to ask for help when needed, and respond with gratitude when it is provided. Her greatest dread is not death but a future of dependency without self-awareness. She does not want to know much about that future "somebody," who will not be capable of knowing herself. Indeed, Mitchell laments not having the means to travel to a country like Switzerland, where physician-assisted suicide is available to those who can afford it. Absent that option, she seems to reach the limits of her chosen form and her capacity to imagine the future. She has little to say about what it will be like to become incapable of self-representation or responsiveness. Grim as it may be, committing a future "somebody" (or perhaps just a "body") to a care facility will spare her daughters from the work of its maintenance.

Where Mitchell's title looks back at a former self, the title of Gerda Saunders's dementia memoir, *Memory's Last Breath*, looks to the future. Her horizon extends beyond the debilitated body's bare dependency to its dissolution and reincorporation into the environment. Like Mitchell, Saunders is unable to imagine her dependent future with anything but dread, but she arrives at a more salutary metaphor by anticipating an interdependency that exceeds the bounded, individual self. In ecology, she finds the image of a more capacious *bios* assembled from elements recycled over the generations: "Imbrications, indeed, stand for the main purpose of my life: being connected, with honesty and integrity, to the mineral, vegetable, animal, astronomical, and cosmological worlds, particularly that infinitesimal subset of the animal kingdom, my fellow humans, with whom I have in common, a wondrously complex brain that gives us access to the 'truth of the Imagination.'"[17]

This notion of life interconnected at a molecular level inspires Saunders's title. Emphasizing continuity over the rupture of an individual life, Saunders imagines the "last breath" of memory destined to be inhaled and incorporated into other living beings. Implicit in this metaphor is an ethics that obliges us to care for one another because, at the level of matter, we are interdependent. "Memory's last breath" provides a lyrical metaphor of interconnection, but it does not make the loss of a discrete self any less devastating. Like Sandy Bem, Saunders was a feminist scholar, employed by the University of Utah until illness forced her to retire. She shares with Bem and Mitchell a feminist sensibility that values independence, productivity, and professional accomplishment. She too writes after a diagnosis of early-onset dementia, in her case caused by cerebral microvascular disease. At age sixty-one, Saunders is an otherwise healthy and vigorous woman accustomed to caring for others, rather than being cared for.

Memory's Last Breath is precisely the kind of memoir that Bem's doctor must have imagined when he urged her to write in the early stages of her diagnosis. But where writing only heightened Bem's sense of loss, Saunders finds a mode to express the more fleeting, provisional self-awareness that comes with her illness. Her subtitle, *Field Notes on My Dementia*, identifies her book as autoethnography. Saunders approaches her former self as a curious participant-observer who is living with newfound vulnerability while also witnessing its arrival. "Field notes" is also the term she gives to the sections of the book consisting of short, disjointed journal entries. Here, the incoherence that Bem found unbearable becomes the genesis of Saunders's form, these seemingly unedited fragments interspersed with more composed narrative reflections on her diagnosis and her past. If notes are typically a prelude, supplement, or commentary on writing proper, Saunders's are reflective of authorial experience.

Long before she reaches the dissolution imagined by the metaphor of "memory's last breath," Saunders knows she will become dependent on the care of others. Saunders is more willing to imagine, and express opinions about the kind of care she wants to receive than is Mitchell. She is less concerned with care as safety or bodily maintenance— typically priorities of dementia care, especially in institutions—than care that enables those aspects of her personhood that endure. One of the most important is her capacity to experience sexual desire. The persistence of sexual feeling is rarely mentioned in memoirs by people with dementia, and when it appears in writing about the condition, it is typically discussed in terms of loss of inhibition that can be dangerous or undignified. For Saunders, the ability to give and receive pleasure is evidence of selfhood that remains, even as other faculties diminish. She claims consensual sex as an integral part of a caring spousal relationship, even when one party is significantly more dependent than another. Her writing is a safeguard against the prospect of overly protective care that would sacrifice quality of life for a one-size-fits-all conception of safety.

Saunders also has strong views on the racialization of dependency and care, which are shaped by her early life as a white South African. Before immigrating to the United States—with its own toxic versions of racial segregation—Saunders came of age under an official regime of apartheid. Her memories of an idyllic childhood are tempered by awareness of living in a culture of state-sanctioned white supremacy. Racial privilege seasoned Saunders's experience of motherhood and the opportunities afforded to her children. She saw Black nannies standing apart from the white mothers at afterschool pickup and knew of live-in caregivers separated from their own children, who were barred from residing in the homes of white employers or attending school with white students.[18] She is aware of how race affected these women's ability to mother, as well as her own, recognizing how all are compromised by caregiving in a context of such inequality. Writing is a way to recognize her privilege—and the injustice on which it rested—before the details vanish from her memory.

Even as dementia threatens to erase her understanding of past inequities, Saunders's newfound dependency brings others into focus. Forced to give up her driver's license, she rides the bus, exposing her to an underclass of disabled people of color. She writes with bitter sarcasm about how the evident misfortune of other passengers puts her own dependency into perspective: "Nothing like being one of the elite on the bus who are not toothless, homeless, in a wheelchair, or on oxygen to take my mind off myself. Nothing to make my troubles seem trivial like the disproportionately large number of African Americans, Native Americans, and Hispanics awakening my racial privilege."[19] Dependency is a spectrum: The decrepitude of fellow passengers makes Saunders aware of her relative fitness. The tragedy of losing the ability to drive her own car diminishes in the company of bodies marked by race for a lifetime of debilitation. The other passengers are likely disabled by slow emergencies of their own, but the versions that disproportionately affect BIPOC people, like the weathering impact of manual labor, inadequate health care, or the absence of nutritious food. These are not people with resources or time to write memoirs. But in noticing them Saunders invites us to read with care, mindful of how race and class shape access to stories about dependencies to come.

No matter how dignified and humane the environment, no matter her relative privilege, Saunders faces the prospect of coming dependency with dread. Like Bem, she is an intellectual, proud of her learning and mental acuity. Like Mitchell, she is a working mother who finds purpose as a provider, rather than a recipient, of care. It is a cruel irony that people who are most gratified by helping others may find it hardest to accept help. Saunders is unable to imagine a scenario in which her becoming dependent doesn't inflict suffering on those who care for her. "I can only guess at the stress that the utterly dependent and exceedingly self centered bundle of need that dementia will turn me into will provoke in [her husband] as my primary caretaker," she writes.[20] Long before she dissolves into matter, Saunders pictures herself reduced to a body that demands without the capacity to reciprocate.

In ending, the dementia memoir confronts a limitation of the genre. Talk about death of the author! The prognosis is a body that persists beyond the capacity for self-representation or meaningful expression of any kind. Where Saunders and Mitchell can imagine only a future of unwanted dependency, they cannot represent what it will be like to exist without self-awareness. Need is unrepresentable because it is an absence, a vacancy that defines the bare requirements of survival. Some authors have used fiction to go there, imagining what it would be like to inhabit the bodymind of a person with more advanced dementia.[21] Sometimes they succeed with great effect, but such narratives do little to illuminate an understanding of dependency and care. At that point the self is so unmoored from its social and physical environment that it is unaware of needing or of being cared for. This unmooring is not where caring activity ends or becomes any less meaningful. It is instead a place where the story of care must be transferred to other tellers.

SLOW EMERGENCIES

Jonathan Franzen has written about dementia from within and without. His 2001 novel, *The Corrections*, devotes an entire section to the interiority of Alfred Lambert, a man with advanced Alzheimer's who is a thinly fictionalized version of Franzen's own father. His nonfiction essay "My Father's Brain" is about that experience from a son's point of view. Franzen finds nothing redeeming about this brutal illness, but that does not make it meaningless. He insists it is worthwhile for caregivers to reflect on the experience, since "senility is not merely an erasure of meaning but a source of meaning."[22] In both novel and essay, he is mindful of being more a witness than a primary participant in the labor and management of eldercare, most of which is done by women.

We do not need Franzen to tell us what it is like to be a woman on the front lines of dementia care. Plenty have done so. From among the many examples, I have chosen Elinor Fuchs's *Making an Exit* and Roz Chast's *Can't We Please Talk About Something Pleasant?* because of their honesty, creativity with form, and view of the wider contexts that embed an individual story. Like all memoirs, their stories are highly particular, as are all caregiving scenarios, but they also tell us something about the societal burdens shouldered by women when there is dementia in the family. As a 2014 report on "daughter care" from

Stanford University's Clinical Excellence Center put it, "the best long-term care insurance in our country is a conscientious daughter."[23] On the face of it, we have a virtuous intergenerational loop in which daughters reciprocate care they once received. If only sons could be so thoughtful, problem solved! But—I repeat—as with all matters care related, such neat symmetries are rare to nonexistent. For Fuchs and Chast, becoming responsible for mothers who never mothered very well is a bitter pill to swallow. Reasonably conscientious daughters, they experience many of the liabilities described in the Stanford report: stress and depression; financial strain; and distraction from work, friendships, and childrearing. More surprisingly, in responding to their mothers' crises, they also find connections unavailable in the past. Ironically, it is at the point when mothers become the "self-centered bundle of need" Saunders imagined with such horror that daughters sometimes manage to join them in an artful and mutually gratifying interdependency. Such treasured, and admittedly brief, moments do not compensate for the burdens caregivers endure, but they do provide readers a vision of how and why dementia care can be meaningful.

This salutary interdependency is nowhere to be found during most of Elinor Fuchs's memoir of her mother's dementia, *Making an Exit*. A theater critic and professor of drama, Fuchs emphasizes the performative aspects of care, describing how she played the part of attentive daughter while feeling none of the sentiments that would ideally accompany caring activity. She feels no innate desire to nurture or protect, nor is giving care motivated by an impulse to return care she once received. Lil was an indifferent mother who pushed her daughter into premature independence. She prioritized career and travel, leaving Elinor in the care of others. She was equally unavailable later, when Elinor struggled to balance her professional life with caring for her own young children. Fuchs thus cannot explain the time put into caring for her mother as repayment of a filial debt. "I have put nearly a decade of my life into this emergency," she thinks resentfully, focusing on opportunities lost. "In that decade my daughters needed more attention, my work was retarded, friendships narrowed, and my last best years to remarry, at least actuarially speaking, expired."[24] Time is not a renewable resource, but it can be an investment in the future. Not so in Fuchs's experience of caring for a person in decline. The output of energy cannot be recovered, nor can opportunities for more satisfying future-oriented self-care or relationships with others.

In frank and often darkly comic detail, *Making an Exit* documents the vast and largely hidden expenditures required to care for a single person with dementia. Fuchs uses the catalogue as a potent formal device. Long lists of needs, professionals, treatments, costs, and supplies emphasize a mounting accumulation of burden, stress, expense. While literary catalogues are traditionally associated with epic poetry and other elite genres—perhaps describing an august genealogy, a gathering of important people, or collection of revered objects—Fuchs does not intend to elevate or impress but rather to connote a piling on of humdrum responsibilities, necessities, and material possessions. Epic catalogues also serve a mnemonic function, listing people and events for posterity. In this Fuchs hews more closely to the genre's original design. Her catalogues have a similarly commemorative purpose, but in this case they record work and workers that would otherwise be unseen and unsung. Here is one excellent example, where Fuchs describes herself as an overloaded circuit in Lil's expanding network of care:

> I am the link to her internist, her cardiologist, her oncologist, her gynecologist, her dermatologist, her lawyer, her bank, her accountant, her insurance agent, her landlord, the IRS, the Social Security Administration, Blue Cross, Medicare, the Wadhwanis, and the helpers. I have left out her piano tuner, her dry cleaners, her hairdresser. The entries in my address book for Mother run to a dozen pages. I am her carapace, a crustacean of memory dragging my mother, my mother the drag queen, the two of us in a single shell.[25]

Care queers Elinor and her mother in ways that have nothing to do with pleasure or sexual activity, imposing atypical intimacies and confounding gender roles. Lil becomes "the drag queen," a dead weight pulled along by her daughter's efforts. In the process, Elinor is transgendered, burdened with the obligations of both a "traditional daughter" and a "traditional son."[26]

Things grow queerer as the catalogue details Elinor's responsibility for the inner recesses of Lil's fragmented and ailing body. Lil can't remember to remove her dentures, requiring Elinor to release and clean them. Elinor learns to change her mother's diaper, and, perhaps most disturbing, she discovers Lil wears a pessary. Forgotten and untended, it gives her "a raging vaginal infection" that requires

> someone . . . to insert a tube of antibiotics into Mother for the next seven days.
> Aiiiieeee! Not me, not me![27]

Elinor's wailing response gets its own paragraph to signal revulsion verging on hysteria at the prospect of ministering to her own mother's infected vagina. Forget about interdependency; she wants nothing of the kind. A different author might describe her mother's suffering with compassion and tenderness, treating all aspects of her body with respect. After all, Fuchs is writing about the very bodily passage that once brought her into the world. In another version, she might protect her mother's dignity by leaving the pessary out altogether. But Fuchs's honesty is valuable in that it denaturalizes a daughter's duty toward her dependent parent. She does the work, but certainly not because she is guided by any instinctual desire to comfort or nurture. There is nothing romantic about care that is urgently needed but also elicits disgust, resistance, and denial. No matter how much she loves her mother, this is not a labor of love; it is the unseen, unremunerated, stomach-churning toil so often demanded of women who have a dependent family member.

When Elinor refuses, "someone" still needs to insert antibiotics into Lil's vagina, along with all the other care required to support a single, frail elder in an environment designed for those who are healthy and reasonable. Fuchs's catalogue lists the numerous medical specialists and other professionals who tend to Lil's appearance and environment and provide more general personal maintenance. Other lists describe just how many people are required to attend to Lil's safety and well-being once she has been moved to assisted living. Lil needs "twenty-four hour everything."[28] Her needs are constant, pervasive, and overwhelming, refusing to obey the clock time of a conventional workday.

To this point I have focused on the negativity of Fuchs's account. As a seasoned complainer myself, I can attest to the virtues of the form. Complaint has the nontrivial function of demystifying women's association with care and exposing the time and expense required of individuals in a society that is not set up to accommodate the needs of dependent elders. And Fuchs does it well, with humor and warmth. But she also finds other, less obvious meanings in senility, or perhaps in the interdependency it occasions between mother and daughter. Among the most important of these are the affective connections that emerge when the dirty work of caring for a dependent body can be distributed to others. Elinor has been depleted by the exhausting, frustrating, and uncompensated toil of managing, and in many cases providing, her mother's care. Once she can delegate responsibility to paid care workers, she has time to develop a newfound intimacy with the mother who had always seemed distant and unknowable. Once Lil becomes dependent—and, crucially, *once Elinor is relieved of Lil's direct bodily and environmental maintenance*—it is easier for her daughter to feel satisfaction, and even enjoyment, in the time they spend together.

The moments of salutary interdependency Elinor finds with her mother are available only within an environment designed to support Lil's changed cognitive state. Living on her own, Lil's lapses in memory and understanding lead to chaos, even danger. Elinor was a reluctant first responder to the crises that erupted unpredictably during that earlier phase of slow emergency. But once she relocates Lil to a more accommodating space, Elinor can see possibility as well as loss: "In this setting [a nursing facility], I think of Mother not so much as ill, but as an original, a zany, an artist, cha-chaing through the corridors, inventing a fractured language that would have excited Gertrude Stein."[29] Like Mitchell and Saunders, Fuchs recognizes that the symptoms of Alzheimer's, as with many other illnesses and disabilities, are produced by an environment as well as by the changing bodymind. What

Mitchell and Saunders could not imagine is that, even well beyond their current levels of reasoned self-awareness, they might continue to thrive and even bring pleasure to others if embedded in the right context. Fuchs witnesses how care succeeds when it attends to the interaction of the bodymind with environmental cues. It is grinding work to maintain a dependent person in an ableist environment. Fuchs provides a vivid illustration of how both caregivers and dependents are served by spaces that slow the impact of disease and emphasize the potential that remains to a person with dementia. We need to create more of them and make them more accessible.

Fuchs is no Pollyanna. Even in a more accommodating environment, the disease takes its course, wearing away at her mother's body and mind. But surprisingly, she does not see Lil as the "self-centered bundle of need" that Saunders imagined with such dread and Mitchell refused to imagine at all. Advanced illness brings mother and daughter to a newfound and welcome interdependency. Surprisingly, in the late stages of crisis, when time is short and meaningful, Fuchs finds something like joy in communing with her dependent mother. "It hardly matters now which of us is the mother and which the daughter," she writes. "Taking care of as good as being taken care of. My job, to keep the little life aflame for just a while, to keep the little spirit in the world."[30] When Lil is most dependent, her daughter unexpectedly perceives their relationship as most *interdependent*, a circuit of attunement in which giving care is as necessary and sustaining as receiving it. Where the awfulness of slow emergency arises from its prolonged and unpredictable unfolding, the perception of time's scarcity means that it becomes precious.

Fuchs survives the slow emergency of her mother's dementia by finding ways to disperse care over an increasingly wide network. Although *Making an Exit* focuses on mother and daughter, Fuchs does bring Lil's care network into view, connecting the maintenance of one frail woman to global chains of labor. Almost all of Lil's paid caregivers are women of color: the "Caribbean lady in a white uniform," who works at her assisted living facility; a caregiver named Olga from El Salvador; others from Ghana, Guyana, Russia and Peru, African Americans, and a

voice that answers the phone with a "West African lilt." Fuchs acknowledges this network with gratitude. "It is astounding how many souls
supported the enterprise of Lil," she writes, "how kind they were, how
genuinely they cared for her."[31] In recognizing these caregivers, *Making
an Exit* becomes, perhaps unintentionally, a portrait of the scandalous
amount of labor and resources required, under current social conditions, to sustain the life of a single, relatively affluent white woman
with dementia. Because of their different relationships to illness, Saunders and Mitchell could only sense this injustice looming on the horizon, while Fuchs witnesses it directly as her own needs conflict with
those of her dependent mother and those of the many Black and Brown
people who are paid to care for her. In this way, the story of a particular relationship is also a more collective portrait of a conflicted
web of care that sustains mother and daughter in a time of slow
emergency.

Roz Chast confronts the racialization of care head-on at one point in
her graphic memoir, *Can't We Talk About Something More Pleasant?*
In the late stages of dementia, Chast's mother, Elizabeth, requires
twenty-four-hour supervision, a level of care that Chast—an only child
who lives in another state, with a family and career of her own—is
unable to provide without professional help. That help comes with a
steep price tag. There is the "phenomenal expense" of hiring a nurse
named Goodie, an immigrant from Jamaica who cares for Elizabeth
with patience and skill. But there is also an emotional cost accrued by
the guilt Chast feels at not "'doing the dirty work' myself." A single
page illustrates the very different forms of labor performed by each
woman (figure 4.1). Divided in half horizontally, a panel showing
Goodie reassuring Roz that she will take excellent care of Elizabeth sits
directly on top of, as if exerting weight on, a panel showing Roz drawing in her studio and taking a walk. Although she pays Goodie a generous salary, Roz recognizes the inequities that allow her to spend her
time on preferred forms of work, avoiding the physical and emotional
exertion of elder care. As she tells Goodie, "Guess I'll go home now and
DRAW!" emanata radiate from her body, the droplets communicating
relief, regret, sheepishness. A text box editorializes, "And once again,

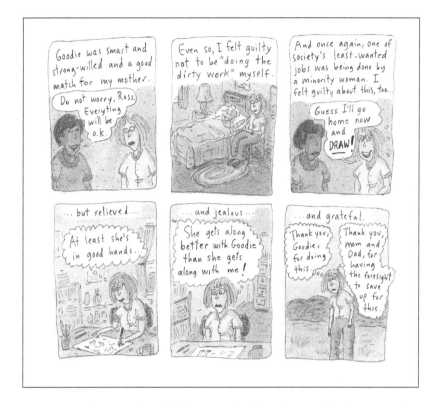

FIGURE 4.1 Two rows of panels from Roz Chast's *Can't We Talk About Something More Pleasant?*

Source: © Roz Chast, 2016, Bloomsbury Publishing Plc.

one of society's least-wanted jobs was being done by a minority woman. I felt guilty about this, too. . . ."[32] The ensuing frames depict Roz experiencing a complex stew of affects that include relief (not at her mother's bedside), jealousy (her mother seems to prefer Goodie's company), and gratitude (for financial means to pay such a competent professional caregiver). Although the racial division of care is not her primary subject, Chast builds her memoir on a foundational acknowledgment of the inequities that allow her to hire a full-time caregiver instead of doing the work herself, and of the emotional slurry that it occasions. Let it also be noted: There are no male caregivers of any complexion anywhere in the book.

The primary subject of *Can't We Talk About Something More Pleasant?* is the gradual onset of age-related infirmities, cognitive and physical, that leave a daughter with the unwanted responsibility for her parents' care. It tells a familiar story in a new form, using comics to portray the gaps, contradictions, and ambivalence that punctuate the slow emergency of parental decline. Like Fuchs, Chast remembers her mother Elizabeth as an inadequate caregiver, leaving her daughter no fund of gratitude or sense of having been nurtured. As seen through a daughter's eyes, the story begins with an aging couple's escalating needs, depicts the events surrounding her father's dementia and death, and ends with that of her mother. Also like Fuchs, Chast tells her story in retrospect, seeking to account for a process that was too incremental to register until it reached a point of crisis and then too urgent an emergency to allow for art. Only after the emergency has passed can she make sense of its unfolding. Lived time marches forward, and there are no second chances to notice earlier, make different arrangements, or care more. But narrative affords an opportunity to reckon with what one was and was not able to do, as well as sharing hard-won experiences that might be useful to others amid their own chaotic experience of slow emergency.

Looking back, Chast can see how the problem of gradually advancing dependency is exacerbated by her parents' refusal to contemplate an unwelcome future. They are certainly not alone. We have already seen how, even for the most practical and organized planners, the care required by Alzheimer's dementia is exceptionally hard to prepare for adequately. Even contemplating what it would be like to have the condition defies imagination. How can a body live on not just in a state of dependency, but unable to know or specify its own needs? The fact that so many families live out the same patterns of slow emergency is evidence of a collective failure of imagination. Here, art can serve a prosthetic function, extending our imaginative capacities through the stories of other people's successes and failures.

Humor is a vehicle that allows Chast to break her family's bourgeois reticence to talk about financial matters and the other unpleasantries alluded to in the book's title. In this, it provides a kind of cathartic accounting that Chast needed but was unable to complete in her parents' presence. Like Fuchs, she recognizes the catalogue as a potent formal device to communicate overwhelming excess, although in her case using images to add affective flavor to words. At one point she records, spreadsheet style, the price of housing, furniture, and extra assistance her parents require to live at "the Place." At another, she lists the many supplies required for end-of-life, the page crowded with words but also illustrated by a drawing of "the depressing aisle," loaded with such supplies as "adult diapers," liquid nourishment "for those who are done with food," and room freshener (figure 4.2). Its shelves are depressing because they hold items to care for a body in decline. We do not see the indignity of human bodies or the messes they produce, but rather a collection of products with ridiculously euphemistic names and packaging. There is nothing funny about the debilitated body of a parent, but we can laugh at the array of consumables designed to meet its needs, reaping profit from erasing its smells and messes.

Chast's grim humor points to a fundamental conflict in modern eldercare: The cost of the Place is massive and unsustainable, but the value of the distributed care it provides is priceless. Taking on the intimate labor of sustaining Elizabeth, the Place allows Roz to redirect energy toward caring about, as well as for, her mother without losing herself entirely. For Chast, like Fuchs, this means having the psychic wherewithal to appreciate the lyrical aspects of late-stage dementia. Because she is not changing diapers, Chast can find the creativity of Elizabeth's demented voice and take on a more appreciative role as scribe, editor, and archivist of these "waking dreams." Chast is a collaborator, organizing her mother's monologues into topics—mother-in-law, real estate holdings, etc.—giving them funny titles ("Ass Full of Buck Shot" or "Unusual Adoption") and illustrations. Chast's favorite story is probably untrue. Elizabeth claims that young Roz ran onstage during a production of *Uncle Tom's Cabin* to yell at Simon Legree for being a "BAD, BAD MAN!" At the bottom of the page, Chast comments, "Needless to say, I am 99.9999999% sure nothing like this ever happened."[33] Regardless of whether this incident happened as described, the story commemorates another truth. A mother who is typically critical

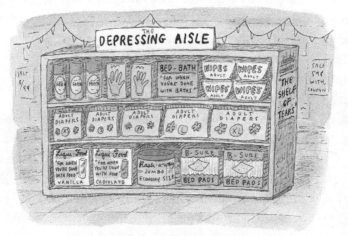

The Place suggested that I get around-the-clock care at this point. I hired two nurses from an outside agency. Each would do a twelve-hour shift. The hospice people were fine, but they weren't there all the time.

My money worries increased. My father's pension was no more. Besides the monthly rent at the Place, there were now these two nurses. There was her medication, and there were all these supplies she needed, now that she accepted her incontinence: bed pads, Depends, extra pads to wear _inside_ the Depends, latex gloves for the nurses, Ensure, baby wipes, bed bath wipes, baby powder, diaper ointment, room freshener. We were blowing through my parents' scrimpings at breakneck speed: about $14,000 a month, none of which was covered by insurance.

THE
DEPRESSING AISLE

A couple of weeks into the around-the-clock care, hospice, etc. I went to see my mother at the Place, filled with dread, fearing the worst.

FIGURE 4.2 "The depressing aisle" is filled with products designed to profit off of those in need of care.

Source: Roz Chast, *Can't We Talk About Something More Pleasant?*
© Roz Chast, 2016, Bloomsbury Publishing Plc.

and unsentimental now remembers her daughter as a brave and defiant protagonist, standing up for the oppressed. The storytelling is real, and Roz is gratified to hear and record it.

Dementia brings out Elizabeth's artistic creativity, and caring for Elizabeth brings nuance to her daughter's art. The predominant ambiance of *Can't We Talk About Something More Pleasant?* is frenetic. Words and images exude anxious energy, racing thoughts, and an escalating crisis. But at key moments Chast uses her art to communicate changes in pace and the affective tenor of the environment. She presses pause on her feelings of resentment and overwork to attend to her parents' needs with compassion. As her tone shifts from grim, neurotic humor to tenderness, it elicits an aesthetic departure from her usual mode. I see these interruptions as an experiment with the art of interdependency, as Chast seeks a form capable of depicting attunement to the needs of another. Sometimes that means allowing empty space, the absence of drawing signaling awareness of the limits of her form.

Comics are a medium that depicts time unfolding as space on the page, so blankness signals a pause.[34] One of the most powerful examples of such blank space is Chast's representation of tending to Elizabeth when she lost control of her bowels on the night of her husband's death. It is hard to imagine a more difficult and necessary act of care than cleaning up your grieving mother's shit. There are no humans in "the depressing aisle" comic, which derives its humor from an accumulation of products and their chorus of jarringly peppy slogans. But here, Chast adopts a far different tone to describe the human experience they are designed to address. Chast explains that she never mentioned the incident, intuiting her mother's need for silence. But sharing it after her mother's death in this muted form does not feel like a violation. Instead, the simple hand-printed text, black on a white page, acknowledges grief with respectful restraint that preserves her mother's dignity. She does the same in announcing the death of each parent, showing the gravity of her loss through the absence of illustration.

Chast depicts Elizabeth's final days with another telling stylistic shift. At that point, the hectic pace of care has slowed to the drawn-out quiet of a deathbed. Elizabeth, who sleeps most of the time, has no immediate needs, and there is little for a companion to do except to be present. Chast passes the time by drawing. "I didn't know what else to do," she explains. "I had been drawing her all summer, since the conversations had been reduced to almost nothing."[35] The style of her sketches is strikingly different from that of her comics. She uses simple black pen against an ivory background, with no additional color and no attempt at humor. In the absence of active care work, they bespeak those aspects of care that require waiting and the kind of quiet, minimally attentive activity—knitting, drawing, magazine reading—human animals do in such scenarios.[36] They also suggest that drawing—which has served through much of the narrative as a cathartic medium for voicing anxiety, frustration, and impatience—can itself be an expression of care, as it helps center the caregiver's attention on her subject, while creating a record of time spent together. As she waits and draws her mother, who also waits, inspiring her daughter to draw, Chast's art becomes an expression of their interdependency.

Dementia challenges some of our best arguments for why care is meaningful work. It requires care that is intensive without any of the future payoffs promised by more hopeful investments. Even under the best circumstances, a person with dementia will not recover. They may not respond with gratitude or even compliance; ultimately they may be unable to complete our care in the sense that Eva Feder Kittay means it, when our caregiving is "taken up by the other as caring."[37] This is why, given an aging population, Alzheimer's and related dementias pose one of the greatest and most pressing caregiving challenges of our time. Reading literature is not going to solve these problems. It is not going to reverse dementia's toll on the brain or find an untapped pool of caregivers or design sustainable environments to meet the needs of dependent elders without inconveniencing a younger generation. But these narratives may help us confront coming dependencies from other angles than our current postures of fear, denial, and crisis. At minimum, knowing how and why things came to be as they are might allow us to do otherwise in the future. An emergency is, by definition, "a serious, unexpected, and often dangerous situation requiring immediate action."[38] The arrival of age-related dependency, both physical and cognitive, may be serious, but it should not be unexpected, even in the absence of an Alzheimer's diagnosis. And its slow pace can provide opportunities, as well as protracted difficulties, for care.

The collective emergency these narratives document is not age-related dependency, but rather an unwillingness to imagine it as part of a lifespan or to adequately value the work of elder care. They speak with eloquence, compassion—and sometimes humor—of the seemingly irreconcilable needs of dependents, their families, and those who are paid to care for them. The populations at the margins of these narratives—the bus passengers, nannies, health care workers, and cleaners—attest to the dire failures of developed nations to care for all people according to their needs. These problems merit the collective future-oriented attention of a society, and we would do well to confront them head-on rather than blundering into them only when we, or someone we love, is in the midst of their own slow emergency. As with other slow emergencies—climate change, extinction, overdevelopment— time is both a problem and an opportunity. Literature helps us stretch the imagination toward temporalities that are hard to imagine at the scale of the self. Sometimes these stretches are hard or uncomfortable, but they also become more manageable when conceived in advance, as preparation for an unwelcome future rather than an unexpectedly calamitous present. Stories can also redirect the temporal orientation of our care from future recovery, cure, or prolonging life to being in the present, while accepting its impermanence. In a world devastated by our inability to act on the many cautionary tales about our planet's slow emergency, I'm aware of how feeble this sounds, even as I feel com- pelled to write it anyway. The stories matter because they speak to a need, even if they don't generate a single, decisive way to act on it.

These narratives are undeniably grim, but they also show why it is worthwhile to care about people with dementia and their caregivers. Those writing from within the experience attest to how its slow, uneven advance may leave pockets of lucid cognition and sometimes expose untapped creativity. They ask us to reimagine a dementia diagnosis from a prediction of unstoppable decline to an unsteady progression that can be mitigated by environments accommodating to a wider range of cognitive styles and abilities. Their caregivers, who tend to write retrospectively, are often surprised to recall moments of mean- ingful attunement amid the wreckage and loss left by a slow emergency. Those moments tend to arrive unexpectedly, and they may acquire value only retroactively. For those facing the awful prospect of becoming "a self-centered bundle of need," perhaps there can be some comfort in knowing that their time of greatest dependency might generate moments treasured by those who live on.

My attention is drawn to those eddies of intimate alignment captured by Chast and Fuchs in which mothers and daughters are simply being together in a profound, nonlinguistic, nonrational interdependency. It is unlikely that those connections will be perceived as they are unfolding, but in hindsight they gain meaning and clarity. They are far more likely to happen when care is distributed so that the person doing the emotional labor is not also required to do the chores of tending to a dependent body and when both forms of work are respected and fairly compensated. It is perhaps too much to expect that those in the throes of their own slow emergencies would be capable of imagining more just alternatives to the inequities they observe. But their stories make apparent a population-wide situation that need not be an emergency. To make it otherwise will require a radical rewriting of current narratives and the social systems they uphold.

II

THE SUBJECTS OF CARE

5

WRITING ON CRIP TIME

Our Dependent Bodies, Our Interdependent Selves

A painting of Christopher Reeve in a massive power wheelchair hangs in the National Portrait Gallery in Washington, DC (figure 5.1). Where a more conventional portrait might prioritize face and torso, here Reeve's lower legs and feet protrude into the foreground so that his knees and shins are monumental, the exaggerated perspective making his upper body appear diminished. Rosemarie Garland-Thomson has praised the artist Sacha Newley for conferring his subject with "dignity and authority."[1] To her, Reeve is a regal figure, his wheelchair a "throne," his respirator and shaved head appearing fashionable and restrained. Where portraits have traditionally sought to conceal disability, Garland-Thomson commends this painting for making its subject's difference visible without stigma. Newley's portrait reflects the politics of disability pride in Reeve's noble bearing, as well as the prominence of his wheelchair. Reeve is not "wheelchair bound," and his device is not a liability to be concealed or ignored; rather, this chair calls attention to its role in enabling uprightness, mobility, and participation.

Thinking about care might draw our interest to those aspects of Reeve's disability absent from the painting, as well as those it reveals. Reeve may be regal, but royal bodies, regardless of ability, require abundant maintenance. As does a person who is quadriplegic and uses a

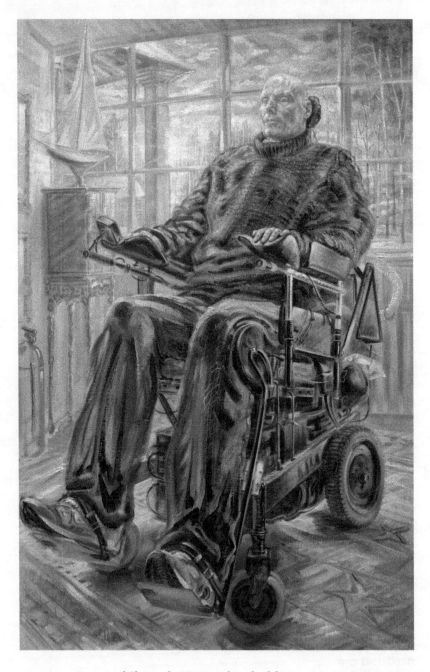

FIGURE 5.1 Portrait of Christopher Reeve in his wheelchair.

respirator. When I look at this picture, I wonder: Where are Reeve's attendants? What about the assistants who clean, arrange, and dress him every day? The therapists who massage his body, work his muscles, maintain his lung capacity and posture? The technologists who service his wheelchair? And the home health aides who complete his bowel program? If, as Garland-Thomson perceives, this portrait attests to Reeve's elite status, one aspect of that privilege is to obscure the signs of vulnerability, as well as the labor of caregiving that goes into ensuring his comfort and well-being. In order for Reeve to sit as a composed, independent subject, his dependency—and the efforts of those who sustain him—must be invisible. If the portrait bespeaks the independence and dignity demanded by the movement for disability rights, it also attests to the erasures that have been required to secure those benefits.

This chapter is about how dependent adults make sense of the care work outside the frame of Reeve's portrait. Where many who fought for disability rights see "independence" as essential to living with dignity, I am interested in those who treat interdependency as an aspect of their lived experience that is worthy of narrative attention. Having devoted the first section of this book to caregiving in the context of family, much of it from the point of view of caregivers, this chapter centers on self-representation by those who need care that extends beyond the unpaid labor of parents, spouses, and other relatives. Of course we all depend on others for daily survival, but I am concerned with the kinds of dependencies that cannot be covered over or forgotten in environments designed by and for the able bodied. In a world where Hollywood movies like *Million Dollar Baby* and *Me Before You* tell us it is better to be dead than dependent, it is a radical act for people living with profound dependencies to make their presence known *with*, rather than *in spite of*, their bodies. And even more so, to insist on being seen in their dependency as other than a tragic spectacle. The life narratives I consider make bodily dependency, and the work of giving and receiving care, central to an account of self.

I focus on literary, rather than visual, portraiture because of its capacity to portray care as a dynamic process. Where a portrait seeks to capture the essence of a self compressed into a single, static image, narrative is an account of change over time.[2] I have already introduced the concept of "crip time," the idea that people with disabilities may move and develop at a different pace or perceive time differently than the clock time of modernity.[3] This term usually implies an individual "crip" out of sync with social expectations, although it can also be used to describe the collective debilitation of a class of people.[4] Here, I am concerned with a crip temporality somewhere between the individual and the population, a scale that encompasses the webs of care surrounding a person living with dependency and those responsible for their maintenance and well-being.

Crip time is rarely limited to a single body, even if it is often discussed as the property of an individual. Bodies do not exist in isolation, so the temporal aberrations of the one have radiating effects that may slow down, speed up, or otherwise warp the timescales of those in their vicinity. To get to my desk, I rode the subway, buzzing with impatience (and aware of my own hypocrisy) as a crip person leaning heavily on a cane made their way up the stairs in front of me. Of course the elevator was out of service, and that person needed to climb at a pace at odds with my need to write in the precious hours while somebody else cared for my disabled son. I am interested in how narratives account for a more interdependent experience of crip time, in which the paces of a dependent body intersect with the labor of those who sustain it. Where the Reeve portrait aspires to suspend time, the monumental body posed in isolation, memoirs move through time, recounting a life and a timescape interdependent with other lives. In what follows, I ask how crip time shapes life writing by and about dependent people, considering how they make sense of the body's highly visible vulnerabilities and integrate care givers and intimate routines into a portrait of self.

Life writing by dependent people presents some intriguing generic challenges. Critics have noted the flourishing of life writing by authors who make experiences of illness and disability the subject of their life story, a genre G. Thomas Couser memorably dubbed the "some body memoir."[5] In addition to diversifying the genre, the some body memoir also has a political bent, as a class of people who have historically been marginalized asserts the right to self-representation and inclusion.

However, sometimes the claim to individual rights involves erasing the body's need for care and, more importantly, those who do the work of caregiving. Christina Crosby and Janet Jakobsen describe how the accessible environments engineered by the Americans with Disabilities Act produce the appearance of independence as Crosby—who is quadriplegic—"seems to come and go as she wishes." But her independence is a performance that depends on obscuring the time and effort of those who care for her. Where the call for disability rights has often led to the backgrounding of care work, Crosby and Jakobsen insist that "the work that produces this illusion about Christina's life is crucial to document."[6] Memoirs by dependent people contribute to this documentary effort, making them an essential component of the archive gathered for this book. And they do more than testify to existing realities. Memoirs are also crafted, and they may use aesthetics to artfully conceal interdependency or to foreground the self's imbrication with others.

In this chapter I am concerned with life writing by those disabled authors who depend on the care of others in order to survive. These authors are not only claiming a place within a genre typically reserved for able-bodied elites, but are also navigating the seeming contradictions among a discrete and autonomous narrative self, a politics of individual rights, and a life of exceptional dependency. Harriet McBryde Johnson, Ben Mattlin, and Christina Crosby are dependent adults who write as participants in, or beneficiaries of, an international movement for disability rights that allowed their voices to be heard. But they take different positions on the rights and obligations of care, which also shape the literary strategies they adopt. While Crosby emphasizes care to recognize the rights and dignity of care workers, Johnson and Mattlin assert bodily autonomy by framing the dependent as a manager and/or employer of others. I conclude by turning to the 1979 *Autobiography of Gaby Brimmer*. Written decades earlier in Mexico, where disability rights was virtually nonexistent, it takes a novel approach to the politics and aesthetics of care, as well as literary genre, with its tripartite, collaborative composition. A different cultural context, and the unprecedented nature of its subject may have inspired exceptional formal creativity, although the work's content and afterlife also reflect the costs of such prolonged interdependencies. Read together, each work offers a distinct version of embodied knowledge as it negotiates the singularity of a narrating self and its simultaneous dependence on others.

CRIP TEMPORALITIES AND NARRATIVE INDEPENDENCE

When Crosby and Jacobsen advocate for the workers who allow them to maintain an illusion of independent selfhood, they speak as relative latecomers to the scene of disability advocacy and activism. Crosby was disabled at age fifty, after a devastating bike accident left her quadriplegic. Imperfect as it was, her access to care and inclusion was the result of decades of political struggle on behalf of disabled rights. This is to say that timing matters. *When* one experiences disablement—the stage of life, as well as the moment in our collective history—profoundly affects attitudes toward care and those who provide it. I will return to Crosby's representation of care work later in this section. But first I look to some precursors, authors with congenital disabilities who came of age before the environment was remade by disability rights and, indeed, who participated in the movement to secure those rights. Their sense of crip identity is shaped by lifelong disablement, as well as a distinct set of political commitments and experiences emerging from the struggle for political recognition. They speak to the extreme vulnerability of the dependent body, while also insisting on the right to dictate the circumstances of their care, sometimes in ways that subordinate the personhood of their caregivers.

The sassy narrative persona of Harriet McBryde Johnson's autobiographical collection, *Too Late to Die Young*, is Exhibit A. Johnson, who was born with muscular dystrophy, pulls no punches about her dependency, describing herself as "Karen Carpenter-thin, flesh mostly vanished, a jumble of bones in a floppy bag of skin."[7] The self-deprecating humor about her appearance does nothing to shake her absolute confidence in her right to the care of others. Johnson—a lawyer and disability rights advocate—finds no contradiction in being a smart, competent, and accomplished professional who also requires assistance for eating, toileting, dressing, and self-care. Care work is essential to maintaining dignified and autonomous personhood coextensive with extreme bodily dependency. These principles are at the heart of Johnson's politics, her insistence that paid care is a right for citizens with disabilities in a world designed for the able bodied. She illustrates these political commitments by making frequent references to hired caregivers in her essays: Norah, the law school roommate paid through a grant and good at "following my exact verbal instructions"; Charlene, who knows to ask Johnson what she wants to wear in the morning; Mandy, who is "entirely and immediately compliant with all my instructions," and numerous others.[8] These caregivers are mentioned with nonchalance, as an ordinary and colorful aspect of her daily life. But the fact that they are mentioned at all highlights their constant and necessary contribution to Johnson's survival.

Johnson's position is consistent with what some feminists have described as "relational autonomy," the notion that all people exist in some degree of interdependency.[9] But she goes beyond this universalizing definition, which would locate a body like hers at the far end of a very wide spectrum, to insist on her right to help in achieving that autonomy. Her needs are exceptional, yet her status as a citizen in a liberal democracy entitles her to the extra resources and protections required to ensure her parity with other citizens. It is also her right to determine the nature of that care, ensuring it is not provided in a spirit of dominance or paternalism. Paid care must be an avenue to autonomy, which is, for Johnson, synonymous with sovereignty. Of her morning routine, she explains, "If it's not Geneva, it's someone else, someone I've chosen, someone following my instructions. It's a daily necessity, entirely practical and matter-of-fact." Here, Johnson performs the politics of disability rights in representing herself as a competent manager of the dependency work that allows her to function in the world. When accorded those services, she has access to the same opportunities and is just as capable of contributing as any other adult citizen. "Self-powered in my chair, self-employed in my office, at large and unsupervised," she writes, proudly living out the political commitments of the ADA, "I am free to spend the morning and the rest of my life as I please."[10] By this logic, it is possible to be free even in a body that is dependent, so long as one receives the resources to which they are entitled and can dictate the conditions of care.

Johnson's approach to dependency is pragmatic, detailing what she needs to function productively. Occasionally, and more surprisingly, she describes care as a benefit, and even a source of pleasure. Physical impairment and vulnerability, so often a source of frustration and anxiety even in her chipper account, sometimes enable unexpected intimacies. Take Johnson's encounter with Peter Singer, the Princeton philosophy professor who infamously advocates euthanasia for infants with severe disabilities. Before she met Singer, Johnson liked to call him "the Evil One," targeting him for protest as part of the disability rights group Not Dead Yet. But then he invited her to a public debate at Princeton, where he was a gracious and accommodating host. At dinner, her elbow slipped out of place, making it impossible for her to eat.[11] She was forced to ask for his help, even while worrying that she was drawing attention to limitations imposed by her physical condition. He responded by adjusting her arm unobtrusively, and the private moment they shared became the basis for a warm and mutually respectful relationship. After Johnson's death, he would write a tribute expressing appreciation for their friendship and admiring her accomplishments.[12]

In isolation, the Singer episode might lead to the troubling conclusion that dependent people have a purpose, which is to teach virtue to the able bodied among us. But Johnson would likely disagree. She finds good in the state of being dependent itself, disputing the idea that she longs to be otherwise. Of her morning routine, she writes, "I sometimes think how strange it would be to do these morning things in solitude as nondisabled people do, and to regard, as many of them do, a life like mine as a dreadful and unnatural thing." To her the able body is strange; what the able bodied consider independence, she describes as "isolation." She denaturalizes the notion that privacy is a universal good by asserting, "To me it is so natural to feel the touch of washcloth-covered hands on flesh that is glad to be flesh, to rejoice that other hands are here to do what I'd do for myself if I could."[13] Being cared for is not simply a necessity, but a source of fleshly pleasure and communion with others. Bodily sensations that might seem unwelcome and intrusive are, for Johnson, a welcome sign of ongoing aliveness.

In his approach to care, Ben Mattlin, Johnson's contemporary, writes more directly about the sexuality of his dependent body. In *Miracle Boy Grows Up*, his story of coming of age with the disabling condition SMA, Mattlin insists that being dependent does not preclude having sexual desires and acting on them. He writes of care as an opportunity, as well as an obstacle, to intimacy. The coupling of care and desire is a delicate topic, given the heightened vulnerability of dependent people to sexual assault. In chapter 2, we encountered Jon Pineda's distress at finding a stranger ogling his sister's naked body as she lies comatose in her hospital bed and Judy Karasik's devastating discovery that her older brother had been sexually abused by staff at his group home. These incidents are echoed with alarming frequency in the news, and I return to the problem of sexual violence in institutional settings in chapter 7.[14] Given the risks, it is tempting to insist that sex and care should never be coupled and that safety should always come first in the care of dependent people.[15] But prioritizing safety can easily be a justification for control and denial, which is perhaps why Mattlin prefers to think of his assistants as valets or butlers, rather than caregivers. "They work for me, I'll say, rather than take care of me," he writes, drawing attention to the transactional nature of the relationship. "And they are never, never nurses."[16] For Mattlin, who is neither a child nor a sick person, a "nurse" carries the whiff of infantilization or debility. As an autonomous adult who depends on others for life-sustaining assistance, he insists that he is also a sexual being who feels desire and is desired by others.[17]

Occasionally, Mattlin's acknowledgment that care can coexist with desire leads him to speak of his male attendants with thinly veiled homophobia. More often, he is comically self-deprecating, especially as he recounts the cringy details of an awakening adolescent sexuality.

These include stories of flirtations, crushes, and inconvenient arousals; obsessive imagining, planning, and attempting erotic contact with female peers; and, eventually, a sexual relationship with the woman who will become his wife, coparent, and caregiver. Anticipating readers' curiosity about the mechanics of his body, Mattlin speaks frankly about masturbation. He finds it a welcome release, but one that requires careful planning, including precise instructions to nighttime attendants about positioning his body in bed, followed by strategic requests for repositioning to conceal the evidence. With characteristic optimism, he finds an unexpected benefit when his posture begins to sag later in life: "I learned I could suck my own dick."[18] Mattlin thus presents himself as a man who is dependent, sovereign, and possessed of a robust, adult sexuality. It manifests in normate activities like masturbation, watching pornography, and adolescent fantasies about attractive women but also in the more unusual kinky autoeroticism enabled by his disabled body.

Mattlin decouples dependency from passivity, insisting that he is an active sexual partner, fully capable of giving as well as receiving pleasure. He came of age watching movies like *Coming Home* (1978), which radically changed the public perception of disabled masculinity. Its story of the affair between an unhappily married woman (played by Jane Fonda) and a disabled veteran (Jon Voight) who "fucks her like she's never been fucked" showed him that "*People In Wheelchairs Can Be Sexy*."[19] In life, Mattlin finds the mechanics of intimacy to be complicated, since he has far less mobility and muscle strength than the character played by an able-bodied Voight. But he turns his dependency into an opportunity for sexy consent by asking—with comic awkwardness—"would it cause too much of a disturbance if I were to ask for a kiss?" His future partner, ML, finds his question funny and exciting, and she answers yes. She confirms the rightness of the match by being unfazed at Mattlin's nightly bedtime routine, which requires the help of an assistant. As their relationship develops, the exchange of care becomes a part of their erotic life. It is gratifying and fun for ML to be Ben's assistant, and he finds her an exceptional caregiver. The reciprocity of their sexual relationship is a paradigm for their marriage, to which each contributes equally as they are capable. Where ML has muscle strength that allows her to assist her husband physically, he reciprocates with attention, advice, and financial support.

Mattlin's coming-of-age story does not end with marriage, as might a more traditional narrative. Instead, it takes a more long-term view of a relationship marked by notable asymmetries of ability, health, and strength. Interdependency is less a status than a process that requires continual assessment and negotiation to ensure that each participant's needs are equitably met. At some points, the marriage thrived on privacy, as both partners found satisfaction in ML serving as Ben's primary caregiver. At others, their insularity became a chafing symbiosis, and they turned to paid assistants to relieve ML of her caregiving duties and provide Ben with the welcome impersonality of a professional attendant. Mattlin describes the dance of their interdependency as mutual, if not always harmonious, with each partner needing a mix of intimacy and individuation. He finds dignity in recognizing his agency and sense of self as consistent with, rather than in spite of, his dependent body. In his portrait of long-term reciprocity, each partner gives and takes according to their capacities.

When Mattlin noticed the absence of information about "interabled romances" like his own, he decided to write a book.[20] My friends and colleagues Janet Jakobsen and Christina Crosby were one of the couples interviewed for his study. At the time he spoke with them, Crosby was also writing a memoir of her own. *Body Undone* is, among other things, an extended love letter to Janet, Christina's partner of six years at the time of the devastating bicycle accident that left Christina quadriplegic, who had become Christina's primary caregiver. Like Mattlin, Crosby speaks frankly about sex, devoting an entire chapter to her physical relationship with Janet. But she finds nothing sexy about her newfound dependency or the life-sustaining care her partner provides. Unlike Johnson and Mattlin, Crosby does not leverage her vulnerability to assert her political right to receive care according to her wishes. Rather, "the profound fact of human interdependence" that is her book's theme leads Crosby to a humbling acknowledgment of the many things she cannot control and the extent to which her survival is inextricably bound to the lives and personhood of others.[21] Crosby's version of disability politics is premised on interdependency rather than individual sovereignty. As with other disability memoirs, *Body Undone* advances an embodied theory, but one that emerges from the experience of disability acquired in midlife, in an environment already significantly remade by the disability rights movement that the earlier authors had helped realize.

Where Ben and ML began their interabled romance by flirting over their differing abilities, Christina and Janet found theirs suddenly and violently imposed. Crosby's accident thrust Janet into the unanticipated role of being her partner's primary caregiver. In chapter 3 we saw gay men fighting to be recognized as family to their partners, but that recognition came at a cost. Janet's new identity was conferred by the bureaucratic language of a hospital discharge that pronounced Christina ready to go home under "the care of one." This welcome sign of repair also cast Janet as the "one," the lone individual responsible for providing and/or managing all of the care her partner required. Where hospital care came at a staggering expense, Janet would do it for free and motivated by love. But Crosby parses the cruel irony of the phrase "care of one" as she details the impossible demands it places on Janet:

> From that point on—in principle—I needed only one person to transfer me from bed to wheelchair and back again, to watch for pressure sores, to dress and undress me, to bathe me and brush my teeth, to feed me and help me drink, to help relieve myself, and to purchase and administer my pharmacopeia of drugs. To keep me alive. The burden of my care was now transferred to private life, where one untrained person was charged with taking over. In most cases this would be a mother or wife. In my case the burden of my care came to my lover, Janet.[22]

Using the word "burden" twice to describe the work Janet is expected to do, Crosby frames care as a decidedly unsexy form of intimacy that has historically fallen to wives, mothers, and other women considered to be "family." It goes without saying that the care of family will be superior but unpaid, because, well, love has no price tag. This passage, which appears in the third paragraph of *Body Undone*, is the end of the story as far as the insurance company is concerned. But it is just the beginning for Christina and Janet. It is also the beginning of Crosby's memoir, an extended reflection on how her sense of self was rearranged by her newly dependent body, its needs and relationship to others.

Crosby's accident forced recognition of a fact that that the able bodied have the luxury to forget "the myriad ways my well-being depends on both the regard and the labor of others." From this ontological claim, Crosby moves to political assertion: "We need a calculus that can value caring labor far differently than we do today."[23] Crosby attempts to account for care's value in the most personal terms. Among other things, *Body Undone* is an extended expression of gratitude and love for Janet, her paid caregiver Donna, and a wider network of care givers, paid and unpaid, that emerged to sustain them. Crosby recognizes that even as her body was unmade by pain and incapacity, an environment of support was made. In this sense her dependency is generative, bringing a web of care into being. At the center is Janet, in her new role as the "one" officially charged with overseeing Christina's health and well-being. This couple is a central node in a network that includes medical personnel, therapists, close friends, and the broader circuits of their university and LGBTQ communities, as well as their many paid helpers. Newfound dependency casts relationships in a different light, and the assemblages of care around Christina and Janet overlap with, but also diverge from, other communities to which they belong. The diverse web of people who offered their support included some already trusted friends, and it turned others into unexpected allies. New friendships were forged; another subset grew more distant or cut ties altogether.

Friendship is not enough to sustain a medically fragile dependent and her lover. This is where the "money" in my title enters the picture. Paid care workers were essential to Christina's survival and well-being, her needs bringing her into intimate contact with people of radically different backgrounds and social positions whom she might otherwise never have known. They "meet at the cash nexus, the labor market" where one party has the ability to work and the other the resources to pay her.[24] There, Crosby recognizes a profound contradiction. The work must be recognized as at once priceless and as a commodity exchanged for monetary compensation. She and her assistant Donna are in a relation of employer and employee even as they engage in the most private and personal exchanges of bodily care. Crosby devotes much of a chapter to Donna, casting a temporary limelight on someone whose profession dictates that she fade into the background. Much as she loves and appreciates Donna, Crosby is also powerfully aware of their differences. Donna is poor, nonwhite, a Pentecostal Protestant, and single mother. Like other certified nursing assistants, who are mostly women of color, Donna's work is low paying, stressful, and physically grueling. In her early forties, she suffers from a painful neck injury, arthritic knee, and frequent headaches.

Crosby knows Donna's aches and pains, and many other things about her, but also acknowledges that certain aspects of her life remain "in many regards, unknown to me and unknowable." This epistemic asymmetry—where Donna's intimate familiarity with the home life and private recesses of Christina's body far outweighs what Christina knows of her—is countered by an economic asymmetry—Christina has money to pay for her care, which grants her a position of power over Donna that should not be denied. No matter how much Christina and Janet respect Donna, their good intentions "are no guarantee against patronage—our intimacy is very real, but it's we who have the money."[25] The ethics of Crosby's project require candid reflection on her uneven interdependence with Donna, grounding her call to improve working conditions for caregivers in embodied experience and the situated knowledge it generates.

Writing from within a web of care—in which one person's needs or contributions ripple outward to affect many others in its radius—requires Crosby to think about agency in more complicated ways. We have seen how Johnson and Mattlin adapt the politics of disability rights, asserting autonomy, if not independence, by directing their own care. Crosby is more hesitant to take on a managerial role, or to assert that her needs take priority over those of others she calls on for help. Nonetheless, she positions herself as an active participant in the exchange of care, rather than its passive recipient. Her contributions include paying her careworkers and treating them with respect and gratitude. She also discovers a more unexpected resource, the willingness to ask for, or make oneself receptive to, help. This is what the anthropologist Danilyn Rutherford calls the "sovereignty of vulnerability" elicited by dependent people, who "institute a web of obligation when they demand a response."[26] People with lifelong dependencies are well acquainted with this form of sovereignty.

Knowing how to ask for help with dignity and confidence is a superpower available to those living with dependency. They are often skilled at enlisting the help they need, but also aware of the satisfaction and even pleasure it can accord those who are willing and able to provide. We don't really need science to prove that it feels good to help others, but there is now abundant data to show the emotional and physiological benefits of giving.[27] By this logic, the problem of care is not with the work itself but the way we imagine it—as unwelcome toil—and the unevenness with which it is distributed. In an ideal world, nobody would live under "the care of one." Care would be apportioned in ways that make it easier to see the ask as a generative rather than an extractive act. *Body Undone* mourns exile from the world of the able bodied, but it also recognizes the generative power of asking for help, among other forms of agency that remain to those who are physically dependent.

Crosby, Mattlin, and Johnson all live with physical impairments that make their survival contingent on help from others, far beyond the typical spectrum of human interdependency. Exceptionally dependent, these authors are also all exceptionally intelligent, well educated, and professionally successful. In writing memoir, they navigate a contradiction, adopting a generic form dedicated to representing a singular narrative persona with a coherent and enduring subjectivity. Even Crosby, who is generally more skeptical about genre, marvels at the continuities that allow her to recognize many aspects of herself even as others were transformed beyond recognition by the traumatic injury to her body. Her narrative voice holds those fragments together, even as it expresses amazement that, somehow, the injured self who writes in the present can still lay claim to the able-bodied self of the past. But what if the interdependency between the disabled subject and their caregivers were built into the structure of the narrative itself? What if the process of negotiating relational autonomy were not simply described but generated a form of its own? In a final example, I turn to a work that is not simply about interdependency, but takes the imbrication of care giving and receiving as its form.[28]

COBIOGRAPHY: INTERDEPENDENCY
AS FORM AND CONTENT

The disability rights activist and titular subject of the book *Gaby Brimmer* lived in a different time and place from the three American authors just considered. She was born with cerebral palsy in Mexico City in 1947 and came of age in an environment that was physically inaccessible and denied any political or economic standing to people with disabilities like hers. Like her Irish contemporary Christy Brown, Brimmer used a wheelchair and had command of only one foot, which she used to type and spell out words on an alphabet board. Also like Brown, Brimmer was intelligent and motivated. Because her comfortably middle-class family had means to travel and maintain contact with relatives in the United States, she experienced the early stirring of the international movement for disability rights, as well as advances in therapy and medical care for cerebral palsy. With the tireless collaboration of her mother, Sari, and her lifelong caregiver, Florencia, she was able to attend college, enjoy a career as a writer and international disability rights advocate, and even become a mother.

When the fruitful, triangulated relationship among these women came to the attention of the acclaimed Mexican author and investigative journalist Elena Poniatowska, she proposed writing a collaboratively narrated story of Brimmer's life. A leftist whose work often had a political bent, Poniatowska had successfully used polyvocality as a device to tell the story of the 1968 massacre of student protestors in *La noche de Tlatelolco*.[29] With Brimmer, she imagined a similar technique to tell a narrower story, but one that spoke to the collective circumstances of people with disabilities and their caregivers in Mexico and abroad. She engaged the three women in conversation, weaving together excerpts from their interviews with selections from Brimmer's letters and poetry, to create a book, which was originally published in Spanish in 1979. Although the English translation, published in 2009, is subtitled *An Autobiography in Three Voices*, the book is not an autobiography but a generic hybrid that I call a "cobiography." Put into dialogue by Poniatowska, whose presence is evident only in the book's framing material, the three women relate shared experiences and themes, often drawing contradictory conclusions and speaking in voices marked by disparities in class, generation, and individual temperament.

I am aware that it is a somewhat odd swerve in my argument to include *Gaby Brimmer* in this chapter alongside the recent life writing of authors from the United States. But stay with me on this necessary tangent: *Gaby Brimmer* is the work that inspired my original quest to write about the narrative forms, as well as the social and thematic problem of interdependency, and it has no literary equivalent that I know of, even almost half a century after its initial publication. Moreover, Brimmer was born just six years before Crosby, making them loose generational peers. Her story allows for a comparative view of how circles of care are shaped by society and built environments, as much as they are by the dependent body.

Gaby Brimmer, like others introduced in this chapter, lived at the speed of crip time, which includes the uneven pacing of an atypical body, as well as the temporalities of those who provide care essential to her survival. Like the memoirs by Crosby and Johnson, *Gaby Brimmer* eschews a continuous, chronological arc in favor of a more episodic and topical organization. But it is more formally inventive than that, its iterative, polyvocal composition reflecting the argument I have been making about crip time. It is a palimpsest of individually experienced temporalities that sometimes operate in sync but often conflict in ways that slow or redirect progress away from a particular goal, including narrative advancement. *Gaby Brimmer* thus builds its form from the strained interplay of individual subjectivity with the synchronous experiences of three different but interdependent people. Instead of moving forward, it revisits the same incidents or subjects from multiple perspectives, each told in a different voice with its own priorities and understanding of past, present, and future. Care is a primary theme, but also generates innovative narrative form.

A vivid example of fault lines within a caring relationship emerges as the three women discuss Brimmer's future. Each speaker's perspective is shaped by her own values and interests. Sari, who is desperate to ensure her daughter's access to long-term care, describes a failed effort to install Gaby and Florencia in a nursing facility in Cuernavaca. Her worries are understandable, given the likelihood that a child will outlive a mother's ability to provide care. By putting her words into dialogue with the voices of the two younger women, Poniatowska shows how a parent's priorities conflict with those of her daughter or her paid caregiver. We witness Brimmer dismissing her mother's worries. According to her, "We [Brimmer and Florencia] protested over and over, but adults never listen to young people. There they were, stubborn as mules, building an apartment in Cuernavaca, taking me out of the university, and moving me and Nana into a depressing environment where you could smell death at every step." Florencia's modulating response reflects her awkward position both as advocate for the happiness and well-being of her charge, and as an employee paid by Sari Brimmer: "I liked Cuernavaca but just to go for a day or a weekend, not to live there for good." The next voice is Sari's, expressing a mother's anxiety about securing the future for her dependent daughter: "I pinned all my hopes on Cuernavaca! I thought the climate was lovely. The Home was surrounded by flowers and plants, and it looked like an oasis—at least that's how I saw it—and I thought, since I'm always looking for a permanent roof over Gaby's head if I die, 'Here she will be safe.'"[30] An environment that Gaby finds bleak and depressing looks like an oasis of safety and permanence to Sari. These statements cannot be prioritized, because each is clearly a legitimate expression of the speaker's desires and needs. Nor can each woman simply go her own way, because their fates are conjoined. Their voices reveal competing temporal horizons that cannot be reconciled: Brimmer's youthful desire to live in the present, in a stimulating environment and the company of peers; Florencia's intermediary position as a confidant and paid caregiver; and Sari's anxiety about the safety and well-being of her disabled daughter. Together, they express discrepant perspectives on the burdens of long-term dependency and care, suggesting the impossibility of fully satisfying any one individual, as well as their intractable entanglement. The irreconcilable nature of their perceptions and desires shapes a narrative that perseverates at key points of tension rather than moving with the forward march of chronological time.

Gaby Brimmer is not the author of her book, but she is the subject. Her spirited, colloquial speech dominates the interviews with Poniatowska, and she is the only one of the three speakers to make a written contribution with excerpts from her letters and poetry. Like other subjects in this chapter, Brimmer negotiates between the need for help to meet the body's most basic needs, and her sense of being an autonomous individual possessed of independent thoughts and beliefs. She claims ideas and values all her own, although part and parcel of a body that requires help in every way. She describes herself as having a "thirst to live my own life," a metaphor attesting to an essential but unfilled desire for independence.[31] Given the unaccommodating environment and the pervasiveness of her need, any degree of autonomy will be hard won. Brimmer fashions herself as a rebel, announcing her leftist politics (a pantheon of heroes that includes Mao, Che Guevara, and Fidel Castro), crushes on fellow student activists, and resistance to maternal authority.

A manual wheelchair is an essential conduit to Brimmer's life beyond the home, an unavoidable stigma, and an impediment to the inaccessible environments of mid-twentieth-century Mexico City. When she writes, in her opening poem, "I'm thinking of / putting a motor / in my chair," she hints at the extent of her dependency.[32] Although the technology was invented some decades before, Brimmer did not have the kind of power chair that allowed her counterparts in the United States to zoom through the streets under their own direction.[33] Even if she had an electric wheelchair, it is likely that the terrain would have rendered it useless. Anyone who has been to Mexico City knows how many of its streets are an obstacle course of cracks, holes, and rubble, and that its lovely historic architecture is frequently elevated by stairs. All of that, at a time when the prevailing mindset was to hide people with disabilities, rather than giving them access to public space. It would require a vast shift in attitude, as well as material resources, to imagine the value of universal design features like ramps, curb cuts, or elevators. In this way, the built environment of Mexico City rendered Brimmer more dependent than the U.S. American memoirists in the previous section. So too, even in 1979, there was already a discernible gap between the services and rights available to people with disabilities in the United States and their Mexican counterparts.[34] Under Mexican law, Brimmer could not have a bank account in her name or manage her own finances, let alone receive resources to direct her own care. Having traveled abroad for treatment and vacations in the United States, Brimmer was well aware of these inequities. They made her all the more reliant on the care of family, which in her case meant her mother, Sari. In *Gaby Brimmer*, the voices of Sari and Florencia attest to the collaborative female labor her sustenance requires.

Sari's voice turns *Gaby Brimmer* from an individual story to a conflicted dialogue. At the time of the book's composition, there would have been few memoirs by authors with disabilities, or their parents, in either the United States or Mexico. Thirty years later, its translation into English coincides with the boom in disability memoir.[35] But even decades after its initial publication, it is distinguished by its polyvocality, introducing a trio of female voices that affirm, contradict, and complain about one another. In her own words, Sari emerges as tortured and anxious, a fierce advocate for her daughter's rights and needs, who sees disability as a defining and tragic aspect of Gaby's identity. "I don't think I've ever forgotten, not even for an instant, that my daughter has cerebral palsy," Sari says. "That thought is with me all the time, like a knife through my heart."[36] Harsh as this may sound, Sari speaks as the household's breadwinner and care manager, as well as the conduit between her disabled daughter and the ableism of Mexican society. There was no question of coparenting in the Brimmer family. Miguel's status as patriarch, combined with the physical frailty caused by heart disease, left Sari to wrestle with the daily realities of domestic life. No one is more aware that her daughter would be helpless without her family, and the strain of this responsibility is evident throughout the dialogue.

The inclusion of Florencia—Brimmer's lifelong, paid caregiver—is the book's most innovative contribution. Her significance is emphasized in the original Spanish-language edition, which includes more photos of her than any other subject aside from Brimmer herself. Although we might expect the book's first image to be the fundamental pairing of mother and daughter, it is a close-up of Florencia holding a young Brimmer, both gazing solemnly into the camera (figure 5.2). There are no corresponding photos of Brimmer with her biological family. Spanning the decades of Brimmer's life, the photographs lend visual weight to the intimate and enduring relationship with her paid attendant, emphasized by the near-absence of born family. What the photographs do not depict are the extreme disparities of wealth and opportunity that led Florencia to become the Brimmers' employee.

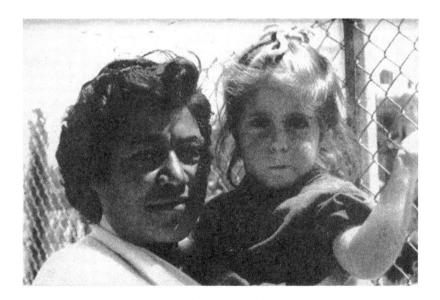

FIGURE 5.2   A younger Florencia and Gaby as a child.

Source: Gabriela Brimmer, *Gaby Brimmer: An Autobiography in Three Voices*, © Grijalbo.

There are no pictures of Florencia's biological family, despite the fact that Brimmer spent time in their home, where she was welcomed and appreciated. It is unlikely that they had access to a camera, given their poverty. Florencia's parents sent her to work for the Brimmers in Mexico City at age thirteen because they could not afford to care for her. She started out as a housekeeper, but her devotion to their baby daughter soon made Gaby's care her primary duty. As Florencia grew into an adult, her energy was devoted to caring for Brimmer, rather than her own development or relationships with her biological relatives. She had no known romantic partner, close friends, or children of her own. Both she and Brimmer speak of the extent to which Florencia's social world and sense of self were rooted in her identity as Brimmer's caregiver.

While it was not uncommon for middle-class Mexican families to have a household staff, it was highly unusual for a woman of Florencia's class and race to have the kind of narrative authority granted her by *Gaby Brimmer*. Poniatowska's commitment to giving voice to the poor and marginalized had already resulted in such innovative works as *La noche de Tlaltelolco* and *Hasta no verte Jesús mío*.[37] Her leftist politics are evident in the form of *Gaby Brimmer*, where Florencia's opinions are given equal weight; her account of the labor of feeding, clothing, and cleaning Brimmer are an essential aspect of the narrative. As she explains,

> [Gaby] can't do anything without somebody's help. I get her out of bed, I take her to the bathroom, and get her dressed.
>
> I'm always carrying her to do everything.
>
> That's right, today I carried her to get her out of bed, give her a bath, get her into the wheelchair, everything.[38]

In a city where nothing is wheelchair accessible and people with disabilities are not welcome in public, Brimmer's mobility is entirely dependent on Florencia's capacity to push, pull, and lift her chair. Interdependent, they move together at the pace of crip time. When Mattlin and Johnson foreground their dependency by describing the assistance they require to complete a morning routine, they also reinforce the politics of U.S.-style disability rights, which entitle them to an aide working under their direction. Note the difference it makes to hear from Florencia, who emphasizes Brimmer's inabilities and the physical exertion her survival requires of a caregiver. There is no question of Gaby and Florencia's mutual devotion, but Florencia's work is tedious, redundant, physically demanding, and emotionally draining.

Florencia's voice contributes to the portrait of Brimmer, but it also says a great deal about the status of self in a long-term symbiotic relationship. Unlike the assistants who work for Johnson, Mattlin, and Crosby, Florencia has lived with her employers since Gaby was a baby, giving her a hybrid status somewhere between chosen family and employee. Perhaps the closest well-known analogue is the relationship of Helen Keller and Annie Sullivan, her teacher/caregiver/friend, which formed at a time when work was understood very differently than it is today. Neither Sullivan nor her employers could imagine the physical and emotional toll of being the exclusive caregiver for a dependent person, nor of being reliant on the care of a single person, as was Keller. As with Keller and Sullivan, the intimacy of Gaby and Florencia is a source of rage, frustration, and conflict as much as it is a cherished bond.[39] When she speaks, Florencia expresses what Eva Feder Kittay calls the "secondary dependency" of the caregiver whose "energies are channeled into the preservation and fruition of another."[40] As Brimmer's conduit to any form of inclusion in the social world, Florencia also loses bodily autonomy and shares the stigma of disability. The experience of discrimination could be the grounds for solidarity between Gaby and Florencia. Instead, it creates shame that forces them apart. More powerfully than any single-authored memoir, *Gaby Brimmer* provides a vivid illustration of the affective burdens of dependency by putting the voices of the two women into dialogue. Although Brimmer sometimes speaks as an activist who turns experiences of prejudice and exclusion into calls for social justice, sometimes she engages in a mutually detrimental transfer of her own shame onto her caregiver.[41]

The negativity experienced by Gaby and Florencia stems, at least in part, from a failure to recognize care as work. In the unaccommodating environment of midcentury Mexico City, caregiving requires brute strength, immunity to the rudeness of others, and the humility to ask for help. Poniatowska's inclusion of these details is deliberate and political, framing care work as a valuable but limited resource that needs to be adequately compensated and replenished with time for respite. The more recent U.S. American memoirists hire caregivers to work in shifts where they are paid by the hour. What Crosby calls "the cash nexus" allows them to exchange money for services, but it also grants the caregiver status as a worker. By contrast, being a caregiver is not only Florencia's livelihood but a primary source of identity, a situation that creates an undue strain on her and also on the subject of her care. The nontrivial rewards of feeling indispensable cannot suffice for the physical and emotional toll of being the sole provider for a dependent person. Or the knowing recipient of a caregiver's back-breaking labor. Florencia's exhaustion and impatience radiates outward to Brimmer, who is all too aware of the strain her care places on others. "It wasn't just that she was physically exhausted from carrying me around," Brimmer says. "She'd get depressed, and on top of that she had to deal with my mother's depressions and, of course, mine." Brimmer's description captures the contagious nature of depression, an affect that spreads among women worried and isolated by the burdens of care. Without respite, both women recognize that care becomes pathological interdependency in which each party is a liability to the other. "[Florencia] didn't do anything to help me out of my loneliness," Brimmer recalls. "I even got to the point of hating her because of this. I felt like I was too tied to her, and the more I clung, the happier she looked. In me she found a substitute for her life without friends, where her only interest was devoting herself to me and making herself indispensable in my life."[42] In this scenario, interdependency is so thorough that it becomes unhealthy rather than mutually sustaining. Dependent and carer feed off of and reinforce each other's suffering. *Gaby Brimmer* thus shows that even the most capable and selfless of caregivers and the most resilient of dependents are affected by relentless interdependency. Rather than attempting to conceal these more negative feelings, the narrative gives voice to the often grueling physical and psychological work of giving and receiving care.

The story of these three women engaged in a mutually sustaining but exhausting triangulation of care takes a somewhat surprising twist with Brimmer's decision to adopt a child. For a woman with Brimmer's disabilities to choose motherhood is a courageous and groundbreaking act. Her collaboration with Florencia is a model of distributed mothering. Even as the identity of mother is defined by care, it is possible to separate physical from affective labor, apportioning tasks according to each caretaker's abilities. This is a point that women with disabilities who are or want to become mothers are still struggling to make known. But choosing to become a mother is also a sign of Brimmer's privilege. Brimmer's ability to mother is contingent on having Florencia to do the physical work of caring for Brimmer *and* her child. But Gaby and Florencia are not coparents. Florencia is not Alma's mother, even as she engages in mothering activity. Her availability to care for Brimmer and her adopted daughter is contingent on forgoing biological motherhood, care for her family of origin, and activities to nurture and sustain her outside of work. This chapter in Brimmer's story thus draws attention to the creative possibilities of distributed mothering, but also the inequalities whereby one woman's experience of motherhood is subsidized by the curtailed opportunities of another, whether for romance, parenting, or other forms of intimacy (figure 5.3).

By including the voices of Sari and Florencia, *Gaby Brimmer* makes interdependence a primary theme but also a guiding principle of its form. Instead of moving forward, matching the progress of narrative time to that of life's unfolding, it uses different voices to exploit time's multiplicity. It is about women living on crip time, but it also crips the narrative tempo expected of memoir. In this, it moves at the pace of care, even as care is also its theme. As one woman's account echoes, diverges from, or complements another, layers of perception emerge from selves that are simultaneously discrete and interdependent. Sari's voice attests to the unequal distribution of care—meaning not just physical labor but its related worries and management—within the family and society, such that the burdens fall almost entirely on women. Meanwhile, Florencia's voice, often recounting the same events, is a reminder that the autonomy of Brimmer and other middle-class people

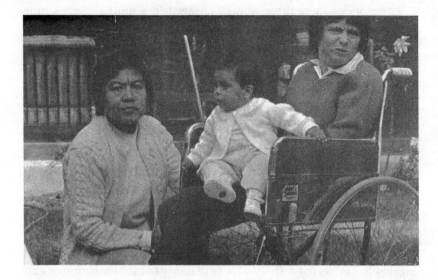

FIGURE 5.3 A family photo showing Florencia Sánchez Morales and Gaby Brimmer, who sits in her wheelchair with baby Alma on her lap, ca. 1978.

Source: Gabriela Brimmer, *Gaby Brimmer: An Autobiography in Three Voices*, © Grijalbo.

with disabilities relies on the work of less privileged supporters whose time and energies are channeled into the flourishing of others. It attests to the fact that, in a society that undervalues the work of caregiving, Florencia becomes as vulnerable and dependent as her charge, sacrificing her own autonomy and well-being to ensure that Brimmer will thrive.

Florencia's story anticipates the growing migration of workers like her across Mexico's northern border. In the late twentieth and twenty-first centuries, many would find jobs as caregivers, and many would sacrifice everything for a chance to mother their own children in the United States, an environment they believed to be safer, richer, and with greater opportunities to flourish. Through its distinctive form, *Gaby Brimmer* affirms sustaining and productive forms of interdependency, the complex personhood of those who are dependent, and the fierce mothering that allows them to thrive. It is also a depiction of the shame, resentment, and animosity that arise when the labor of care is unrecognized and undercompensated and when care giver and recipients are bound in pathological symbiosis.

Interdependency is hard work that takes time and changes over time. The relationship between Brimmer and her collaborator, Elena Poniatowska, was central to the book's design, execution, and promotion. As the guiding presence who elicits and organizes her informants' stories, Poniatowska manages an artful negotiation between their independence and her own authority. The introduction lays out her personal and professional stakes in the project: One reason she was drawn to Brimmer's story was that she had witnessed her nephew Alejandro endure prejudice and exclusion after he was disabled in a car accident. She committed to finish the project even when her friends questioned whether it had any literary merit. Having established her investment in Brimmer's story, Poniatowska vanishes from the narrative proper. Her disappearance might seem disingenuous, since she is so clearly the book's architect. Yet we can also see it as a form of narrative modesty that allows her informants' voices to take center stage. Perhaps this is a model of artful editorial care, one that subordinates the hard work of composition to allow its subjects' autonomy.

In life, Poniatowska was less successful at managing this balance between controlling her subject and granting her autonomy. Her relationship with Brimmer took an inharmonious turn in the years following the publication of *Gaby Brimmer*. Thanks in part to the success of the work that bore her name, Brimmer would publish two books of her own—a chapbook, *Gaby, un año despues* (1981), and a collection of letters, *Cartas de Gaby* (1982)—and become a vocal leader in the movement for disability rights in Mexico and abroad.[43] Poniatowska gave her blessing to her collaborator's newfound independence. But disputes arose when the director Luis Mandoki decided to make a film about Brimmer's life.[44] Initially, Poniatowska declined offers to participate, stating that Brimmer should have opportunities to speak for herself. Once production began, however, Poniatowska complained of not being invited to the set and demanded that her work be mentioned in the credits. Through a lawyer, she argued that film would not have been possible without *Gaby Brimmer*. She asserted that Brimmer was merely the book's coauthor and thus had only partial authority over the use of her story, half of which rightly belonged to Poniatowska.

This conflict revealed the limits of Poniatowska's willingness to grant Brimmer's autonomy or to relinquish ownership of her story. For their part, Mandoki and Brimmer asserted the independence of *Gaby: A True Story* (1987) from Poniatowska's authorial hand. They claimed that the film—which tells a more conventional story of love, loss, and personal growth than Poniatowska's book—is based on Brimmer's own account of her life. Where Poniatowska had devised a life story that deliberately complicates the model of authorial autonomy established by traditional autobiography, Brimmer herself opted for more a traditional generic form. In doing so, she gained authority over her own narrative, but only by subordinating interdependency. These later events are a fitting coda to *Gaby Brimmer* because they attest that even the most artful interdependency evolves over time. Interdependency is a process that requires constant, and often difficult, negotiation.

This chapter has focused on memoir, a genre some have criticized for its preoccupation with the individual, seeing it as the expression of a liberal preference for the independent subject over the collective.[45] In this sense, an autobiography is the very antithesis of interdependency, a form that values individual accomplishment, progress, and overcoming at the expense of entanglement with others. But this is to greatly oversimplify the affordances of the genre we have explored in this chapter. Memoir has proven an elastic form that can do many things, depending on the aims of its teller. Instead of denying entanglements with others, the authors discussed here make the complex negotiation between bodily dependency and a sense of self their subject and, in the most interesting cases, a problem of form. Admittedly, literary memoir is a rarified outlet available to those people with disabilities who not only have access to good care and education but also to avenues for writing and publication. In addition to their accomplishments, it is a welcome development that people with disabilities are now telling their stories in many different media, including film, video, dance, TikTok, social media, blogs, and performance art, which make narrative accessible to a wider range of authors and audiences. But literary memoir may be the best place to document and work through the profound tension of an individual self in interdependency with the care networks that sustain it, all moving at the pace of crip time. And the book is a vehicle that captures the paradox of the lone person's story bound into an artifact that countless people contributed to shaping, producing, and circulating. We should be wary of generalizing too much from any one person's story, and yet, the singularity of each experience attests to a collective insight: How one manages being dependent in a culture that values independence, and successfully and justly coexists with a caregiver must always be specific. The terms of coexistence can never be settled once and for all but require a constant process of negotiation by the parties involved. Recognizing the contradictory status of the self-in-interdependency does not mean letting go of collective struggles to make the world more respectful of dependent people or to compensate their caregivers better, but it does acknowledge that, in addition, there is considerable psychic work that each set of people engaged in a node of interdependencies must imagine anew.

III

PROFESSING CARE

6

THEORY OF MINDS

The Irreconcilable Temporalities of Paying
for Care and Caring for Work

When the journalist Megan Stack became a mother, she left her job as a foreign correspondent to focus on domestic matters. Her subjects were domestic in the most literal sense: Working from home turned her attention to the women she hired to watch her two young children. Unable to make progress on the novel she hoped to write, Stack pivots to journalism, the genre she knows best, to explore and document the lives of women who work as paid caregivers. Accustomed to navigating war-torn landscapes and tense political diplomacy, she finds this investigation frustratingly blocked. Her nannies are reluctant informants, obfuscating her efforts to understand their thoughts and motivations while at work or enter their lives beyond. They simply refuse to make their private time and space fully visible to their employer, even while politely inviting her into their homes and answering her questions. Published in 2019, *Women's Work: A Reckoning with Home and Help* is as much a story of failed collaboration across the gulf of class and culture as it is about the life circumstances and emotional landscapes of childcare workers.[1]

Stack found herself unable to write a novel, but other authors have used fiction to probe the obscure worlds of women who work as caregivers in other people's homes and have few opportunities to tell their own stories. In this chapter, I am interested in literature that seeks to represent what Leila Slimani describes in her novel *The Perfect Nanny* as "the details of a life that will never be recorded."[2] Fiction excels at illustrating, and training the development of, a theory of mind, the ability to explain observable human behavior as an attribute of another person's thoughts and motivations.[3] "As a sustained representation of numerous interacting minds," writes the critic Lisa Zunshine, "the novel, in particular, is implicated in our mind reading ability."[4] It can facilitate recognition, if not understanding, of voices that might otherwise remain unheard. It can also represent the silences and vacancies where marginalized people cannot be, or refuse to be, heard. The outcome of such imagining is ethically complex, sometimes making way for mutual recognition that could be the precursor to more just working conditions and sometimes reinscribing familiar misunderstandings about the nature of domestic care work and the people who do it. The project of imagining the minds of those engaged in a caring relationship that is also a financial transaction is all the more knotty when more than two people are involved. Often care within the home is triangulated by a third party who is responsible for and deeply invested in the well-being of the dependent and also mindful of a household budget. Multiple selves entangle in a caring exchange that is also a job.

What Christina Crosby calls the "cash nexus" where dependents, care workers, and those who employ them (the latter two almost always women) meet is the starting point for this chapter.[5] As we will see, the intimate and necessary tenor of the work can create powerful affective bonds among dependents and paid caregivers in excess of their financial obligations. The affective nature of care, especially in a domestic setting, often means that terms of employment are arranged informally among women who may see themselves as partners, confidants, or allies, as well as employer and employee.[6] But their self-understandings don't always align: I may see you as a confidante, while you see listening as an obligation, adopting a demeanor of attentiveness as you also watch my child or wash the dishes. Such circumstances can pit the needs of vulnerable groups against one another, while obscuring the connections between care work and those more public-facing, economically productive workers who are its beneficiaries.[7] Narrative cannot resolve those questions at the level of policy, but it can help us understand the unique nature of paid domestic care work and the profound ambivalence underpinning the triangulated relationship among caregivers, the recipients of care, and the third parties responsible for a dependent's well-being. At its most hopeful, it represents artful caregiving, making apparent through stories those priceless connections among givers and receivers that are often unseen or unacknowledged by outsiders. At its worst, we see the psychic and sometimes physical violence that results from being forced to care.

This chapter is a departure from earlier chapters in its attention to the "money" in my book's title: care exchanged for cash. It emphasizes the kinds of transactions that are almost always informal, and almost always involve a third party who is responsible for the care recipient and for paying the care provider. After considering a number of documentary sources, I decided to focus exclusively on fiction because of its unique capacity to portray multiple points of view. I was less interested in hearing one side of the story or another than in a theory of minds, the dense, invisible, and deeply meaningful webs of affect that undergird the repetitive daily routines of dependency work and the efforts of participants to probe the thoughts and feelings of others in a shared space. This chapter begins by looking at childcare and the triangulated relations among mothers, nannies, and their charges in three novels: *The Perfect Nanny* by Leila Slimani, *My Hollywood* by Mona Simpson, and *Lucy* by Jamaica Kincaid. It then turns to representations of care for dependent adults in Lila Savage's novel *Say Say Say* and Rebecca Brown's *Gifts of the Body*. While it might seem perverse to lump together childcare and the care of adults with illness or disability-related dependencies, doing so reveals unexpected commonalities between these forms of dependency and the work they require of others. Both are intimately connected with the problems of time and care we have been following throughout this book. When care work is paid, the time of the clock is measured against the needs of a worker, a dependent, and, in some cases, their guardian. Where the clock imposes a consistent standard for measuring time, the parties involved in a caring relationship are likely to perceive and value the passage of time very differently according to standpoint. Behind the walls of home, domestic dramas play out among caregivers who turn time into money, the people who pay them, and the needs of a dependent person.

The narratives I consider engage the fraught seams where the temporalities of care, need, and cash unevenly align: the tension between paying someone according to hours worked when the work she does seems impossible to quantify in terms of time, the porous boundaries dividing the time of work from its Other, the varied ways "time off" matters to the exchange of care, and the uneven fit between the duration of a given dependency and an employee's need for a job. While each fictional work has a different emphasis, all probe the interiority of women's minds and private time that proved inaccessible to Stack's investigative journalism, and, even more importantly, they use creative forms to portray relatedness among dependents, employers, and paid care workers. In what follows, we will see a range of fictional strategies for representing individual subjectivity, as well as moving beyond it to portray the affects that radiate among those engaged in giving, receiving, and managing care. Narrative helps us see the value of the work and the complex personhood of those who do it, but it also shows why the particular problems that care presents are so tenacious. As we follow the webs of care outward from the family, our perspective on the forms of class, gender, and regional inequality that subtend them expands proportionately, and we will see the direct exchange of cash for care as a disruptive undercurrent in even the most artful interdependency. Its unseemly presence is also a prompt to reflect on those aspects of care that have no price, as well as what it would mean to justly compensate those who provide it.

NOT LIKE ONE OF THE FAMILY

Like One of the Family is the title story of Alice Childress's collection of vignettes told in the voice of a sassy, worn-out domestic worker. It aptly captures the contradictions, sometimes veering into hypocrisy, of employment situations that claim to value a worker as much as a family member, meaning they are compensated with gratitude and affection rather than a living wage.[8] Taking Childress's lead, I consider paid home care as a historical and cultural phenomenon before turning to the differences between childcare and care for an adult dependent. The forms of paid care work that are our subject emerged in the twentieth century, as families began to have fewer children and employ fewer, if any, live-in domestic servants.[9] Later in the century, rising numbers of women working outside their own homes created the need for paid help to care for their dependents, whether those were children, aging parents, or other family members.[10] The domestic care industry continues to expand, one of the few sectors with a consistently rising demand for workers. A 2018 report estimates the proportion of caregivers in the global workforce at 11.5 percent. It finds 19.5 percent of working women are employed in domestic labor, which accounts for 2.5 percent of all jobs around the world.[11] As the numbers suggest, the majority of domestic care workers are women, whose duties may be shared with a household's unpaid family and friends and who often care for families of their own. This work is considered unskilled and compensated accordingly, typically through informal arrangements that provide none of the benefits or protections afforded in recognized places of work. Paid care is rarely understood as productive, even as it subsidizes activities that are valued as work because they contribute to economic growth. And it is virtually never described as an art, although it requires a combination of talent, creativity, and skill we associate with aesthetic acts.

Care is a special kind of work because it involves the sustained and sometimes genuine production of affect. Paid caregivers often care *about* those who depend on their labor for comfort, safety, and survival.[12] They are also likely to develop close relationships with their employers, who may or may not be the recipients of their care. When they work in a home, they also become familiar with other people's intimate spaces, stuff, and habits. Paid home care falls into the category of work Arlie Roth Hochschild calls "emotional labor," meaning that it requires the performance of affects like friendliness, cheer, or concern.[13] Some jobs in Hochschild's account require a time-limited expression of affect. The emotional labor required of home care workers (who fall into the category Hochschild calls "marketized domesticity") is much more sustained. Over time, the performance of affect may grow into a genuinely felt attachment. Sometimes, the evident vulnerability of a dependent elicits caring feelings, and not just their performance, from the start. Care for a baby or a frail elderly person might be extended with more affective sincerity than the solicitude offered, say, to a business person traveling in first class. Physical gestures of maintenance that are offered to a dependent with gentleness, affection, and generosity are likely to generate responses of gratitude, kindness, and affection in kind, creating a feedback loop of positive affect. Unlike the time-bound work of a server, flight attendant, bank teller, or manicurist, the affective currents of home care do not easily align with the clock time that regulates the exchange of caring activities for a salary. The timing of a dependent's call for comfort, help with toileting, or pain management might not coincide with the caregiver's scheduled shift, but she is unlikely to turn away from a vulnerable person in need.

The affective tenor of care is one of many reasons domestic workers have required different organizational strategies than most other workers.[14] Although they constitute a significant proportion of the workforce, they have been left out of most major labor legislation over the past century. Caregivers tend to work in isolation, making it difficult to build alliances of the kind that have enabled other workers to organize. In the United States, domestic workers, along with agricultural laborers, were excluded from the 1935 Wagner Act, which protects the rights of workers to unionize, as well as the Fair Labor Standards Act of 1940, which provided such benefits as old age insurance, unemployment, minimum wage, and a cap on hours worked.[15] When it was amended in 1974, an exception called the "companionship rule" continued to exclude jobs like babysitter or companion to the elderly and disabled from federal minimum wage or overtime pay requirements. The overtime exclusion continues to extend to those who provide "fellowship and protection for an elderly person or a person with an illness, injury, or disability who requires assistance in caring for himself or herself" and are employed directly by a client or their family.[16] The 1970

Occupational Safety and Health Act also excluded those working in private homes.[17] Thus, paid home caregivers labor with few of the benefits or protections that have been secured for other workers.[18]

Home care workers have been seen as the next frontier for the SEIU (Service Employees International Union), and efforts to organize have met with some limited success. In 2007, the same year that the Supreme Court excluded companions from overtime pay, the National Domestic Workers Alliance formed in an effort to secure full access to the rights accorded to other workers. Yet despite such progress, new organizational efforts and the regulations they secure will bypass many home care workers because they are so often paid under the table, at the behest of employees as well as employers. Embedded in the private space of somebody's home, approximately 80 percent of paid domestic care arrangements are informal, meaning that employers do not contribute to any kind of social security nor are they subject to legal requirements for overtime pay, vacation, and sick leaves.[19] The improvisational nature of these transactions, combined with the domestic setting and affective tenor of relationships, further contributes to the muddy terrain of such work. This is where narrative steps in, giving voice to those aspects of care that cannot be organized or regulated, that reside less within an individual than in the ambiance generated among participants in an exchange, but are nonetheless crucial to identify if we are ever going to adequately value care as work. Although each care exchange is unique, there are categorical differences between caring for a child, whose dependency is an ordinary developmental stage experienced by all human animals, and a dependent adult. These differences matter enough to divide these two kinds of care into separate sections.

NATIONS OF NANNIES: CHILDREN, HOME, AND PAID CARE

Children are the crux of our most hopeful narratives about care. As we saw in the first chapter, those narratives also implicate mothers, holding them responsible for ensuring a child meets their full potential.

When unable to provide their children with constant care, mothers become managers of other, less-privileged women, who are sometimes also mothers working to support themselves and their dependents. Such strained but necessary interdependencies are informed by race and the legacy of colonialism that separates women who have resources to pay for childcare from those who provide it, a theme often brought into the foreground in recent narratives about nannies. Another notable feature of these works—as opposed to almost any others in this book—is that they have relatively little to say about the dependent child (or children) at the crux of a caring network. The child tends to be bland and uncomplicated, a minor character whose needs and desires are easy enough to address, while serving as the locus for the nuanced, deeply ambivalent, and emotionally complex dynamic between mothers and paid caregivers. And where are men in all of this? Most of the families represented in these narratives include a male parent. But even when sensitive and involved, he is virtually immune to the affective tensions between mother to paid caregiver. Men pay the bills, participate in family life, and sometimes stray into infidelity. But gender somehow inures them from the longings, anxieties, and guilt borne by female counterparts who manage and provide care for their children. I don't say this to let men off the hook. Their capacity to absent themselves from the affective slurry of paid childcare is a glaring problem, one I continue to dispute with my own very kind, very caring husband and coparent.

In my family, I am the working parent who does the hidden administrative labor of finding, arranging, and paying for childcare. I am also the parent who *feels* intensely the uneasy mix of gratitude and anxiety about the women (and very occasionally men, usually actors, usually queer) who care for my children. My most prolonged and intense relationship is with Angela, who has cared for my two sons since babyhood. She is ten years older than me, with a husband, children, and grandchildren of her own. I know she arrived in the United States from the Dominican Republic as a teenager, but I don't know exactly how much education she received except that she didn't graduate from high school and struggles to read and write fluently, especially in English.

She is also a brilliant caregiver with bottomless reserves of patience and affection. When we first met and I asked her why she wanted a job caring for my son, she said simply, "I love babies." She has never been big on verbal language, but her body, tone, and gestures speak volumes. She seems to find the company of young children utterly absorbing, without needing the distraction of a screen or an adult companion that many other caregivers require to stave off numbing boredom.

I love Angela deeply, but we are not friends, and even after all these years, we are not comfortable around each other. I imagine the work that I do and many of my parenting choices make little sense to her, while aspects of her personality and interests remain opaque to me. Mostly we enjoy a productive coexistence triangulated by our shared commitment to caring for my children. Henry is the target of her affection and interest, and I am just a necessary conduit to his attentions. When I first met Angela, I thought about Doris Sommer's *Proceed with Caution, when Engaged by Minority Writing in the Americas*, which I had read some years before.[20] I remembered finding Sommer's thesis— that some writers, particularly from marginalized groups, deliberately obfuscate and block their readers' understanding rather than trying to facilitate it—surprising and persuasive. It opened my eyes to all the ways a literary work can resist a reader's probing, drawing attention to, without satisfying, her attempts at more intimate knowledge. I have come to a similar understanding about Angela, who discloses to me on a need-to-know basis. When I greet her with rote politeness by asking how she is doing, she says she is "good" and then tells me what matters: She isn't feeling well, has an appointment, or needs to leave early for her granddaughter's birthday party. Instead of asking how I'm doing, she asks, "How is Henry today?" He is the overlap in the improbable Venn diagram that causes our lives to intersect.

The ambivalence between Angela and I has no effect on her relationship with Henry. I know her love for him is deep and genuine, and she is his favorite person in all the world. At some point my older son and most of Angela's other charges outgrow her, rejecting her gentle motherly companionship for rougher play with friends. But Henry's attachment continues in his teenage years. Unlike those other children, who will likely forget Angela as they mature, Henry does not seem to grow apart from her, and I imagine a lifelong relationship, changing over time along with their needs. Their special interdependency is real; once in a while I catch sight of them on the street or come into the apartment quietly and overhear their banter. Other people sense it and tell me how the sight of this odd couple, Henry and Angela together, radiates intimacy and comfort in each other. Neither is very good with words. Both excel at deliberate and strategic unknowing. They understand each other.

None of this affective grout obviates the fact that I pay Angela and that she relies on and expects payment for the time she spends with Henry. I believe I compensate her generously, showing appreciation in cash, as well as felt gratitude. Still, her evident affection for Henry and the pleasure she clearly takes in being with him make it easy to forget that I am also paying her for that time. Once she called after leaving on a Friday to tell me that I had undercalculated her pay for the week. I was mortified, apologized profusely, and arranged to get her the money. But I also felt a jolt at being reminded that, in addition to the genuine feelings she has for Henry, caring for him is also work. Her time must be properly compensated. That arrangement extended through the pandemic era, when we paid her to stay at home. As I wrote about care work, I also recognized the effort involved in not working, and knew that time had to be paid for even with the world on pause. The uneasy mix of care with work, the seemingly impossible reconciliation of affect with paid time, and the strained relationships that often triangulate the exchange of money for care are central concerns of this chapter.

My experience of Angela's withholding is partly a facet of our particular relationship, but it is also a structural phenomenon arising from disparities in opportunity and social status between childcare workers and their employers. Nannies and nurses are often written about, but they have far less access to self-representation than those who hire them. I don't think Angela will ever write a memoir. When my older son, Noah—whom she has known since he was born—tried to interview her for a Spanish project in school, she eagerly agreed but then offered only the most minimal answers to his questions.

Fiction grants access to the lives of others, and the history of Western literature includes such memorable caregivers as the servant Eurycleia in Homer's *The Odyssey*; the eponymous Jane Eyre; and the housekeeper, Dilsey, in William Faulkner's *The Sound and the Fury*. In the twenty-first century, the bestselling novel and film *The Nanny Diaries* (and its less well-known counterpart about a Jamaican immigrant protagonist, *Minding Ben*) captivated audiences by taking the nanny's point of view to expose the bad parenting of wealthy elites.[21] These works entertain with an underlayer of social criticism aimed at cartoonishly awful mothers and, sometimes, the rich more generally. But satire is not well suited for representing care with any nuance. Exploitation and abuse of domestic workers are real problems that demand our attention. But the way these novelists portray care work obscures the complex affective terrain that can radiate between a nanny and the woman who employs her, even under the best working conditions. To learn something about care, we need stories less invested in moral dichotomies, moving away from extreme cases to those where the competing needs and interests of women who triangulate the paid care of a child remain unresolved.

Care is often described as a relation between two parties, but it usually involves more, especially when it centers on a dependent child. Fiction can enter the subjectivity of women engaged in care to explore the affective and material circumstances that sometimes occasion, but more often obstruct, a shared dedication to the child's nurture and future development and the well-being of all involved. Picking up where the previous chapter ended—with the tripartite dialogue of Gaby, Sari, and Florencia—I am particularly concerned with works that show relatedness, offering a theory of minds that toggles among the perspectives of women from very different social and economic backgrounds. Uneasy collaborators, sometimes they manage and sometimes they fail to resolve irreconcilable conflicts among the needs of the three parties in a caring triangle. In the narratives I consider here, relationships among women in the present are informed by the history of colonialism and racial capitalism that turned some countries into "nation(s) of nannies" (in the words of Mona Simpson's Filipina protagonist) to be employed as care workers by women in more affluent regions of the world.[22] I turn first to two novels—Simpson's *My Hollywood* (2010) and Slimani's *The Perfect Nanny* (2016)—that use the conventions of genre fiction to bring imagined resolution to those conflicts, the plots wending toward opposite poles of comedy and horror. The third, Kincaid's *Lucy* (1990), refuses these more generic options, instead staying with the discomfort and irresolution that the novel summons up in its account of the relationship between a teenaged au pair from the Caribbean and the affluent U.S.-American mother who employs her.[23]

My Hollywood is the right title for Mona Simpson's novel, which brings picture-perfect closure to the seemingly irresolvable dilemmas of paid domestic childcare it introduces. It could be set nowhere other than Los Angeles, moving between the posh neighborhoods that house the most successful culture workers and underserved areas where migrant women live crowded together. The book's chapters are alternately narrated by Claire, a new mother and professional composer, and Lola, caregiver for Claire's son and mother of five, who supports her family in the Philippines with remittances from her weekly pay. Simpson's characters are not villains or heroes; instead the novel grants each woman the emotional complexity of realist fiction. Claire is a classic professional mother, desperate for time to herself, but anxious that her creative work is not lucrative enough to merit it and guilty about paying another woman to care for her baby. Perhaps it should go without saying that the man who is Claire's husband and William's father does not share her angst about the value of his work or the well-being of their child while in another woman's care.

Claire is a familiar character; what makes her story interesting is its juxtaposition with Lola's. In chapters that alternate between the two women, we learn how Lola thinks of her employers, her genuine affection for her charge, "Williamo," and the life she left behind. Lola's chapters also follow her into the diasporic community where she spends her time off. In giving equal time to Lola's world and making her a dynamic, fully rounded character, the novel attempts to rectify the epistemic asymmetry built into a relationship where the nanny has intimate knowledge of her employer's home and private life while her own life remains opaque. So too, by embedding Lola in a community, it fills out the story of one relationship with the compound portrait of a cohort of migrant care workers. All of these women have chosen to leave their families in the Philippines, caring for them from afar by earning money through caring for others. This investment pays off only for some. Lola's story of nearly unmitigated success is complicated by examples of other women migrants who fail or come to harm.

Having given each narrator an inner life and exposed the uneasy seam where they meet, My Hollywood creates a problem, then smoothes it over with an implausibly happy resolution. First, Claire fires Lola, having decided a nanny can no longer meet her son's developmental needs. This gesture instantly transforms a relationship built on mutual affection, respect, and exigency to one that is about an employer's power over her employee. However difficult it is for Claire to let Lola go, the transition is far more materially and emotionally consequential for Lola. Whatever affection she feels for her charge, her work is still precarious and contingent on informal, private arrangements. Insecurity is baked into the job itself, a problem the beloved fictional nanny Mary Poppins solves by simply vanishing when she is no longer needed. Lola signals her distance from this fantasy when she says, "Disney did not draw me. And I refuse to dissolve into sky."[24] Instead of allowing Lola to vanish when Williamo goes to preschool, My Hollywood stays true to Lola's promise by pursuing her into a new job and, eventually, return to her country of origin.

Expanding its terrain beyond Southern California, the novel accompanies Lola on her homecoming and reunion with her family in Tagaytay. The Philippines, a place imagined by the novel's affluent white characters as "a nation of nannies," is given reality as a geographic locale embedded in the history of American colonialism. This part of the novel has a clear political design aimed at illustrating the personhood and agency of diasporic women. In her nonfiction writing, Simpson cautions against seeing migrant care workers as victims. Where a privileged Western audience might be tempted to pity, Simpson asserts the volition of women who deliberately choose to seek work abroad, benefiting themselves and their families.[25] Her Lola, like other nannies she knew or interviewed for her research on the book, finds dignity in her work, enjoys the comforts of living in the United States, and appreciates the earnings that support her family of origin. She is a woman with purpose and autonomy, the primary wage earner for a household, and a leader within her diasporic community.

In Simpson's portrayal, the relationship between a nanny and her employer has the potential to be mutually beneficial. The history of colonial injustice that creates inequalities of status and opportunity can be redressed by individual mothers who treat their nannies with respect and compensate them fairly. Simpson's novel also resists the idea that care is, by definition, compromised by the exchange of cash. Lola loves her work and she loves making money. It turns out that even when she can afford to retire, she would prefer to be working as a caregiver. Having relocated to the Philippines, Lola soon feels bored and useless. She longs to be needed, and her desire is satisfied because as soon as she leaves her former employers discover she is indispensable! Claire travels to the Philippines to beg for Lola's return. This implausible discovery of mutual necessity allows employers and employees to reconfigure their relationship in a way that is beneficial to all.

My Hollywood's vision of domestic care work is not entirely rosy. Lola is embedded in a community of migrant women, many of whom are less fortunate or canny than she. Their unhappy trajectories also belong to the story of global care chains that serve the needs of more affluent Western families. Still, Simpson gives her an ending worthy of Hollywood's most famous industry. Later, she would echo that penchant for happy endings in a *New York Times* essay on migrant childcare workers. "I attended a wedding a few years ago," she wrote in the last paragraph. "The nanny who stayed with the family for years stood next to the two parents (by then long divorced) for the marriage of the girl they had all raised."[26] In this pleasing image, biological family is broken and remade around practices of distributed care. The wedding is an occasion to celebrate the collaborative effort involved in raising a child, even as it marks the initiation of a new generation into the gendered burdens of marriage. But I stumble over the description of the nanny who "stayed with the family." The time, the questions about membership and obligation evoked by "the family," and the ambiguous agency of staying speak to complexities unresolved by this simple phrase. Like other Hollywood-happy endings, it seems too good to be true. I turn now to an equally extreme alternative, a vision of how the unresolved contradictions of paid childcare can culminate in horror rather than comedy.

The horrific crime related by Leila Slimani's bestselling French novel, *The Perfect Nanny*, is the merger of two notorious real-life cases where children were murdered by the women charged to care for them.[27] There is no suspense about how this story will end. Where Simpson's novel follows a forward chronology, Slimani is proleptic, beginning with the sentence "The baby is dead." A sibling was found alive but succumbed soon after. The eponymous nanny survives her self-inflicted wounds, although her testimony confounds the detective who attempts to plumb "her rotting soul" and is unable to explain her motivations.[28] Where a rotting soul suggests individual corruption, Slimani's novel embeds the nanny's crime in a corrupt social context. It does not justify her actions, but it exposes the irresolvable contradictions more successfully repressed by other care workers and the women who employ them. While a reader might put down Simpson's novel feeling better about hiring other women to care for her child, she is likely to feel deep discomfort after reading Slimani's.

Beginning with an atrocious crime, *The Perfect Nanny* circles back to a familiar origin story of maternal discontent, hired help, and the seemingly ideal relationship that developed among working parents, their two young children, and a paid caregiver. Like Simpson, Slimani shifts between the perspective of the nanny and that of her employers, recounting a widening gulf of misrecognition that preceded the crime. Nobody in this novel is very good at theory of mind; their failures form the backbone of its tragic story. From the employers' perspective, all is well. Paul and Myriam are an affluent Parisian couple who begin their journey into parenting with the plan that Paul will continue to work outside the home, while Myriam will take time off to care for their young children. Myriam soon grows unsatisfied with this arrangement, and they hire a nanny. Like Simpson's characters, Myriam and

Paul are decent people, doting parents, and generous employers. They also have the good fortune to find Louise, a nanny who is the envy of their social circle for the loving, attentive care she provides their children, all while keeping their home neat and well stocked.

Like others in their situation, Myriam and Paul's professional success is enabled by forgetting about the work taking place at home and deliberately not knowing about how Louise spends her time off the clock. Perhaps their ignorance about her living situation or state of mind shows respect for her privacy but also, perhaps, a disinclination to probe the circumstances that leave their nanny so eager for their children's company and affection. Only when they catch sight of Louise unexpectedly—while driving through an unfamiliar neighborhood—does Myriam realize how little she knows about her nanny. It is an employer's privilege not to imagine her employee's private life, save a vague wish that it would be restful, replenishing Louise's energy to care for their family. Ideally—as I believe, I hope, accurately, is the case with Angela—the nanny would like it that way and, as long as she does her job well, be entitled to that privacy. But if a worker's ability to care is compromised by circumstances outside of the workplace, the dynamic of unknowing becomes much more complicated.

The Perfect Nanny pierces the employer's deliberate forgetting by showing "everything Louise is when she is not with them."[29] An ironic seam opens between the revelations made available to the reader and Paul's and Miriam's unknowingness. Louise may be the perfect nanny, but she also lives in a squalid apartment where she is behind on her rent, harassed by the landlord, and contending with mounting debts left by her dead husband. To her employers' children she is an energetic and doting caregiver, but she is estranged from her own teenaged daughter. Instead of finding time off restorative, Louise is impatient to escape from her troubles by returning to the comfortable and orderly world of her charges. But these boundaries are hard to maintain, and her own unmet needs seep into the relationship to her employers' family. Instead of neglecting her job, she takes it to excess, consumed by desire to be indispensable. When her efforts to nudge Paul and Myriam to have a third child are unsuccessful (she is no better a mind reader than they are), murdering her charges is a desperate effort to ensure they will never grow apart from her. Her ghastly crime indeed makes her unforgettable. It permanently arrests the children's development before it is possible for them to move beyond or forget the caregiver they once depended on.

The Perfect Nanny represents Louise's crime as the act of a pathological individual. But it also shows that this one "rotting soul" is embedded in the deeply contradictory social logic and history of paid care work. In the margins of Slimani's story of a single family we find unsubtle vestiges of a colonial past that destined some women to be caregivers and others their employers. Where Simpson takes U.S. imperial relations with the Philippines as a backdrop, Slimani obliquely engages the colonial history of French Morocco. Slimani herself is Franco-Moroccan and worked as a foreign correspondent during the 2011 Arab Spring in Tunisia, where she witnessed mass dissent against political corruption and economic inequality.[30] Her fictional counterpart is the working mother Myriam, rather than her nanny. Louise's whiteness sets her apart from the other nannies. She witnesses, without fully belonging to, the ad hoc global community these caregivers form in the park where their charges go to play. "Around the slide and the sandpit [Louise] hears snatches of Baoule, Dyula, Arabic and Hindi, sweet nothings whispered in Filipino or Russian." These voices form a global chorus of "languages from all over the world." They "contaminate the babbling of the children, who learn odd words and repeat them to their enchanted parents." The description of their language as a contaminant suggests Louise's reserved, disapproving view of peers, however enchanted their employers might be. These women, who have fled poverty and oppression, taking traditions of care with them, transmit the history of European colonialism in the words of endearment and delicious foods they prepare for their employers' families. The children—who "all look alike, often wearing the same clothes bought in the same shops"—eagerly assimilate the tidbits of cultural Otherness offered by their caregivers, only to lose them with time and maturity.[31]

Like so many childcare workers, it is the nannies' fate to be forgotten by the children they nurtured to independence. Many of these migrant women endure a worse possibility, of also being forgotten by the bio-logical children they left behind in their countries of origin. Mean-while, they do not have the luxury of forgetting. Most carry memories of past violence and hardship that drove them to seek work abroad, although their talk focuses on easier topics like entertaining their charges and the strange habits of their employers. Most work under precarious conditions, since the care they provide a developing child will eventually render their job obsolete. Even while harboring resent-ments and sometimes scorn for the parents who employ them, they shower the children they care for with love and affection. They know the intimate details of their employers' lives, even as their own lives remain unknown. And these nannies will remember the children they nurtured even as they are destined to be forgotten. Louise differs from the other nannies in being consumed by the contradictions of her labor that other women more successfully repress. Slimani makes the weighty conditions of their lives visible in the background of her novel, even as she focuses on the exceedingly rare incident where a care worker snaps under the pressure.

Does that exposure have consequences, beyond making the reader uncomfortable? I once met one of the real mothers whose horrific experience is a basis for Slimani's fiction. I learned who she was only after our very pleasant and mundane conversation in the kitchen of somebody else's apartment during a party. It is hard to describe the mix of shock and compassion and revulsion I felt on learning whom I had been chatting with. Later, I hugged my children a little bit longer, until they squirmed out of reach. I told Angela, one more time, how much I appreciate her. Did that awareness of my own good fortune, and its proximity to the tragedies of others, change the world? It did not. But I am writing about it here, believing that perhaps the accu-mulated weight of such stories and their circulation brings us to a better and more just appreciation of the value of good care. Beyond the shock value of her subject, I think Slimani shares such motivations.

One of the challenges of a narrative centered on childcare is that it is most effective when very little is happening. Children thrive on the mundane and repetitive, when environments are small and consistent, one day very similar to the next. Slimani and Simpson manage that challenge by adopting the modes of comedy and horror, emphasizing plot over inner subjectivity and focusing on protagonists who are exceptional rather than ordinary. Jamaica Kincaid's 1990 novel, *Lucy*, is a precursor to these twenty-first-century works that contends with the seemingly humdrum activities of its protagonist by building them into its form. Instead of outward-facing drama, it adopts a more modernist focus on interiority, relocating the primary site of conflict to the domain of thought, feeling, and affect. Narrated in first person by the eponymous protagonist, it tells the story of a teenage au pair from the Caribbean during the year she spends working for an affluent U.S.-American family. Unlike Simpson and Slimani, Kincaid makes no attempt to create an equitable narrative space by entering the subjectivity of the American characters, who remain opaque to the reader as well as her protagonist. Readers see that Lucy spends relatively little time thinking about the children she cares for. She is far more preoccupied with their mother, Mariah, a decent, loving, and oblivious woman who triggers Lucy to remember her own experiences of being mothered, as well as the many ways her mother's care fell short, merging into neglect and harm. Kincaid renders Lucy's interior consciousness far more vivid than any interactions taking place in the external world, making her subjectivity the narrative center, rather than that of the woman who employs her.

Kincaid embeds her story of paid care work in the history of empire, anticipating the patterns of migration that would later concern Simpson and Slimani. Critics who have written about this aspect of the novel often focus on a scene where Lucy first sees daffodils. Mariah loves the flowers and wants to share their beauty with Lucy as a way of introducing her to a new world. But Lucy, whose previous knowledge of daffodils came only from a Wordsworth poem she was forced to recite in school, cannot share Mariah's joy. A symbol of the gulf that divides the two women, the flowers fill Lucy with rage and bitterness, and summon up "a scene of conquered and conquests; a scene of brutes masquerading as angels and angels portrayed as brutes."[32] Where critics have noted the daffodils' obvious association with colonial education, I am interested how colonialism shapes aesthetic sensibility.[33] As we will see, the history of empire informs not only each woman's capacity to feel that something is beautiful, but also whether and how she feels care and how it infuses her caregiving activities.

In this passage, the word "love" is repeated three times in the space of a few sentences. A vague and loaded term, it describes the affective bond between the two women but also the very different feeling evoked in each. Mariah is the beneficiary of empire, its privileges imbuing her with an uncomplicated willingness to give and receive love, a word she uses often and unproblematically in reference to her children, her husband, and Lucy. Much as the daffodils displease her, Lucy has the emotional intelligence to develop a theory of mind, understanding that they represent an expression of love on Mariah's part, a well-meaning effort to share her experience. "This woman who hardly knew me loved me," Lucy acknowledges, "and she wanted me to love this thing—a grove brimming over with daffodils in bloom—that she loved also." Mariah's desire for Lucy to feel as she does, and Lucy's inability to do so, brings the two women to an affective impasse. When Mariah reaches out to hug her, Lucy resists, refusing to complete the gesture of care or to separate the aesthetic experience of the flowers from the politics of conquest. And although Lucy feels something for Mariah that she also calls "love," her version is shot through with animosity. Her mixed feelings about love are rooted in childhood experience that led her to perceive her own mother's love as a "burden," since it came with the expectation that Lucy, by virtue of gender, would follow in her footsteps, becoming a harsh, self-sacrificing, upright woman worn out by caring for others.[34] Kincaid imbues love with these varied meanings, while suggesting that all are genuinely felt. Where love becomes coercive is when one person attempts to force another to share her aesthetic experience or devalues the perceptions and feelings of another. The different connotations evoked by the same word help explain the distance between these women. Writ large, such different emotional valences also inform how Lucy and Mariah approach the shared work of caregiving, sometimes functioning as collaborators and sometimes—at least in Lucy's perception—as antagonists or competitors.

This complicated relationship between the caregiver and her employer is far more important to Kincaid's novel than the dependent children who receive their care. Lucy expends almost no mental energy on the children or the work required to maintain them, except to note her particular affection for the youngest child, Miriam. When Lucy describes her feelings for Miriam as "love," she means something far more effortless and instinctual than her feelings for Mariah or her own mother. "I loved Miriam from the moment I met her," she explains. "She was the first person I had loved in a very long while, and I did not know why. I loved the way she smelled, and I used to sit her on my lap with my head bent over her and breathe her in." Although Lucy claims not to know why she loves Miriam, the child's unabashed dependency and her willing uptake of Lucy's care seem likely contributors. And Lucy responds in kind, her love underlying caring activities like getting up in the night when Miriam has a bad dream, coaxing her to eat, and carrying her on their trek to the lake. Seeing Miriam as a double for her younger self enables Lucy to imagine the child's needs, taking a better version of her own mother as a model: "I treated her the way I remembered my mother treating me then."[35] Caring for Miriam is a way for Lucy to mother herself and to recapture more positive memories of being mothered.

While all human animals had to receive some mothering, its extent and quality can vary dramatically, and Lucy's strict, withholding mother left her with a deficit. She arrives in the United States as a teenager pushed to early independence, with her own talents and aspirations for the future still to be explored. Even as she cares for Mariah's children, Lucy is undergoing her own youthful coming of age, creating tension between her job, which requires her to subordinate her needs to those of her charges or her employers, and her desire for self-development. Ultimately, she makes the bold and reckless decision to prioritize herself over care of or about others. This is a radical place for *Lucy* to end, but not a happy one. Raised on the weighty expectation that women are born to care for others, Lucy wants to be "alone in the world." But she finds her solitary life sometimes small and melancholy, and she longs for Mariah's seemingly infinite capacity to care for others. An astute mind reader, she recognizes that other people have feelings that are inaccessible to her. "I wish I could love someone so much that I would die from it," she laments in the novel's last paragraph, before bursting into tears.[36] In my reading, Lucy's cries express the irresolvable contradiction between desire to care for herself and the expectation that she will sacrifice herself to the care of others. Where women like Mariah can give with seeming abandon because they have had so much, Lucy's upbringing and temperament provide no such resources. Being "alone in the world" is different from being independent, since Kincaid recognizes the fact of human interdependency, the tragic, difficult, and sometimes rewarding need for support from others. Choosing to be alone is an especially hard path for women who are positioned as caregivers by history and society. Lucy's story thus ends not with triumph but with struggle, as she confronts the incredible difficulty of resisting the obligations of care and the vacuum left by their absence.

Lucy does not quit because she is dissatisfied with a particular job but rather with the idea that she is destined for a lifetime of care work. Having been steered toward a career in nursing, Lucy resists, imagining a future self who is "a badly paid person, a person who was forced to be in awe of someone above her (a doctor), a person with cold and rough hands, a person who lived alone and ate badly boiled food because she could not afford a cook."[37] She objects to the low pay, lack of respect, and humble circumstances this kind of work affords, regardless of whom she is caring for. When Lucy envisions her superior as "a doctor," she helps make this chapter's transition from the care of children to the care of the ill and dying, from a population whose dependency is appealing and optimistic, to one that is burdensome and unwelcome. What might seem like a perverse pairing of dependency at its most hopeful and most unwanted extremes makes more sense when seen from the perspective of the care worker and the precarious circumstances of her employment. These continuities make it possible for Lucy to reject, in one fell swoop, her work as an au pair and her future in nursing, and they also explain why Lola, in Mona Simpson's happier version of the nanny's story, can easily segue from caring for a child to caring for a grandmother with dementia. It is to home care at this opposite pole that we turn in the final section of this chapter.

PASSING TIME: DEPENDENT ADULTS, HOME, AND PAID CARE

As with Kincaid's *Lucy*, the inner life of a home care worker is the primary subject of Lila Savage's 2019 novel, *Say Say Say*, although in this case the dependent client is a woman with dementia.[38] Reading these works together illuminates common threads in the experience of a home caregiver, a job that involves being present as much as it does a proscribed set of tasks, and whose duration is contingent on the development (whether growth or decline) of the recipient of her care. Savage's protagonist is Ella, a hired caregiver for Jill, a woman with dementia resulting from a traumatic brain injury. The plot is minimal, unfolding mostly while Ella is in the home Jill shares with her husband, Bryn. Unlike Lucy, she is in a stable relationship with her female partner, Alix, at a life plateau where she is neither coming of age nor undergoing any other meaningful transition. Ella's work days are very similar, and her tasks are narrow: to keep Jill safe and relatively clean, while giving Bryn a break from her care. The novel's primary subject is thus the vivid interiority of a care worker and her subjective relations to the dependent she cares for, her employer, and others in their small social world.

How to care for a person who is both unwilling and unknowable? Ruminating on this question, Ella finds herself unable to develop a usable theory of mind regarding Jill. This is a challenge for Ella but also for the novel, since Jill cannot be relegated to the narrative margins in the manner of a young child. She has a full history, an identity, relationships, and a lifetime of experiences before her current dependency. She is also suffering. She is physically robust, but her judgment and awareness are impaired to the point where she may harm herself or others, resists basic hygiene and other self-care, and has minimal ability to communicate. The desperate unhappiness of her demeanor suggests that she is at least somewhat aware of the enormity of her loss, but lacks the ability to express herself or participate in the activities she once found meaningful. Ella recognizes that to care for Jill respectfully, she will need a theory of mind that acknowledges her history, as well as Jill's misery in the present. The problem is that Jill does not want to be cared for or comforted, and her mind is unreadable to Ella. Jill's disability renders her incapable, or uninterested, in reading Ella's mind. She greets Ella's attempts at connection with blankness, resistance, and sometimes physical violence. Her days pass in a circuit of melancholic activities like folding and unfolding towels and turning the sink on and off. At best she tolerates Ella's company, sometimes seeming not to notice her at all but more often rejecting her gestures of help and sociability. What Jill is "surprisingly, painfully able" to communicate to Ella is "her loss of self, her impenetrable solitude," along with enough self-awareness to recognize its absence.[39]

Jill's opacity and her fervent refusal to accept Ella's attention make her different from the dependent adults represented in the previous chapter, who were fully capable of self-expression and, in different ways, welcomed the care of others. They saw care as essential to their dignity and well-being, took an active role in managing their routines, and built relationships with those hired to assist them. But certainly not all adult dependents are as lucid and accomplished as our group of memoirists. Care is not a social contract where each participant is a rational, consenting contributor. In a just society, care must be given according to need, and often those who need it most are nonresponsive or actively resistant. Eva Feder Kittay describes an ideal where even the most dependent care recipient can contribute by engaging in the "subjective uptake of another's actions as caring." However, even when the dependent is unable to "complete" the exchange of care, Kittay argues, the caregiver is obligated to act as if "the cared-for could understand, then she would endorse my actions as CARE."[40] This ethical position works well in Kittay's example of a dependent in a comatose state. But

Jill is vigorous and capable of expressing her unwillingness to be cared for. A considerable amount of the novel is taken up with Ella's inner deliberations about how to manage her relationship to a dependent who does not want her attention.

Ella's job, like that of a nanny or babysitter, is to provide care, whether it is wanted by the recipient or not. She must find ways to fill the time with a dependent who does not appreciate her or want her around, while also satisfying her employer that she is indeed working in exchange for her salary. One option would be to overlook Jill's unappealing presentation, attempting to cultivate love and concern in spite of her external demeanor. In a just world, all dependent people would have the care they need, regardless of their ability to reward the caregiver with affection or gratitude. But Savage gives us a more realist literary world where Ella's good intentions are rattled by Jill's verbal and physical violence. Another option is to try to see Jill otherwise, by imagining her life before the accident. Ella attempts to imbue Jill with history by studying family pictures and listening to stories about her life as a wife and mother, her husband and children providing a connective thread to the person she once was. Ella also tries to care for Jill by developing a theory of mind that would penetrate the mysteries of who she is in the present. Mostly she fails. Ella perceives Jill as "beyond self-consciousness, outside the seductive passageways of her capable mind," and finds herself unable to imagine what it would be like to inhabit that position. Sometimes, she gives up on understanding altogether, simply joining with Jill in crying or uttering short, declarative incantations, since "it was perhaps only in this state that she and Jill could occupy the same isolating plane of being: that is, feeling minus the perpetual buzz of thought."[41] Having failed to meet Jill on the terrain of reason and sociality or to soothe her tormented inner life, Ella tries to enter her lonely world by echoing her gestures and sounds.

More often than joining with, Ella is beside Jill, coexisting in space without entering or connecting to her inner world. In this capacity, her care is less targeted at fulfilling Jill's needs than those of her husband, who desperately needs respite from his own caregiving duties. One of Ella's primary activities is to take Bryn's place beside Jill during long stretches of the day. This is where the ambiguities of care as paid work are most pronounced. Her job is literally "passing the time," something she sometimes does by "staring listlessly into space, watching the clock tick through the minutes."[42] We have already seen many instances of care that involves waiting, withholding, or doing nothing.

When a caregiver is being paid for their time, new questions arise. Ella is relatively content to pass, rather than fill, the time she spends with Jill, making sense of it as a service to her employer. But her position is complicated by others who occasionally enter the household. However brief and innocuous their interventions, these visitors trigger a cascade of feeling in Ella. Her discomfort at being watched suggests her own irresolution about the nature of her work. Some visiting relatives perceive Ella's companionship as inactivity, giving her lists of chores like maintaining Jill's hygiene and cleaning the house. Ella responds with a mix of resentment and understanding. She recognizes the desire to be "helpful" that underlies their recriminations and acknowledges that a demeanor of calmness or patience might look to some like "laziness." Their suggestions also stir up her own guilt at not doing more with her time or being more helpful to Bryn. Other visitors seem concerned for Ella's well-being, given the tedium and inactivity of her days. Jill's daughter-in-law, Lisa, offers a magazine, "as though Ella's boredom were an unsafe working condition and OSHA required them to provide reading materials." The intrusion she finds most objectionable seems, on the surface, the most insignificant. When Jill's son finds Ella reading the paper and tells her, "you don't have to hide it. I know you've got a newspaper. I don't care if you read," his words fill her with rage.[43] However well-intentioned, she takes them as a display of power that presumes his right to decide what she is or is not allowed to do while at work. The vehemence of her response also signals her own ongoing uncertainty about the terms of her employment. In the absence of clear tasks requested by her employer or her dependent client, what is she being paid for, and what does it mean to provide good care? These uncomfortable questions get at the contradictions of paid care work, especially when it involves less physically active forms of care.

There are other ambiguities in Ella's status as a worker. As is the case with childcare, when an adult in need of care is cognitively, as well as physically, dependent, care work must be triangulated by a third party who is both an employer and a guardian. Often that managerial relationship is far more complicated and fraught than that between caregiver and recipient. In Savage's novel, care work is tinged with gendered, quasi-sexual tension, with Ella imagining herself as something of a winsome Jane Eyre and Bryn, the dashing husband of a madwoman, as her Rochester. But this is not a Victorian novel, and its more muted modernist registers leave ambiguity about whether the emotional depth of the relationship—including its sexual tension—is experienced by Ella alone or shared with Bryn. A different literary work might use sex or romance to resolve some of the difficult realities of work, care, and human frailty that it introduces. In that case, Ella would be an adept mind reader, acting on desires she knows Bryn to harbor. *Say Say Say* rejects such a soothing fiction, its uneventful ending leaving the fraying edges exposed. The novel's third-person-limited narration leaves no doubt about Ella's preoccupation with the gendered and sexual dynamics of her relationship to her male employer. But even as Savage gives us prolonged access to Ella's theory of Bryn's mind, Bryn's own mind remains opaque.

Savage's insight here is about the insurmountable difficulty of caring for the spouse, parent, or other closest intimates of a dependent who is suffering. Tending to a dependent person's pain and dirt seems easy by comparison. This is why, in her final days of caring for Jill, Ella fantasizes about consummating the desire she imagines radiating between her and Bryn. Perhaps that is the one strategy she can think of to soothe Bryn's devastation. As a gifted, if imperfect, caregiver, it is easier for Ella to imagine having sex with her employer than being unable to help him feel better. It is a virtue of Savage's novel to draw attention to these predictable gender dynamics, while punctuating them with the unexpected and the queer. Ella is attracted to Bryn but also in a satisfying long-term relationship with a woman. Bryn mistakenly assumes "Alix" to be a male name, and Ella fails to correct him, feeling a mix of pleasure and shame as she plays at belonging to a heterosexual couple. Ella is also a queer mix of gender attributes, combining such conventionally feminine qualities as compassion and restraint with a hatred of housework that looks like "laziness" when seen through the eyes of Bryn's visiting relatives. Despite her perception of Bryn's attitudes and bearing as "masculine," he complicates her view of gender with unexpected tenderness. His version of masculinity includes patient and uncomplaining attention to his wife's needs.

The novel closes by reasserting the powerful ambiguities of care at the cash nexus. Ella's work is done when it is no longer possible to care for Jill at home. Some months after Jill is moved to a nursing facility, Ella returns to visit Bryn and he gives her an envelope of money. The exchange of cash, which he clearly intends as a gesture of gratitude, strikes Ella as a dismaying confirmation of the transactional nature of their relationship. It ruptures the sense of her special power and importance, reducing her to the status of former employee, a person who can use money that Bryn has to spend. This ending reinforces Ella's transitory status as a paid care worker, rather than a friend or a family member. Despite her participation in the emotional economy of the household during a time of crisis, the cash nexus ensures the separation between care and love. The melancholy of paid care is that no matter how much emotional capital a worker invests in her dependent charge, when that dependency evolves, it often also abruptly severs her ties to the people and spaces involved in its social web.

There is no exchange of cash in Rebecca Brown's 1994 short story collection about a home care worker, *The Gifts of the Body*. Where Savage's protagonist works for a single family, the unnamed protagonist in Brown's work is itinerant, serving a caseload of clients with AIDS at the height of the epidemic. And where the work of other home care providers in this chapter is informally managed by the family of the dependent, Brown's character works through an agency called Urban Community Services. The centralized organization of care work alleviates the frisson of the cash nexus where caregivers and their employers improvise the arrangements considered earlier in this chapter. Despite these differences, I include Brown's novel because of its domestic settings and concern with the interiority of a professional care provider. *Gifts of the Body* allows us to consider home care at a different scale and tempo, moving from the focus on an individual family to a case load of dependents who are overseen by a single care worker whose movements are coordinated by a centralized manager. In this sense, *Gifts of the Body* serves as a makeshift bridge between this chapter's focus on care within the home and the institutional care that is the subject of the final chapter.

Gifts of the Body is structured episodically, its stories of individual illness unified by the first-person narrator, a care worker who travels from one client to another. The shape of the novel echoes the uneven rhythms of the work she does, with some clients reappearing in multiple chapters, others mentioned only in one. These stories can be read individually, as snapshots of patients in advanced stages of AIDS and their intimates, but they are designed to be read together, providing a more collective view of illness and the weathering effect of care on one woman who witnesses it all. Brown's minimalist language communicates the narrowness and redundancy of the work, which may involve tasks as simple as hand holding, washing dishes, making tea, or sitting quietly at a bedside. These gestures are a powerful source of comfort and sustenance, but also so small, fleeting, and private that they are easily forgotten. In making them the subject of a book, Brown grants visibility and permanence to expenditures of time and effort that would otherwise be overlooked. *Gifts of the Body* thus preserves a record of the things people do and say and the unusual groundswells of emotion or its repression that occur in the moment when care is exchanged, details that are often written out of our practiced memories of the past.

The motif of gifting runs through the book, emphasizing why care work is so hard to quantify in monetary terms. Brown's caregiver does basic household chores and nursing, but she also engages in inactivity. Repeatedly, these stories emphasize the importance of knowing when *not* to speak or act. Being silent, restrained, or waiting are all forms of work, involving an expenditure of energy equivalent to, and sometimes greater than, cleaning or tending to the body of an ill person. Brown excels at describing subdued emotional labor, the invisible work that takes place behind the caregiver's placid, self-effacing demeanor. Some of this work is intuitive—this protagonist seems exceptionally sensitive to others—but it is also cultivated through deliberate practice and thought. Sometimes it is merely a façade required by the situation, covering over anger, aversion, or sadness. Sometimes care simply involves not speaking, not showing disgust, not doing a thing until asked, pretending not to hear a client vomiting in the bathroom. Sometimes it involves a state of mind, such as remaining present when the imagination longs to flee to something more pleasant. Always, the carer's own feelings and needs are subordinated to those of her clients: She eats to keep a sick person company whether or not she is hungry, she watches the client's chosen TV shows, takes the elevator because a client is too weak for the stairs, cooks food that won't be eaten, cleans, and comforts at the client's direction.

Brown communicates the tremendous effort such care requires with restraint, her narrative style echoing the small scale of her protagonist's work. The speaker describes her actions with such simple subject-verb constructions as "I washed," "I held," "I took," "I cleaned." She frequently uses physical perceptions to communicate the emotions of the cared for—"his skin . . . felt cool and clean," "I could feel him shaking," "I could feel his hands tremble."[44] We have seen how caregivers develop a theory of mind to help them imagine the personhood of another. In *Gifts*, the caregiver senses the feelings of others through bodily contact. Her body responds to discomfort and pain with its own physical sensations: "I felt my skin crawl" or "all of a sudden my face felt hot."[45] A gifted reader of minds and bodies, sometimes she is so attuned to her clients that she simultaneously experiences a feeling and imagines the other's response to it: "I saw him recognize the look on my face" or "I didn't want him to feel ashamed of how he looked."[46] Heightened empathy generates strong reactions to the plight of others, but also an equally strong impulse to repress the signs of emotional excess: "I made myself not say anything, but I couldn't hide how I looked"; "I was ashamed of how I thought, of how I tried to think myself away from the terrible sight of his sickness"; "she saw me wonder how long she had to live."[47] Witnessing suffering repeatedly does not inure the caregiver, but it does give her practice at concealing her emotions behind a façade of composure.

Initially, the work of composure seems justified if it helps calm frightened patients and their loved ones. These stories erect a clear divide between the sick (home or hospice-bound, suffering, cared for) and the well (mobile, attentive, care providing). The narrator adopts an emotional reserve, projecting an aura of calm professionalism appropriate to her job. Although she works with multiple clients, she aims to treat each as if they were the sole focus of her care. This preserves the client's privacy and is also a protective measure for the caregiver, who might be paralyzed by horror or sadness if she were to think about the epidemic in its totality. But the massive effort required "not to add them up" registers as the narrative continues and the narrator carries the burden of witnessing repeated scenes of loss, suffering, and grief.[48]

As the stories in *Gifts* unfold, we see the costs of maintaining the boundaries between the professional and her clients, as well as one client and another. Over the course of the collection, the carer becomes increasingly bogged down by the accumulated tragedy of the epidemic. Roles start to blur when a beloved supervisor, Margaret, discloses her own seropositive status and the lines separating healthy from ill, caregivers and receivers, become confused. By the end of the collection, the narrator has progressed toward acknowledging her embeddedness in a spectrum of dependencies, meaning that she, too, has needs for care and comfort. *Those who are obligated or paid to give care also need care themselves.* This axiom underpins all of the stories considered by this chapter. But cash transactions may make it harder to see. Brown avoids those compromises by making relatively few references to the monetary aspects of care in favor of attention to its emotional economies. Putting her work in conversation with others allows us to see how the absence of a direct cash nexus brings other elements of caring into focus.

Dying and growing up are very different milestones in the history of an individual life, but both mark an endpoint to a period of interdependency between caregivers and a care recipient. When the needs of the dependent and provider are no longer aligned, usually the paid worker is required to move on; the job is done even if a worker's need to earn money or find purpose in employment is not. For the caregiver who works in another person's home, these are also spatial transitions. She no longer belongs to a domestic environment that may have become so familiar it feels like her own. When the pandemic forced us into lockdown, signs of our suddenly disrupted intimacy with Angela were everywhere: her clothes in a drawer, food she left in the refrigerator, a glass of water on Henry's dresser. Over Zoom, she showed Henry all the reminders of his presence in her home, holding up a sweatshirt, toys, a box of snacks. Each of the works considered in this chapter takes a different approach to this moment of separation, but all recognize it as a key transition for those who are paid to care, their employers, and those who rely (or once relied on) their work.

This chapter has focused on the time of interdependency, that period when a dependent who has financial resources (or, in the final example, access to services paid by an indeterminate source) to exchange for care align with those of a care worker who has labor to offer. Paid domestic work is a necessary chapter in our evolving understanding of care within and beyond the family. We see how the exchange of cash complicates care, on the one hand requiring us to consider the value of work we might otherwise take for granted and, on the other, crudely diminishing relationships that seem like they should be priceless. We see how paid care work brings together people who might otherwise never meet, as a class of mostly women shaped by a history of racial and imperial inequity to perform work-considered-to-be-unskilled enter the homes of a class of mostly women shaped to be more than caregivers for children and other dependents. Although writing about end of life complicates the gender dynamics of those who employ and manage care work, the work itself continues to be done primarily by women. Care that occurs in an environment that is one person's home and another's place of work is further complicated by the ad hoc, personal nature of most agreements between employers and employees. Excluded from the regulations that protect other workers from abuse and the safety nets designed to sustain them in the event of their own dependency, the terms of the work must be invented anew and constantly renegotiated.

Paid domestic work also introduces new understandings to the temporalities of care. Paying for care and caring for work contain a timely paradox. How to put an hourly wage on the work of tending to needs and desires that cannot be dictated by the rigid schedules of clock time? And, given the inchoate, subjective, and relational nature of care, how to define the tasks that constitute work? To what extent can activities that appear to be forms of inaction or passing time—waiting, being present, not speaking, not doing—be considered work, and how can such duties be equitably assigned and managed? How to recognize and compensate the unseen and unquantifiable emotional labor involved in repressing sadness, boredom, anger, or disagreement as well as building reserves of love, patience, and kindness? When the relationship between a dependent and a caregiver is triangulated by a third party, how to reconcile different ideas about how the paid time should be spent? Focusing on the caregiver's needs introduces yet another set of questions having to do with her time off the clock and how and if that should matter to her employers. Once we acknowledge a relation of interdependency, is the desire to know about where and how a caregiver spends her unpaid time an ethical imperative or a paternalistic invasion of privacy? And what about the caregiver's future? To what extent is the employer obligated to consider the long-term well-being of a care worker beyond the duration of a job? And how do those who make a living as care workers juggle the requirement of absorption and attunement to a particular dependency relation and the awareness that the need for work will likely outlast the dependent's need for care? Or, sometimes, that the need for care is so physically or emotionally tasking that it will wear out the caregiver's reserve of labor even as she continues to depend on the income?

Fiction offers a nuanced vantage on these complexities because it has the ability to imagine the lives of others, to build and reflect on theories of mind, and to represent the affects generated between and among different parties. While the safety, equity, and compensation of domestic care workers are increasingly being addressed by organized labor, fiction is better suited to access the underlying needs, desires, and fantasies of the women (and occasionally those of other genders) at all points of a caring triangle and its extended networks. We have seen a variety of formal strategies employed by literary fiction to give voice to the otherwise unheard stories of care workers, as well as the affective relations generated among those workers, the dependents and their care work, and the people who manage and pay for it. These include entering the subjectivity of care workers either through first-person or third-person-limited narrative, alternating between the perspectives of caregivers and their employers, and following out temporal arcs different than those of the workday, either by moving with the care giver into her time off the clock or her life beyond the ending of a particular job. We have also seen fiction draw attention to the strategic unknowing deployed by care workers to reclaim privacy and personhood beyond a workplace. In exploring how understanding is alternately built or blocked, fiction can help us recognize the value of care work and appreciate the lives of those who do it. But it also exposes how deeply present injustice is embedded in histories of gender bias, racism, capitalism, and colonialism in ways that shape a particular person's ability to give or receive care, another person's sense of entitlement or discomfort at paying for care at home, and yet another's willingness or reluctance to do care work for money.

Paid domestic care is a key segue from the uncompensated care work of family to care in institutional environs, which is the focus of the next chapter. Having seen just how snarled and tenacious are the problems with care work in domestic space, the final chapter turns to organizations that have sought a different kind of solution by relocating the scene of care outside of the home, scaling up the individualized and particular exchange of care to the size of a group. The possibilities and failures of institutional care, as illuminated through stories about asylums, hospitals, and nursing homes, are the subject of the final chapter.

7

COMMITTED

Asylum as Care and Its Opposite

"Time ticks by differently next to the sickbed: Nothing's happening—or maybe it's everything that's happening, or is about to," writes Amy Hoffman near the beginning of her AIDS memoir, *Hospital Time*. If you have ever been in a hospital, you'll recognize this sensation. Time feels different because it is profoundly unnatural, guided not by the body's needs, movement of the sun, or the routines of daily life but by rounds, shift changes, and dosages of medication. Hoffman is not writing about just any sickbed but a bed in the ICU, an environment designed to provide medical care, not solace or rest. Above it all looms the clock, with its "big black numerals. One hand that moves in sudden ticks, minute by fucking minute."[1] Hoffman establishes the clock's authority, her profane adjective suggesting that it is not a welcome presence. She hates the impersonal way it measures out the boring, sad, and uncomfortable duration of a friend's suffering. Minute by fucking minute, hospital time feels redundant, sterile, and utterly antithetical to care.

Why is it that institutions dedicated to care so often cause us to feel uncaring and uncared for? And conversely: How and why do institutions of care succeed? How have stories helped expose the terrible harms that have taken place under the guise of institutional care? And do they ever show how and why institutional spaces facilitate care?

How are narratives shaped by, and how have they shaped, the caring institutions that are their setting? These seemingly paradoxical questions are the subject of my final chapter. Residential institutions are the Other to home and community, places that have centered my discussion of care to this point. This chapter begins with the premise that institutions are essential, if deeply flawed, nodes in the networks of care studied throughout the book. They are critical to offering the distributed care required in a modern world where gender relations have been rearranged, families are diversified and dispersed, and strangers live cheek by jowl. Under such conditions, institutions provide a necessary coordination of time and space: The hospital time that Hoffman finds so fucking awful also allows for a division of caring labor in which some workers treat the sick and alleviate pain, others clean and prepare food, all while she sits at the bedside, offering companionship and comfort. She has time for her friend because she is not providing, or directly paying for, the care work performed by others in the institutional ecosystem.

Institutions distribute caring responsibility and effort beyond the family. Residential institutions remove care from the home, the primary location of unpaid care work, and relocate it to a communal setting where some people work—often paid, but sometimes volunteer—to care for others who are dependent. I believe institutions are essential to a just world where care is not a privilege only for those lucky enough to have families or communities that can provide it, but a human right. But they often fail miserably, harming as much as healing, causing anxiety and work for family and friends, concealing suffering and wrongdoing. Even as they redistribute the responsibilities of care, institutions also replicate patterns of social inequality, leaving the lowest paid and most taxing care work to the same devalued classes who have always done it. Narrative helps us peer behind gates and walls to better understand how institutions fail to care, as well as where they succeed. It has also helped mold collective perceptions of institutional care, occasionally showing what it does right but also exposing its worst excesses to galvanize change. As we look to a future where more of us live into age- and disability-related dependencies, more people are born with disabilities that require ongoing care, and fewer are available to care for them, figuring out how institutions can care better and more sustainably could not be more important.

"Institution" is a general term that needs sharper definition to be of any use to critical thinking about care.[2] Institutions can have many different functions, but I focus on those that claim care as their central mission, including hospitals, nursing homes, and residential facilities for people with disabilities. For the purposes of this chapter, "institution" will refer to an organized (usually residential) environment dedicated to care and set apart from home and family. Institutions are spaces where care is distributed among workers who are hired, trained, and paid by a central administrative authority. Although a stay may be costly—whether paid by an individual, health insurance, or the state—institutions eliminate the intimate cash nexus and its many contradictions, as described in the previous chapter.

The institutions of care that are my subject are adjacent to but different from residential institutions like prisons, schools, and the military. Some will find this distinction controversial. The editors of the essay collection *Disability Incarcerated* begin with Foucault's rhetorical question: "Is it surprising that prisons resemble factories, schools, barracks, hospitals, which all resemble prisons?"[3] The implication is that it is not at all surprising, since all institutions share the prison's investment in surveillance, discipline, and control. For people with disabilities, these oppressive mechanisms have often been imposed in the guise of care. Without denying the continuities, my analysis seeks out differences as well as resemblance. If you think that the differences are irrelevant, ask the person with mental illness who has been prematurely released from the hospital, where they went for treatment, onto the street, only to wind up in jail. Institutional differences matter if we are to find spaces and organizational modes that redistribute the work of care, and that care more sustainably for dependent persons and those who support them.

Institutions are good at making themselves invisible, both by literally erecting gates and walls and with routines that become so ingrained they recede beyond notice.[4] Narrative is a device for making the familiar strange, for drawing attention to what happens behind closed doors, as well as logics that have been habituated into obscurity. When it comes to institutional change, stories have decidedly made a difference. In the past century, narrative has been essential to revealing the horrific failures of institutions that claimed healing, education, or respite as their mission. In its capacity to make strange, narrative can also identify the more unexpected ways that institutions *succeed* in caring for dependents, enabling communities to form, and providing meaningful work for those they employ. Beyond documents of existing reality, narratives by those who have resided in or worked at institutions of care communicate subjective experiences of time and space, as well as the affective texture of relationships, caring, abusive, and everything in between. The very existence of these narratives—which give imaginative shape to experiences of those who have often been hidden and voiceless—testifies to the sometimes generative nature of the congregate settings from which they emerge.

In what follows, I consider two sets of literary narratives, representing distinct eras in the evolution of modern institutions of care. The first are a trio of influential literary works I call the "asylum classics." Set in the 1950s and 1960s, all focus on a particular kind of institution, the environs, staff, and residents of the psychiatric hospital. Ken Kesey's *One Flew Over the Cuckoo's Nest* (1962), Sylvia Plath's *The Bell Jar* (1963), and Susanna Kaysen's *Girl, Interrupted* (1993) were all widely read and critically acclaimed at the time of their publication. They set the terms for subsequent narratives, as well as broad cultural understandings, of institutional care. In their day, Plath and Kesey marked a new openness in speaking about mental health and psychiatric treatment. Their protest against its abuses dovetailed with other social justice movements of the 1960s, laying the groundwork for institutional reform. Although these works are well known, I hope that my attention to care offers a different perspective, while also establishing a foundation to understand more recent asylum literature. A second set of literary works, Therese Marie Mailhot's *Heart Berries* (2018), Thomas Gass's *Nobody's Home* (2004), and Susan Nussbaum's *Good Kings, Bad Kings* (2013), attests to a new diversity of voices and perspectives on institutional care in the twenty-first century. These narratives reflect on a more recent moment in the history of modern care institutions, marked by the twinned forces of deinstitutionalization and privatization. They include the perspectives of staff, as well as residents, and they broaden the range of institutions to include a nursing home and a residential facility for disabled teens, as well as a psychiatric hospital. They also introduce new formal variety, pushing at the boundaries of memoir and the novel.

Across all of these literary works, the contradictory temporalities of care and clock time that we have seen within families and domestic space are amplified and complicated by the consolidation of dependents and care workers within congregate settings. These include the tensions between the official time of the clock and the individualized needs of workers and residents, between work that can be measured in hours—and compensated accordingly—and the inchoate effort of giving and receiving care, between time that is unbearably slow, tedious, and empty and time that is a source of respite and repair. Ultimately, residential institutions may be the place where we most vividly see the connections between care and time, the necessity of time to caring successfully, and the harm done when the time of care gets out of whack.

INSTITUTIONALIZING CARE

The history of institutions of care has been told by Foucault, Jacques Stiker, and others as a continuous effort to segregate, contain, and normalize those who are different, but it can also be seen as a history of more uneven change. I prefer the latter because it avoids an overly congratulatory or gloomy take on the present, while also recognizing the variability of institutions at any given time. Such a view is more consistent with the narratives explored in this chapter, which speak to varied experiences rather than making a singular case for or against the institutionalization of care. Even individual works, perhaps with the exception of *One Flew Over the Cuckoo's Nest*, portray the benefits, as well as liabilities, of institutional care for those ill enough to need it, weighing them against the alternatives of home, family, community, or no care at all.

One place to begin this more uneven version of history would be with the contradictions of the Enlightenment era. That period's new emphasis on reason, independence, and self-government amped up the stigma of dependency, particularly for those with cognitive or physical disabilities.[5] But it also drew new attention to care, education, and healing. Until that time, the majority of care for ill, disabled, and elderly dependents took place at home. Those who did not have families or charities to provide for them were often deemed a nuisance and a burden. However, their fate varied depending on where they lived. Historians of the early United States say that there was no equivalent of the "Great Confinement" of the mad that Foucault has claimed for Europe. Even problem individuals were often allowed to roam freely, mostly because it was too expensive to confine them. It was work to house, guard, and care for those whose behavior was unusual or eccentric and often deemed not worth the effort.[6] On both sides of the Atlantic, the nineteenth century saw increasing efforts to distinguish among various kinds of dependency, separating out those deserving of care from those who merited punishment or warehousing.[7] This was also the moment when institutions of all kinds emerged and began to flourish, along with a system of professionalization that would train and certify a class of experts to manage them. There were institutions of punishment, of course. But there were also institutions with a more salutary mission of care, like hospitals, asylums, and homes that developed alongside those dedicated to learning, culture, and religion.[8]

Modern institutions were more specialized than their precursors, and they conceived of care in therapeutic terms. Their design was informed by a new optimism that intellectual disability and mental illness could be cured with the right kinds of treatment.[9] The eighteenth-century French physician Philippe Pinel, along with the British philanthropist William Tuke, are credited with reforming approaches to mental illness with their concept of moral therapy. Instead of punitive confinement, they advocated for a humane protocol oriented toward psychological understanding of the motivations and needs of the ill.[10] What Pinel and Tuke did for mental illness, the educator Edouard Seguin accomplished for intellectual disability. He believed that cognitive defects of all kinds could be remedied with carefully regulated environments, individualized psychological treatment, and the right kinds of education. Exposure to culture—theater, music, literature, and the arts—was seen to have therapeutic benefits, along with art making, writing, and performing.[11] Under these more progressive influences, residential institutions emerged in the United States and Western Europe, aiming to create total environments for the reform and training of the ill and disabled, before releasing them as more productive and self-sufficient members of society.[12]

The rise of the residential institution was accompanied by a new professionalization of care. Once care for the intellectually disabled or mentally ill had been an obligation of family, folded in with the other work of maintaining a household. Now, it became the domain of experts, requiring special training, professional oversight, and dedicated environments.[13] Walter Fernald, superintendent of the Massachusetts School for the Feeble-Minded—the first public institution dedicated specifically to the care of people with intellectual disabilities—saw the purpose of the asylum as alleviating what he called the "burden of feeble-mindedness" on family and society.[14] He argued that families, regardless of economic means, did not have the expert knowledge required to care for their dependent relatives. "Home care of a low grade idiot consumes so much of the working capacity of the wage earner of the household that often the entire family becomes pauperized," he claimed heatedly. "Humanity and public policy demand that these families should be relieved of the burden of those helpless idiots."[15] Modern residential institutions would benefit society as a whole by freeing the able-bodied to engage in economically productive activity, while providing their defective family members with expertly administered care.

The idea that institutionalization was not a punishment but an opportunity, and indeed a necessity, for both the dependent and their family persisted well into the twentieth century. In his poignant home movie *Think of Me First as a Person*, Dwight Core Sr. depicts the process of institutionalizing his cherished son with Down syndrome in the 1960s.[16] Core's voiceover explains that his family would prefer to raise the boy at home, but experts advised that sending him away is best for all involved. The camera says otherwise, panning over severe institutional architecture and peering into barred windows, as Core expresses his concern about the forbidding environment where he has just left his boy. He had good reason to worry; by the time his son was born, institutional conditions had declined. The optimistic promise that the right kinds of care could lead the feebleminded and mentally ill to be independent and even productive had fallen short. No matter how enlightened their treatment, many institutional residents failed to meet expectations for reentering an ableist society. Under a medical model of disability, they were the problem, and their freedom was contingent on showing that they could be productive and obedient citizens. As they proved incapable of rehabilitation, the agenda of care increasingly shifted from education and reform to custodialism. Absent evidence for success, funding for residential institutions declined, as did the prestige of working with clients who were seen as unredeemable. The failures of reform, manifest in growing numbers of aging, long-term residents, led to crowded conditions. Low pay and chronic understaffing meant inferior care, neglect, and abuse.[17]

Eugenics also contributed to declining conditions at residential institutions.[18] The new science saw defects like idiocy and mental illness as heritable, meaning that the stigma of diagnosis expanded to include the entire family of an affected individual. "The normal members of a definitely tainted family may transmit defect to their own children," warned Fernald in his 1912 presidential address to the Massachusetts Medical Society. Those of good heritage should forgo marriage with defective partners, as "the immediate sacrifice is less painful than the future devoted to the hopeless care of feeble-minded children."[19] If the only goal of care was normalization, then care for or about a degenerate child was a hopeless pursuit. Even worse, that child reflected a tainted genealogy. Where an earlier generation of families had maintained close contact with loved ones, residential institutions became a place to warehouse shameful relatives.[20]

Eugenic measures went beyond the suggestion that bad marriages be avoided, introducing compulsory sterilization as a method to stop the perpetuation of inferior bloodlines.[21] Beginning in the 1920s, such practices were widespread at institutions in Western Europe and the United States, where they remained legal in many states into the 1970s. Female promiscuity, in particular, was viewed as a symptom of degeneracy that could be mitigated by preventing the transmission of hereditary defects to future generations.[22] The legacy of this logic, if not the practice of involuntary sterilization itself, is evident in the narratives I consider, where female promiscuity continues to be cast as pathology. Under the guise of care, institutions engage in repressive management of female residents' sexual activity even while leaving them vulnerable to abuse.

By the early 1960s, when Ken Kesey and Sylvia Plath published their influential novels about psychiatric care, conditions at state-run institutions had deteriorated to an appalling degree. The antipsychiatry movement began to protest the overuse of medication and confinement to treat mental illness, its activism dovetailing with efforts to expose the scandalous conditions of institutions for people with intellectual disabilities.[23] On gaining entry to facilities that were allegedly caring for the most vulnerable people with disabilities, investigative journalists found horrific scenes of neglect, violence, and mass death. In his reporting on Willowbrook State School, Geraldo Rivera described the naked, emaciated bodies of residents. He called them "freaks" to communicate the total loss of humanity that confronted him.[24] After touring institutions for the mentally ill and disabled in the Northeast, the researcher Burton Blatt and the photographer Fred Kaplan published a similarly scathing photo essay called *Christmas in Purgatory*. Blatt wrote, "It is difficult for 'uninvolved' people to believe that in our country, today, human beings are being treated less humanely, with less care and under more deplorable conditions than animals."[25] These exposés revealed that institutions, despite being labeled "Hospital," "School," or "Village," had become little more than warehouses for unwanted dependents abandoned by their families and social services.

The result was "deinstitutionalization," a movement to shutter large, state-run facilities, shifting funds to smaller centers that would house

and serve dependents in their own communities. Deinstitutionalization aimed to provide dependent people with disabilities more autonomy, flexibility, and social integration. In doing so, it recentered care
on home, family, and community, creating the conditions of possibility
for many of the caregiving arrangements discussed earlier in this book.
Some benefited from deinstitutionalization, but its progress has been
halting and sometimes backward. In 2004, the *New York Times* told the
story of Migdalia, a survivor of the Willowbrook State School, who
moved in with her mother after it closed in 1980. She thrived for twenty
years, but when her mother died, she was transferred to a group home
in the Bronx. There, she was one of several Willowbrook survivors to
be abused and neglected, despite the promise that extra safeguards
would be in place after the trauma they had endured.[26] Her experiences
reflect the uneven effects of deinstitutionalization, which resulted in
greater levels of autonomy and inclusion for some, while leaving others
in equally bad or worse conditions. Often its promises were unfulfilled,
as was the case with the special protections pledged to Migdalia and
other survivors. Her story also shows that the care of newly released
dependents continued to fall disproportionately to women and people
of color. Migdalia had a loving parent who welcomed her home, but not
all were so lucky. And the precarity of her situation became clear after
her mother's death, evidence of the vulnerability of dependents who
rely on a single caregiver, particularly an aging parent.

Deinstitutionalization has also been incomplete. Residents who were
most capable of independence or had family resources to support them
were the first to be released. Meanwhile, thousands of people with
intellectual disabilities still remain in confinement, with no available
alternatives. Sometimes deinstitutionalization has simply meant down-
sizing residents into smaller and equally harsh environments.[27] There
is no guarantee that a group home will provide better care than a hospital or asylum, and its small scale makes it easier for abuses to go
undetected.[28] According to a 2012 report by the National Council on
Disability, over one hundred thousand Americans continue to live in
restrictive settings such as nursing homes or smaller congregate housing units.[29] Many such facilities, which were once managed by the

government, have been taken over by private corporations that promise improved safety and efficiency. But they also seek profit, answering to shareholders rather than the needs of residents and their families.[30] We have already seen that good care is often inimical to the capitalist values of productivity, profit, and efficiency. In this chapter, the authors Susan Nussbaum and Thomas Gass explore the damaging impact of a profit-oriented mindset on those who inhabit and work in residential care institutions and who rarely have opportunities to speak of their experiences.

Where deinstitutionalization has resulted in ongoing confinement for some, it has diminished access to needed residential care for many others. Classic asylum narratives tend to focus on involuntary confinement, but today a more common problem is premature release or having no care at all.[31] As is so often the case, defunding measures are much better at cutting back than redistributing money to more favorable alternatives. The point of deinstitutionalization was not to curtail government spending but to redirect support from large hospitals and asylums to community-based clinics and smaller residential facilities. But resources have been woefully inadequate. Many survivors of institutionalization were not moved into supported living that had been promised or recommended but simply turned onto the streets or jailed as criminals. A 2016 report released by the Treatment Advocacy Center declared that prisons had become the nation's "new asylums," with far more restrictive conditions and fewer resources than the hospitals that preceded them.[32] Patients who do manage to gain admission to residential facilities find that the duration of their stay is determined by cost rather than the care they require. As we will see, in *Heart Berries*, her memoir of mental illness, Therese Marie Mailhot chafes under the constraints of hospital care, but she also recognizes the privilege of having health insurance that will cover her stay, while an equally needy friend is released prematurely.

These pages are a sketch rather than a comprehensive history of caring institutions. My intention is to identify some key places where the mixed motives and consequences of such institutions are in evidence, showing uneven change rather than steady progress or decline. Among the most important changes were efforts to humanize and redistribute care so that family would no longer be the first and only resource for dependent persons. Those have come at a steep price that is both financial—proving, yet again, that care and profit are unseemly bedfellows—and social—resulting in confinement and loss of autonomy for dependent persons. Too often, the mission of care has been abandoned, resulting in abuse, neglect, and degradation of vulnerable populations. At any particular moment, the quality of available care has also varied widely, correlating with broader economic and social inequalities of its time. Throughout this history, narrative has played a key role in rationalizing the need for institutions of care, as well as galvanizing reform and abolition. So too, it has personalized the stories of those who might otherwise be treated as an anonymous cohort and peered behind walls and gates that may offer shelter and privacy but also conceal terrible wrongs. The asylum classics examined in the first section made an influential contribution to public understandings and efforts to reform residential psychiatric care. They also created a foundation for subsequent writing, which would introduce new voices and forms, as well as different institutional settings. This chapter is not intended to be an apology or a condemnation of institutional care, and its placement at the end of the book should not be mistaken for a solution to the problems of care in domestic and/or familial settings. I consider institutions to be one essential part of a broader fabric, a flawed but crucial component of the stories told by and about those who are dependent, their caregiving networks, and the practices and relations that emerge among them.

ASYLUM CLASSICS: PSYCHIATRIC CARE
AS REFUGE AND PUNISHMENT

Ken Kesey's bestseller *One Flew Over the Cuckoo's Nest* may be the most influential asylum narrative of all time. Based on Kesey's experiences as an orderly at the Menlo Park Veterans' Hospital in California, it captures a transformative period in psychiatric care, as talk therapy was supplanted by psychotropic drugs and electroconvulsive therapy (ECT). Kesey's novel would remain in the public eye for over a decade, first as an international bestseller, then a Broadway play and an Academy Award–winning film. The title of a 2011 article in the *Daily Mail*, "Jack Nicholson Did for Shock Therapy What Jaws Did for Sharks," captures its lasting impact on social understandings of psychiatry.[33] "There is probably no fictional story that so haunts our consciousness of a medical treatment," writes Jonathan Sadowsky, author of a book about ECT, who also notes that it had little resemblance to reality.[34] Kesey did not aim for realism, although he must have witnessed patients undergoing treatment. In his novel, ECT is a symbol of the institution's failure to care, its use of psychiatric pseudoscience to suppress dissent and punish nonconformity, turning men into passive, drooling automatons.

In Kesey's vision, the mental hospital is antithetical to care, but he is also skeptical about care in general. He is less concerned with improving care than nudging it out of the conversation altogether. The word "care" rarely appears in his novel, a strange omission for a story set in a hospital. When it does, it is synonymous with domination, never in reference to nurturing and sustaining those in need. The hospital is a microcosm of a society that emasculates with crushing expectations of productivity and obedience. To be "cured" means accepting submission, agreeing to rejoin the world as a self-regulating and docile member of society. Kesey's solution to the problems of psychiatry is not better forms of care. His hero, the strident nonconformist Randall McMurphy, boasts that he has "no one to care about," stirring up fellow inmates to break rules and shed their sense of obligation to care for others.[35] If McMurphy had his way, they would form a band of rugged outsiders, unfettered by commitments to other individuals or society. Not caring is essential to a natural order that defines manhood by freedom and self-sufficiency. That order has been violated by the institution, a machine for subduing male rebellion and restoring conventional standards of behavior.

Kesey's critique of the hospital is inextricable from his portrait of 1950s-era gender trouble. In the asylum, a pathological role reversal has put women in charge, when they should be providers of care and keepers of domestic space.[36] His tyrannical Nurse Ratched is cold and bureaucratic, exhibiting none of the feminine ideals associated with her professional title. Kesey salts his misogyny with a dash of racism. He expresses no sense of solidarity with the Black male orderlies who respond to her beck and call, doing the actual dirty work of securing the premises, suppressing the residents, and cleaning up their messes. Under her control, days run "like a smooth, accurate, precision-made machine," but there is no comfort in a routine that seems designed only to induce submission.[37] Kesey's antipathy to psychiatry and psychiatric hospitals is thus inspired more by his protest against effeminate and conformist society than by its failure to care for those who are ill and dependent. Dependency itself is a symptom of social malaise that will be remedied only when men become radically free individuals. This solution is modeled at novel's end, when its narrator, Chief Bromden, escapes into the night.

Like Amy Hoffman, Kesey perceives time as a key element of the hospital's tyranny, although in his case the point of time management is not to facilitate care or healing but to enforce homogeneity. In an early chapter, Bromden provides an hour-by-hour breakdown of the hospital's daily schedule, his extended description giving a sense of time as monotonous and rigid but also whimsical, since the "Big Nurse" can manipulate it at her will. Tightly controlled time is a prominent feature of life in a residential institution, where communal conditions often require coordination of movement and activity. Assuming that predictability is always oppressive, Kesey's novel begs the question of why, aside from crushing the souls of patients, hospital time might be so organized. As we will see, while some other authors feel similarly constrained by institutional time, some find that it introduces a soothing regularity to a world that seems dangerously chaotic. Sometimes relinquishing control and allowing oneself to be cared for can be healing. And sometimes tedium can be reparative or even a pathway to creativity.

Many of the objections to psychiatric care voiced by Kesey surface in other influential asylum classics, including Sylvia Plath's *The Bell Jar*

and Susanna Kaysen's *Girl, Interrupted*, which center on women's stories of mental illness. In their view, women are more likely to be psychiatry's victims, diagnosed as delusional for wanting something other
than marriage, motherhood, and predictably feminine forms of paid
work. But their protagonists also suffer from debilitating symptoms
that cannot be explained away as youthful rebellion, the product of
misogyny, or generational madness. Neither suggests that mental illness is *just* a social fiction or that the hospital is *merely* a technology of
social control, even if it often has that effect. Rather, a hospital can
sometimes serve as an asylum—in the sense of a refuge and a source of
care—for those in need. Although both authors are sharply critical
of some aspects of institutional care, their protagonists emerge from
confinement having experienced repair, if not cure. I realize this is an
unconventional take on authors who are usually read as decidedly
skeptical about psychiatry. They are. But it is worth reading further
into their narratives because they do not seem entirely ready to throw
out the baby (in this metaphor, an apt figure for necessary care) along
with the asylum's admittedly contaminated bathwater. The care it
offers is often compromised, but sometimes it also soothes and restores,
offering a much needed antidote to the toxic environs of home and
family for women who do not have the liberty to simply break free and
run off into the night.

The more nuanced view of institutions offered by Plath and Kasen is
as much about class as it is gender. Residential care has always been
segregated, replicating the economic inequalities of society at large.
Even in the heyday of Enlightenment-era optimism, when progressive,
humane, and individualized treatments were revolutionizing hospitals
and asylums, such concierge-level care was far more accessible to those
with means than to the poor.[38] In noting these authors' differing views
on psychiatry, it is important to acknowledge the material difference
between the state-run facility that houses Kesey's characters and McLean
Hospital, the expensive private facility that treated Plath and Kaysen.[39]
Even among elite institutions, there was a particular cultural cachet
associated with McLean, whose clientele included such literary celebrities as F. Scott Fitzgerald, William Styron, Anne Sexton, and Robert

Lowell, as well as Plath and Kaysen. Writing of her own mental illness in the twenty-first century, Daphne Merkin looked back, only slightly tongue in cheek, at "the glamour days of nuthouses, when wealthy patients—'thoroughbred mental cases,' as the poet Robert Lowell described them—strolled across two hundred acres of manicured grounds at McLean Hospital in Massachusetts, a site chosen for its beauty by Frederick Law Olmsted."[40] Plath and Kaysen are the beneficiaries of such refinement, and they know it. However much they wish not to be in the hospital, both allude to its steep cost, the privilege of those it serves, and the fate of those without means to pay for such luxurious and attentive care.

One sure sign of the differences between Kesey and Plath is that residents of McLean Hospital, as portrayed in *The Bell Jar*, are not beholden to a communal schedule. Its refined atmosphere allows for a less standardized experience, with care tailored to individual needs. Residents not only seem to have more control over their time; they also have access to pleasurable activities to relieve the numbing tedium of hospitalization described in most other narratives. There is talk of golf, maid service, strolls on the grounds. Plath, who stayed at McLean for six months after her first attempted suicide in 1953, was far more concerned with the *price* of the time she spent in residential care than the structure of her days. She is well aware that her middle-class family—living on the income of a single mother after Otto Plath's death in 1940—could not have afforded her stay at McLean. In *The Bell Jar*, Plath's semiautobiographical character, Esther Greenwood, escapes a "cramped city hospital ward" only thanks to the beneficence of the same wealthy patron who sponsored her scholarship to Smith College. At McLean she is served breakfast in bed, where she reflects that without her benefactor, "I'd be in the big state hospital in the country, cheek by jowl to this private place." The proximity of the two hospitals attests to a healthcare system segregated by race and class. In a grim fantasy, she imagines the cost of long-term dependency to her family, who would first "sink all their money in a private hospital like [McLean]," then, "when the money was used up, I would be moved to a state hospital, with hundreds of people like me, in a big cage in the basement. The more hopeless you were, the further away they hid you."[41] The distance from breakfast in bed to a cage in the basement encapsulates the wide disparities in available care at the time.

Plath's vision of a forgotten population living in mass confinement, caged rather than cared for, accurately describes the conditions of public hospitals that would be exposed in the decades to come. Ten years later, Senator Robert Kennedy would use a similar image to describe Willowbrook State School, where he found "rooms less comfortable and cheerful than the cages in which we put animals in the zoo."[42] Plath's reference in *The Bell Jar* suggests that the impulse to confine and conceal, rather than to care for, the mentally ill was an open secret. But note that she does not imagine that she would be released "when the money was used up." Her complaints do not lead to thoughts of escape or early discharge. Rather, her anxious fantasy is also an acknowledgment of her own need for hospitalization, as well as her good fortune in having access to high-quality care.

In Esther's nightmarish vision, the state hospital is grim and overcrowded. But she also learns that it is understaffed, a problem that further diminishes the quality of care for its residents. A nurse who works at both facilities tells Esther, "You wouldn't like it there one bit, Lady Jane." Compared to the state hospital, she says, McLean "is a regular country club." By contrast, "over there they've got nothing . . . Not enough em-ploy-ees." The chatty nurse explains that she is holding down two jobs until she can afford a new car. After that, she will take "only private cases."[43] The implication is that private clients provide better working conditions and perhaps better pay, presumably more like the home care arrangements described in the previous chapter. Even as the nurse describes the higher quality of care available to those with means to pay, the boundary between the two institutions is porous. Underpaid staff carry their stress and exhaustion from one job to the other, and Esther worries that she is one unpaid bill away from being sent "over there."

In addition to the hospital's material luxuries, Esther also has a feeling of being cared for. She genuinely likes her psychiatrist, Dr. Nolan, who earns her trust by speaking honestly and respecting Esther's needs and preferences. Even the doctor's more restrictive orders seem motivated by concern for Esther's well-being. When she prescribes ECT, which Esther found torturous under a previous doctor, she gains Esther's confidence by communicating with her rather than simply digging in. And, unlike previous treatments, this course of ECT seems to work, temporarily lifting "the bell jar" of stifling ennui that was a symptom of Esther's illness.[44] The representation of ECT as a tool for healing, when used properly, is a striking contrast to the blunt trauma it exerts in Kesey's novel.

Esther also finds comfort in the environment: In bed she feels "warm and placid in my white cocoon"; when she wakes abruptly, a nurse brings hot milk that she enjoys, "luxuriously, the way a baby tastes its mother"; she sits in "sisterly silence" with an unspeaking fellow resident.[45] To be sure, these sensations are cozy, childlike, regressive. But sometimes the appropriate care is simply to satisfy such basic, animal needs. The hospital feels familial in the sense that it is dull and unchallenging. It also protects Esther from her actual family, particularly her mother, who tends to worsen rather than soothe her symptoms. Hospital care is expensive, but family care incurs an emotional debt that may be even harder to pay off.

Care that is warm, cocooning, and maternal does not lead Esther to lifelong dependency, despite her anxious vision. She emerges from the hospital "patched, retreaded, approved for the road."[46] The tentative language suggests nothing so decisive as a cure; whatever healing has occurred is provisional and, perhaps, temporary. But patching and retreading are gestures of care for something that has been injured or worn out. Time in the hospital has prolonged Esther's life. And survival appears a better alternative than the fate of her friend Joan, who was released from the hospital only to commit suicide. The period of asylum—involving attentive talk therapy, a community of similarly affected clients, and perhaps even ECT when correctly administered—has resulted in repair. Esther may not be well, but there is no doubt that she has been cared for, at tremendous cost, and that her stay in the hospital has provided some relief from the most debilitating symptoms of her illness, care she could not have received at home.

Some fifteen years later, Susanna Kaysen, another aspiring writer, was also committed to McLean Hospital. By that point, it feels a lot less like a country club. There is no breakfast in bed, movement of the residents is more restricted, and she finds the environment shabby and sterile. *Girl, Interrupted* is Kaysen's bestselling memoir about the two-year hospitalization that followed her own attempted suicide.[47] As its title suggests, the disruption of time—the period of life "interrupted" by an involuntary hospital stay—is a central concern of Kaysen's work. And hospital time, as it is managed and experienced, is far more important to her account of care than it was for Plath. However, she feels similarly ambivalent about the effects of her involuntary hospitalization, which sometimes seems like a healing respite from a violent and demanding world and sometimes a punitive obstacle to experiencing it.

Kaysen's time in the hospital is controlled, agonizingly slow, and tediously empty. Long stretches of unoccupied time—perhaps meant to be restful or protective—are experienced by residents as profoundly boring. They are also sometimes antithetical to care, since they tend to produce disruptive behavior that leads to punishment and confinement. Boredom also allows Kaysen's thoughts to spiral into unhealthy rumination. While she will eventually transform those experiences into some of the book's more lyrical and formally innovative chapters, in the moment she finds them deeply uncomfortable. Meanwhile, official time marches forward on a predictable schedule of treatments, medications, shift changes, and safety checks. An awareness of life going on outside the hospital makes the time of healing feel wasteful. Youth is finite and precious; time spent, squandered, or "murdered" in the hospital cannot be recovered. In the guise of care, the young women at McLean, much like the inmates at Kesey's hospital, are being robbed of a precious and irreplaceable resource. But amid the criticism are quieter suggestions of the asylum's reparative function. Even as she perceives it as a place that steals, murders, and empties time, Kaysen also sees the hospital "as much a refuge as a prison." The timed surveillance she hates so much is "sour" and wasteful, but she also likens it to a "lullaby" and a "pulse," primal, life-affirming descriptors.[48]

An affirmation of hospital care is certainly not the primary agenda of *Girl, Interrupted*. Kaysen's particular target is the psychiatric tendency to pathologize female rebellion. Still, she does not dismiss the reality of mental illness or the need for psychiatric hospitals. Under the right conditions, institutional care may be necessary, and it sometimes has the capacity to repair or to save lives. It can provide a community where residents care for one another, even as they chafe under the care administered by hospital staff. And institutionalization—with its numbing routines and limited activities—can interrupt behaviors that are harmful to self or others. When family is a source of suffering and bad feeling—as it is for Kaysen and as it was for Plath—being cared for by professional strangers can be soothing. In contrast to the blanket critique of institutions offered by the antipsychiatry movement, Kaysen acknowledges that "though we were cut off from the world and all the trouble we enjoyed stirring up out there, we were also cut off from the demands and expectations that had driven us crazy." By this account, institutions are not an extension of an oppressive society but a shelter from it. Institutional care is an unwelcome and unpleasant interruption, but it also presses pause on crazy-making "demands and expectations." To underscore the point, Kaysen, like Plath, includes a negative example in the story of Daisy, a resident in her cohort who commits suicide after being released. Kaysen does not affirm life at any cost, recognizing that death brings an end to Daisy's evident suffering. But she also acknowledges that her own experience was different: "I got better and Daisy didn't and I can't explain why."[49] Whether this means healing or simply being more capable of functioning in society, to emerge from hospital time "better" than before connotes improvement, however tentative.

Kaysen, like Plath, is aware that good care comes at a steep price, and it is not available to all who need it. Plath's reliance on a wealthy patron reflects a time when individuals were more directly responsible for the costs of their own care. By the time of Kaysen's hospitalization in the 1960s, health insurance had emerged as an intermediary between the patient and the institution providing them with care. Insurance was a safety net that protected against financial ruin in the event of illness, but it also placed new limits on care, prioritizing cost-cutting over the needs of the patient.[50] Kaysen was already identifying its inadequacy in 1967 in a way that sounds remarkably prescient. "Ninety days was the usual length of mental-hospital insurance coverage," she explains, "but ninety days was barely enough to get started on a visit to McLean. My workup alone took ninety days." Psychiatric treatment takes time, and the stay covered by insurance may be out of alignment with the standards of care or the requirements of an individual patient. When insurance runs out, patients are responsible for their own expenses. "If our families stopped paying," Kaysen writes, "we stopped staying and were put naked into a world we didn't know how to live in anymore."[51] The utter vulnerability conveyed by this image of being "put naked into a world" is very different from Kesey's resourceful escapee. Kaysen does not give an example of a patient being released because her money has run out, but she makes clear that this is an unwanted outcome. Her hypothetical also anticipates the scarcity of more recent mental health resources. The limits on insurance coverage for inpatient care, as well as the unequal distribution of health insurance and the corresponding inequities in care received, will become an increasingly prominent theme as we move toward the present.

A consistent feature of the asylum narrative is that it depicts the unlikely community that forms in a mental hospital, where people with similar needs are confined for prolonged periods. For Kesey and Kaysen, social bonds are the most redeeming feature of institutional life; in grim and controlling environments, residents entertain, commiserate, and sometimes care for one another. And for Plath and Kaysen, whose books were based on personal experiences of psychiatric care, a sheltered space where time is predictable and undemanding provides an opportunity for repair. Compared to the unhealthy environment of home, the hospital is a salutary alternative, a place where staff dispense care for a living rather than because it is a familial obligation. Even if the price of care is high, at least its monetary costs are clear compared to the inchoate costs of a family's forced, unpaid labor and the unwholesome effects of being cared for by the very people who make you sick.

These themes are echoed by more contemporary narratives, in which ill people find solace among others in shared circumstances, as well as in the sheltered, impersonal, and controlled routines of institutional life.[52] In her memoir, *The Scar*, Mary Cregan describes the care she received for melancholic depression at Bellevue Hospital in the 1980s. Initially, the hospital fails her. Left unattended in the shower, Cregan makes a near-fatal attempt at suicide that left the scar of the book's title. The scar is a permanent symbol of the breakdown of care in the very place intended to protect her from harm. Still, Cregan distinguishes between this particular incident and the overall success of her treatment at the hospital. There is no magical cure for her illness, but her time in the institution allows her to manage its most debilitating symptoms. "The hospital took us in when we could no longer function in the world," she writes, emphasizing the more affirming connotations of "asylum." A key part of healing is the community Cregan finds with other patients. "Thrown together as strangers in terrible circumstances, we had no choice but to share our suffering, but we shared our humor and resilience too."[53] Without minimizing the terrible suffering of severe depression, Cregan identifies the aspects of residential care that facilitated healing. The total environment of the institution allows her to find companionship among those in similar circumstances, it (mostly) keeps her safe during a dangerous episode, and it relieves her of demands imposed by home and the world beyond.

Reading these authors with an eye to care reveals a view of institutionalization that is critical but nuanced. All condemn the practice of involuntary commitment that was common for people with mental illness, intellectual disabilities, and others whose nonconformity was deemed socially disruptive. And all are aware that institutions reflect broader patterns of inequality, providing good care to those with means and its opposite to those without money, insurance, or advocates. The deinstitutionalization movement that began later in the twentieth century intended to correct those problems, avoiding unnecessary confinement, embedding care in local communities, and making treatment more flexible and individualized. But the realities fell far short of those ambitions. The combined impact of institutional closures, the rise of managed care, and the shift toward privatization has made good residential care increasingly inaccessible, without providing adequate resources to care for dependents at home or in their own neighborhoods. Today, dependent people are less likely to be confined against their will than to be denied the care they need.[54] More recent complaints about residential care tend to be that it is too short to be effective. The families of psychiatric patients are called on to fill the gaps with unpaid labor, while those without family are released into the streets. As we will see, the experiences of care recounted in the asylum classics discussed earlier are historically and culturally specific. This becomes more evident when they are compared to narratives produced about the more recent era of deinstitutionalization that are the subject of the next section.

BORN TOO LATE: INSTITUTIONS IN THE ERA OF PRIVATIZATION AND MANAGED CARE

Writing of her hospitalization for severe depression in the twenty-first century, Daphne Merkin laments that she was born too late for the "plush bedside service" offered to earlier authors. "With the advent of managed care, drastically shortened hospital stays, and increased pressure to medicate rather than listen," she writes, "private psychiatric hospitals, like so many other things in life, weren't what they used to be." Based on the history of a prior generation, she had imagined the hospital would be a nurturing cocoon. Instead she finds it impersonal and bureaucratic. Yet despite its disappointments, Merkin ends up feeling cared for and sheltered. There is comfort in sharing a space with others in similar states of need. "I wasn't lonely, for one thing, which I often was at home," she observes. "Although I wasn't living among friends, exactly, no one around me appeared to feel much more hopeful than I did, which was a form of company."[55] Home is familiar but isolating and unhealthy. Hospitalization is surely not a vacation, but it is also not a prison. Somewhere in the tedious insomniac nights in front of the TV, the ping-pong games, bland environment, and disengaged staff, Merkin receives the care she needs to return to her life.

Merkin knows that her experience, however imperfect, is better than most. We have already seen that the quality of hospital treatment received by patients in the United States is directly related to the ability to pay. But by the time Merkin entered the hospital, the combined forces of deinstitutionalization, managed care, and privatization had eroded the quality and duration of residential treatment for almost everyone. Where an earlier generation had protested involuntary confinement, Merkin describes a world where there is not enough care to go around and where those in need are often punished instead of being cared for. There is abundant data to support her claim, but I can also see it with my own eyes, people who are visibly ill, suffering, and in need of care on the streets I walk every day. Some are there by choice, driven by the awfulness of available housing alternatives, and others because they have simply run out the clock on their allotment of institutional shelter and care. All endure the stigma of being seen as a problem, unwelcome in public space, and frequent targets of violence. Instead of residential care, they often end up in jail simply for sleeping or sitting in one place.

Narrative helps us further understand—at an individual, subjective, and highly particularized level—the consequences of these failures for dependents, their families, and those who are on the front lines of care work. Narratives also attest to a growing diversity of voices speaking about experiences of institutional care and the creative literary forms they adopt to do so. While Plath, Kaysen, Cregan, and others represent the care available to those with means,[56] more recent authors represent the minor voices of those who have historically been unheard and uncared for. New perspectives and forms offer opportunities to better understand, and possibly reimagine, current practices of institutional care. They bespeak the urgent need for sheltered community, respite, and nonfamilial care provided by well-designed institutions, the grave violations of care that take place at many others, as well as the consequences of mixing care with profit.

Therese Marie Mailhot (Seabird Island Band) adds a distinct perspective on psychiatric care in her memoir, *Heart Berries*. While it would be perverse to call her book a revisionist *Cuckoo's Nest*, it certainly evokes Kesey's novel in its story of an Indigenous person who is a narrator and patient in a psychiatric hospital. While she does not mention Kesey by name, she writes critically of the prevailing stereotypes of "the Indian" and of Native women in particular. Care's absence is everywhere in her story of childhood poverty, a worn-out, alcoholic mother, an abusive father. The abuse continued in various foster homes where she lived as a teen. After her first marriage ended, she lost custody of her older son, and another relationship ended in a disastrous breakup. At no point is there a person or place that serves Mailhot as a refuge or reliable source of care. So she checked herself in for residential treatment.

Mailhot's diagnoses—similar to those of her literary precursors, if updated for the twenty-first century—include PTSD, disordered eating, and bipolar II. But her treatment took place in an unnamed mental health facility in New Mexico, not the storied McLean Hospital. Instead of being committed involuntarily, Mailhot actively sought care, at least in part to prevent her young children from witnessing her suffering. And unlike some earlier female authors, Mailhot was encouraged to write when she entered the hospital, which supplied her with a notebook and pens. The desire to write was seen as healing, not a symptom of illness. In this sense, the hospital is something of an ironic foil to a cherished writing residency she is awarded over the course of the narrative. Despite its many limitations, it *is* like the residency in that it encourages productivity, respite, and attention to self in a world where Native women are expected to care for others until they simply die of exhaustion. When they give Therese rudimentary materials and a rote set of exercises, the hospital staff present writing as a path to self-discovery and healing.

At first, the institutional space Mailhot describes seems unlikely to inspire creativity, let alone repair. The space is bland and impersonal, eroding differences that matter in the world outside while also making Mailhot feel Othered. The coloring of the interior, with its "stark white" rooms and "large pink book" for therapeutic writing, strike her as symbols of psychiatric care designed by and for people unlike her. In group therapy she is alienated by "white culture," with its belief that "forgiveness is synonymous with letting go." By contrast, she claims an indigenous cultural tradition in which "we carry pain until we can reconcile it through ceremony."[57] Echoing a critique often leveled by BIPOC people against the modern medical-industrial complex, Mailhot alleges that methods of care intended to be generic are, in fact, shaped by culturally specific assumptions that she finds alienating. The hospital's ambiance and focus on individual treatment seem ill-suited to care for someone oriented toward collective rituals of healing.

But something more interesting and complicated is going on here. Despite her initial qualms, Mailhot eventually comes to feel cared for in the hospital. She realizes that at least some of her feelings of exclusion are symptoms of illness. Becoming more receptive to and comfortable in her environment might be signs of repair. "It was nice to feel at home in that odd place," she writes. "I tidied my room like I never do at home." Home can be both a feeling and a place, and sometimes these two meanings conflict with each other. When they do, they complicate the notion that "at home" is always the best setting for care. When the home is a place of violence or neglect, as it has been for women in Mailhot's family, it is antithetical to the safety and comfort associated with feeling "at home." By contrast, the hospital environment, which Mailhot perceives as bare and confining, eventually generates the more affirmative sensations of being cared for. "I like these walls," she thinks. "It feels artificial but good." And later, when she struggles with the difficulties of life outside, "for comfort, I remember my hospital bed and the neutrality of the room I had. I was safe from myself and from you [her partner]."[58] Sometimes, feeling cared for means being contained, secure, and anonymous; home is a feeling of belonging and comfort rather than a specific place. With this account, Mailhot helps us imagine that a caring institution could generate the feeling of being at home when one's actual home is inimical to caring.

Perhaps the most important attribute of Mailhot's hospital stay is time. Care can be slow and inefficient: She needs time apart, time to heal, and time to herself. In an ideal world, the length of a hospital stay would be determined by the needs of the ill, whether for sustenance, treatment, or rest. But in an era of managed care, the privilege of time is unevenly distributed. The poor and uninsured are forced to wait for the care they need, as if they have too much time and it is worth less than that of more affluent consumers. When it comes to the duration of care, the same disadvantaged population gets less time than others. Mailhot comes from a class of women whose time is seen as having no value. She describes her mother as a woman who wore herself down by attending to everybody else's needs, using alcohol as an escape. Mailhot bucks this inherited self-image by committing herself to the hospital. The time she spends there is hers alone, and she feels cared for, emerging more capable of facing the world than when she entered.

One important difference between mother and daughter is that Mailhot has good health insurance. She learns its value by negative example, when she befriends another patient. If anyone needs time in the hospital, it is Laurie, a drug user, victim of incest, and attempted suicide; she embodies the hardships and abuses endured by women living on the margins. If released from treatment, she will have nowhere to live. This is America, so it almost goes without saying that she has no health insurance. In an era of deinstitutionalization, she is the kind of ill person who routinely winds up in prison when she should be in a hospital. When Laurie has to leave involuntarily, Therese understands "they're keeping me longer because I have good insurance."[59] Good insurance means there is at least some correspondence between prognosis and care; it allows her psychiatrist, rather than an accountant, to determine the extent of her stay. In an unjust society, there is not enough time and space to care for those who need it. Laurie is Mailhot's literary double, a counterexample for whom care has failed and who helps bring the ingredients of the author's more successful repair into relief.

To this point, the narratives under consideration have focused on psychiatric care and have been narrated from a patient's point of view. This is in part because there is a robust tradition of writing about psychiatric hospitals and treatment to draw on. But there are many other kinds of caring institutions and other types of dependency that require residential care. And when I looked beyond canonical literature, I found their stories. The final two examples will further expand the range of voices, types of institution, and creative forms used to represent residential care. The first introduces the perspective of a nursing aide, the least well-paid and most physically demanding job in an institutional hierarchy. When the nurse in Sylvia Plath's *Bell Jar* complains that the state hospital does not have "enough em-ploy-ees," her voice is channeled by Esther Greenwood. But *The Bell Jar* is not the nurse's story. She doesn't even have a name, and we learn nothing further about her working conditions, thoughts, or feelings, except that she needs two jobs to afford a new car. In *Girl, Interrupted*, we hear the kind and sometimes stern voice of Valerie, a favorite nurse on the ward, but she too is focalized through Susanna Kaysen, the memoir's protagonist. It is unsurprising that such women have not written their own novels or memoirs, given the grueling, low-status jobs they work for a living. But in 2004, Thomas Gass did precisely that when he published *Nobody's Home*, a memoir about his job as an aide in a nursing home. While a nursing home has a somewhat different purpose and clientele than a mental hospital—given that most residents are there because of age-related dependency—both are total environments where dependent people live together under the care of paid staff. As such, nursing homes share many aspects of institutional care already introduced by this chapter, while expanding our scope to include those with age-related dependencies and their caregivers.

Nobody's Home begins with a meditation on form: How to tell a story where little happens and where time is so redundant, predictable, and structured? As Gass puts it, "long-term care just rambles on without clear purpose or direction." In the familiar pattern of institutional life, the same sequence of events repeats day in and day out. But in a nursing home, residents also lack the kind of trajectory we associate with character development, one at least loosely followed by narratives considered earlier. Even under the best care, frail nursing home residents have little promise of growth or future accomplishment; when change happens, it tends to be in the direction of decline rather than improvement.

"If I were a totally faithful writer," Gass confesses, "this project would end in bits and scraps, some half-words, and then perhaps a lot of blank space."[60] I would like to see that project, which might look more like a modernist experiment than a memoir. The book he writes instead is a kind of portrait gallery, a series of intimate and textured character studies that accumulate—much like the assemblage of residents in the home itself—rather than unfolding a story in chronological time.

Compared to nursing home residents, who are depicted as individuals, Gass represents the staff as a collective, with shared routines, attitudes, and life circumstances. As such, they stand in for a broader class of people who end up working at demanding, low-status, low-paying jobs like nursing aide. Gass describes them as "a group of very caring people," "good and decent," who have chosen work that requires them to "give their lives away to strangers." They also tend to be one step away from dependency themselves: poor, with little access to education or other forms of social or economic capital, "people who would love nothing more than to work their way up into the lower middle class." The work they do is physically and emotionally exhausting, leaving little reserve for self-care. It takes its toll on their bodies as they seek out small pleasures like eating junk food and smoking; they "drive old cars and suffer bad teeth." Still, he insists, "this is a low-class job, but that does not mean it has no moral value."[61] Gass's project is to make that work visible and communicate its worth. There is good in caring for those in need, and there is something wrong with a workplace where carers are so unappreciated and underpaid.

Nursing home staff members confront the daunting task of caring for "an entire population in emotional peril." Frontline workers—who are themselves poor, undernourished, and under-cared-for—are the clients' primary and often only source of emotional sustenance. In their "style of caring," staff can communicate intimacy and comfort, or its opposite. "Normally it is the aides who are left to touch and nurture the residents, if the residents are to get touched at all," Gass explains. "Intimacy is built into the aide's work, and loss of intimacy tears the most aching void in our residents' lives. It is up to us on the front lines to make our touch meaningful or cursory. . . . We are closer to them than anyone else on a daily basis. So our style of caring comes to represent all of humanity to them."[62] This kind of emotional labor, which is so crucial to his clients' quality of life, is also exceedingly difficult to see, document, and gauge in the ways that work is typically measured. Residents who are alone in the world have nobody to witness and recognize the care they receive, which is also unacknowledged by institutional management concerned primarily with cleanliness and safety. Gass's book commemorates work that is invisible and unrecognized and provides a firsthand account of how badly we misuse those who do it for a living.

Writing as a professional caregiver, Gass makes a more concerted attempt to identify the ingredients of good care than do most narratives written by patients. In a nursing home, good care recognizes the dignity of those who are old and dependent. And it focuses on the now, rather than investing in future development. Gass and his colleagues are good caregivers because they find meaning in a stage of life many see as pointless and burdensome. Accumulated life experience enriches the personhood of his clients, but it also has benefits for the caregiver. "Sometimes, when people have nothing more to lose, they become liberated," Gass explains. Prolonged interdependency with his clients sometimes allows him to share in that liberation. "Maybe some of that freedom rubbed off on me. Witnessing a spent life as it unravels is like staring into a campfire in the dark of night: endlessly fascinating, heartwarming, and beautiful to behold."[63] Where often we value old age by looking to prior accomplishments or status, Gass finds purpose in the present lives of his clients. In his best moments, Gass practices the art of interdependency, seeking to care with attunement that is rewarded by opening him to the affect of "freedom" communicated by its recipients.

When Gass calls old age "heartwarming, and beautiful to behold," he risks the kind of sentimentality sometimes associated with writing about care. But then there is the shit. Shit features abundantly in nearly every portrait of an aging resident in *Nobody's Home*, and managing it drives much of the work done by nursing staff. Shit is the paradigmatic symbol of pollution, influentially defined by the anthropologist Mary

Douglas as matter out of place.[64] Shit out of place is also an unavoidable sign of dependency, one that demands immediate attention to its author and the surrounding environment. It can be a last-ditch expression of resistance from those who feel powerless, devalued, and forgotten. It can also represent the ultimate loss of control, dignity, and selfhood. And attending to it with dignity can sometimes be the most compassionate, loving, and selfless form of care. Recall that Roz Chast's mother lost control of her bowels on the night of her husband's death and that Roz showed respect by cleaning it up without comment. So too, Christina Crosby wrote of her intimate bond with the nurse who performed her bowel program and the deep shame her disabled brother experienced when he soiled himself.

Shit out of place is sometimes a limit case, demarcating the caregiving line a loved one is unwilling or unable to cross. When the anthropologist Arthur Kleinman's wife, who had dementia, was no longer able to use the toilet independently, he knew it was time for her to go into a nursing home.[65] Some kinds of care are better done by strangers. Shit unattended can also symbolize the depths of uncaring. Geraldo Rivera sought to capture the horrors of Willowbrook State School by describing its stench; it "smelled of filth, it smelled of disease, and it smelled of death."[66] And when Susanna Kaysen visits a friend who has been moved to the more restrictive ward at McLean, it is a sure sign of her decline that she has smeared her own shit on herself and her surroundings.

When Gass describes what nursing home residents do with their own shit, the effect is not to degrade them but to recognize personhood, as well as to detail, in blunt terms, the daily tasks of a nursing aide. To remain silent about shit is to be complicit in the practice of hiding unwanted people and their carers in institutions, allowing their desperation, loneliness, and rebellion to remain invisible. In a space that threatens to reduce care to bare physical maintenance, shit is one sure way for residents to assert needs in excess of those minimal requirements. Perhaps, in a society that so powerfully equates personal worth with the ability to work, incontinence represents a final expression of productivity. Residents no longer make anything of economic value, but they make something that demands attention, requiring an interaction between care giver and cared for that simply cannot be ignored, dealt with en masse, or put off until later.

Gass's accounts of shitting say something about the character of the dependent person but also about the interdependency they share with the caregiver. Care workers are affected by the constant exposure to shit in a variety of ways. When one person attends to the toileting of multiple residents, they may develop a pragmatic ability to see "feces as 'just stuff.'" Shedding its taboo aura, Gass writes, shit becomes simply "undifferentiated matter, seminal, stinky peanut butter."[67] Absent the distancing effects of disgust, the caregiver has more energy to approach a person in need without hesitation or recoil. This is why, when it comes to toileting, a paid care worker—inured to shit, impersonal, equipped, and trained to dispose of it—is often preferable to a family member or other intimate.

But Gass's nonchalance toward shit is also a sign of overwork, of staff so pressed for time that they can no longer invest their job with feeling. The same demanding environment that might numb a worker to the presence of shit might also wear away at such desirable faculties as compassion and empathy. When nursing homes are managed by private corporations, as is the case with Gass's facility, staffing decisions are likely to be directed by the imperatives of profit and efficiency, rather than the needs of clients. Understaffing creates time pressure that forces Gass to depersonalizing calculations. "There are twenty-six residents on my hall," he reports. "Seventeen are incontinent. . . . On average, we are allowed fifteen minutes to get each resident out of bed, toileted, dressed, coifed, and wheeled or walked to breakfast."[68] Each resident gets a modicum of care, but there is little time for more. Communal conditions meant to facilitate care can easily become harmful to clients and staff when the ratio is so out of proportion that there is no flexibility to address individual needs or preferences. Workers cannot adopt a "style of caring" when their duties are so strictly proscribed, their time so limited. Not only is nursing care among the most physically dangerous of all jobs, but it also has emotional risks.[69] Low-wage care workers who "give and give until they give out" rarely have opportunities to write about their experiences, but also, more immediately, they lack the reserves to care for themselves or their own families.[70] Gass's book gives one person's view of what it's like to work in a place where there are "not enough em-ploy-ees." We see a care worker who respects his dependent clients and knows the value of good care, even when it is unseen and holds no promise of future independence or productivity. But we also see the devastating mismatch between the temporalities of corporate profit and the needs of staff and residents. Making their shit visible is Gass's effort to disclose what institutional walls have concealed.

Heart Berries and *Nobody's Home* are an unusual pair, with little overlap in style, purpose, or narrative voice. They are written from very different standpoints, and the institutions they describe are also different, one a hospital and the other a nursing home. I put them together to create a dialogue about residential care, seeing their variety as a resource: Each introduces the perspective of someone who has not historically had narrative authority that would grant credence to their stories. Each contributes something to an emerging portrait of what makes institutional care work and what causes it to fail. A final narrative builds polyvocality into its form, using fiction to represent the voices of multiple care givers and receivers, each with a different perception of a shared institutional environment.

Susan Nussbaum's novel *Good Kings, Bad Kings* is set in and around the fictional Illinois Learning and Life Skills Center (known by its appropriate acronym, ILL-see). The vague designation "Center" indicates that this is neither a hospital nor a nursing home but a residential facility for poor, multiply disabled teens who do not have families or friends to care for them. Managed by a for-profit corporation, ILLC is a representative byproduct of deinstitutionalization, which turned dependency work into a major economic driver. The burdens of care have become a big business, fueled by the needs of dependents and their families.[71] ILLC leadership makes new claims to efficiency, safety, and individualized treatment, while clients and staff experience many of the same abuses that were rampant at their larger, state-run predecessors. In Nussbaum's novel, the narrators are the "good kings." Having a narrative voice means having personhood, interiority, and a perspective that, however imperfect, merits time and recognition. Chapters alternate among multiple tellers, including adolescent residents; exhausted frontline staff, who are "scraping the underneath of the bottom of the barrel"; and, more surprisingly, an employee of Whitney-Palm, the company that runs the facility.[72] Working in the tradition of social reform literature, Nussbaum's criticism is often a blunt weapon, and her attempts at adolescent and working-class voices verge on cliché. But her novel is interesting because of the chorus that emerges among these speakers; its more subtle recognition of the social conditions that produce dependency; and its depiction of the rarer moments of attunement, compassion, and unlikely alliance that form when vulnerable people are brought together. Its silences are also telling, affording no voice to such "bad kings" as corporate bosses, rule-bound supervisors, and abusive staff.

Good Kings, Bad Kings provides an unsubtle laundry list of all the ways an institution of care can harm its residents. Like the nursing home where Gass works, ILLC is designed for security and maximal profit. Nobody lives there if they have a better option, although there are worse places to end up. Residents are often punished and neglected when they most need attentive care. And when they need opportunities to grow and test their independence, they are infantilized. Liability is the primary concern in determining rules of conduct among residents and between staff and residents. A character named Mia is strapped in "like a baby" to a manual wheelchair she cannot operate, unable to move herself because nobody has bothered to get her an appropriately sized power chair. Rebellious Yessenia rails against "the most stupidest rules" that require her to pass a test before she can use the elevator or leave the building. Teddy vents his sexual frustration at being "twenty-one years old and never been laid" when he is shamed by nurses for getting an erection during his care routine. "Kids like this are trained to stay helpless," observes Joanne Madsen, a wheelchair user who works in the office. "So they have to stay institutionalized."[73] In an era of privatization, where companies profit by keeping beds full, there is little motivation to encourage the autonomy of residents or direct them toward less restrictive living environments. And because these teens are a captive audience without resources or supporters to advocate on their behalf, ILLC has no incentive to provide them with more than a minimal level of care.

The stories of residents who come to serious harm belie even the institution's minimal promise of safety and cleanliness. One unintended consequence of deinstitutionalization was to reduce the population in congregate care to those who were neediest and least capable of self-advocacy. Residents with mobility, cognitive, or verbal impairments are particularly vulnerable because some literally cannot speak, as was the real-life case of a comatose woman who was raped and impregnated in an Arizona nursing home in 2019.[74] Those who do speak out are treated as unreliable narrators. Fiction allows Nussbaum to tell these stories in first person, narrated from the point of view of victims who would rarely have the opportunity or capacity to represent themselves, and leaving no doubt that they speak the truth. Mia Oviedo is repeatedly raped by a staff member who threatens to kill her if she tells anyone. Even after her attacker is fired, she suffers from lapses in memory, an inability to speak, and ongoing fear and depression. Her boyfriend Teddy is fatally scalded after being forgotten in a shower. ILLC management issues an anodyne statement that portrays him as an anonymous victim. Corporate officials emphasize "the fragility of the population we serve," as if Teddy's disability were the cause of his death, rather than neglect.[75] But the novel has given Teddy personhood, describing his quirky preference for dressing in suits, love of practical jokes, kindness, and modest desires to drink beer and lose his virginity. The voices of Teddy's friends and supporters identify the accident as a failure of care resulting from overwork and understaffing that compromises even the most well-meaning employees and puts their clients at risk.

The novel's narrators also include frontline staff, creating a dialogue among care givers and recipients while also showing that care workers have worries, needs, and dependencies of their own. Knowing that a worker is worn out or depressed does not make their robotic demeanor more pleasant, but it does ground it in circumstances rather than character flaws. Staff speak of low pay and rules that limit the care they are able to provide for clients. A new hire named Jimmie Kendrick, recently homeless herself, describes the litany of chores she must do after personally attending to residents: "You have to clean up. Wipe down their shower chairs with alcohol, pick up, collect the laundry, collect the garbage, all of that. There are not enough hours. No, that's not true. There just aren't enough aides."[76] Like Thomas Gass, Jimmie complains of too many duties crammed into the time allotted, an untenable balance of emotional and physical labor and too few staff to share the effort. These burdens compete with worries about her living situation and future security of the kind that preoccupy low-wage workers.

Jimmie's account reads like a laundry list of chores that any staff could do. But when it comes to the center's human residents, she is one of several artful caregivers in the novel, characters Nussbaum uses to embody virtues that are not fungible and cannot be accounted for in a training manual or set of daily tasks. Jimmie speaks of her clients with compassion and respect. She knows that caring for people is an activity that cannot be rushed and demands her full attention. "All of them need your time. I don't care who the kid is, he or she is going to want to talk about their day, ask you questions about any and everything. They might be upset about something or not feeling well. I mean, it's more than just going through the motions. You have to be there, be present."[77] Jimmie understands the affective requirements of a good caregiver, the need for patience, attention, and intuition that may not align neatly with the hours and assigned duties of a work shift.

Another artful caregiver is the bus driver Ricky Hernandez, who determines to build personal relations with his charges. "I like to take each kid at face value," he explains, resisting the institution's tendency to classify and diagnose. "I don't want to memorize someone's file or chart or whatever they got and think I know them by that. That's bullshit."[78] Ricky's care for his teen clients is repeatedly undercut by demands that he restrain and punish, such that his acts of kindness often require him to break the rules. He and other dedicated staff use covert tactics to subvert restrictions that obstruct their ability to care. Under bleak and demanding circumstances, they practice artful caring, finding ways to connect, comfort, and attend to the needs of the residents who depend on them. They are guerilla caregivers who sneak in hugs and snacks, bend the rules about curfew and outings, and steal company time to listen. These kindnesses are rarely recorded in reports of job performance, and, when noticed, they usually result in a reprimand. Rescripting official accounts of the center's mission and activity, the staff tell the story of institutional life otherwise, commemorating small gestures that would otherwise be unknown or forgotten but also noting the piling up of slights and indignities that wear away at everyone involved.

Good Kings, Bad Kings is critical of institutional care, while also recognizing it as a symptom of social inequalities further upstream that debilitate the poorest and most vulnerable dependents and their caregivers. Even as characters loudly denounce ILLC's dehumanizing regimes and speak of many ways it could be otherwise, they recognize the absence of good alternatives. ILLC is not keeping these teens from a good life outside but rather is a manifestation of their grim standing in a society without adequate resources to care for the dependent poor. All of the ILLC residents have disabilities that require extra care. Their dependencies could be mitigated, but not erased, by appropriate accommodations. Some come from loving families that are unable to support them; others have no families to advocate or provide for them. Abandoned by her parents, Yessenia was committed to ILLC when the beloved aunt she considered her "real mother" died of cancer.[79] Cheri's family threw her out after blaming her for being sexually assaulted. When she runs away from ILLC, she ends up in a mental hospital, where she is medicated beyond recognition. Pierre is a disabled and emotionally distressed tween who has been cycled through one foster home after another. Teddy has a devoted father who lacks the money or understanding to get better services for his son. The family of his roommate Bernard, a wheelchair user, lives in a third-floor apartment with no elevator. He doesn't live with them because he isn't able to leave the building unless siblings are available to carry him up and down the stairs. His mother is disabled by diabetes, which makes her unable to provide him with physical care.

In the happiest outcome, Jimmie arranges to take Yessenia permanently into her home. They have built a promising interdependency
with mutual benefits: Jimmie rescues the teen from institutionalization, while Yessenia brings welcome stability to their life together. Their
story has a reassuring sense of closure, but it arrives through an ad hoc
tactic rather than a systemic fix for the social problems introduced
by the book. There are not enough kindhearted surrogates to care for
all the disabled teens and young adults without families or communities to support them. In the absence of happily-ever-after, Nussbaum
does allow for the possibility of more modest reform. After Teddy's
death, an impromptu protest by residents and staff leads to some positive changes. Whitney-Palm and its top executives are under investigation. There are rumors that Mrs. Phoebe, the condescending and controlling housemother, will retire. The center hires a new psychologist to
tend to the teens' emotional needs, and Mia is approved for a power
chair. Far from a revolution, this uneasy ending represents Nussbaum's
recognition that, in the absence of broader social transformation, we
can still aspire to better versions of currently existing institutional care
and greater attention to the victims of its failures.

How to do institutional care better is a question that preoccupies
this chapter, but it is also an increasingly personal question. My disabled son is the same age as the characters in ILLC, with similar levels
of dependency. When Henry was a baby, it was easy to celebrate the fact
that he lived at home. We were committed to raising him as part of a
family and a community, like any other child. And we felt lucky to live
at a time when inclusion is valued, allowing him to learn, play, and
grow alongside children of many different abilities. But inclusion does
not mean the erasure of meaningful differences. Now Henry's class-
mates ride the subway independently and have cell phones. He is
approaching the age when many typical children leave home to go to
college, take jobs, and develop social circles apart from the family. Living at home under parental guardianship will no longer be a sign of
inclusion but of difference. All people are interdependent, but some
have the capacity for what we collectively describe as independence,
while others live in continued dependency. According to those terms,

Henry is unlikely to have the same level of independence as his typically developing brother. As his father and I age, it is also unlikely that we will want to or be capable of providing him with lifelong care in our home. I would like to imagine that, when the time is right, his care will be distributed in ways that allow him to thrive, and that those who care for him will be fairly compensated for the work they do. As I write, this is little more than a fond wish for the future. I know that making it happen will be hard, time consuming, and expensive. I am lucky to have time to devote, but those are hours I will not be able to spend working at my job or tending to my own well-being or to the world's many more severe problems

The disability activist group Self Advocates Becoming Empowered (SABE) defines institutions broadly as "any place, facility, or program where people don't have control over their lives."[80] What they mean by "control" is ambiguous, perhaps deliberately so. If it means something like "autonomy," I would like Henry to have it, to be able to make choices about his life, where and when he is capable of doing so, perhaps with the support of others who know him well. Working with his father (my husband), I will do my best to help him secure a future where his agency is not unduly restricted. But by most definitions, Henry is likely to live in an institutional setting of some kind, whether that is a private house with a support staff, a group home, or some more innovative communal setting. I don't expect him to have the financial autonomy, freedom of mobility, and some other forms of self-determination we associate with full adult independence. Where I might once have found that tragic, I now have a more expansive understanding of flourishing that can coexist with dependency. Writing this book has given me ample opportunities to see how, under the right circumstances, dependency is consistent with a good life and how caregiving is valuable, dignified, and important work. I am more concerned with recognizing the personhood of those who are dependent than I am with trying to force independence on those who genuinely need care and support, or with buying what looks like independence on the back of full-time workers who aren't recognized or justly compensated.

Most of all, I aspire for Henry to have dignity, contentment, and opportunities to thrive. His thriving cannot depend on an individual caregiver, no matter how generously paid. And that is where institutions come in, since, at their best, they are social machines for distributing care, removing the direct cash nexus that can be so compromising to workers and dependents alike. Good care takes work that is valuable but not priceless. In an economy driven by wage labor, creating conditions where care workers are treated with dignity and paid fairly for their work is more important than locating care within any one kind of setting. If there is a lesson in this chapter, it is to school us in the need for institutions that distribute the care for dependent people, tending to their needs while promoting autonomy and allowing them to flourish, while also providing appropriate compensation and good working conditions for those who support them.[81] That sentence is a mouthful because it makes a tall order, but it is one worth the aspirational energies and fullest resources of a just society.

The story of Judith Scott provides a final object lesson. Scott is the well-known artist whose picture graces the cover of Eve Sedgwick's memorable last book, *Touching Feeling: Affect, Pedagogy, Performativity*.[82] It features a portrait by Leon Borensztein, in which Scott embraces one of her famous sculptures, a human-sized bundle of found objects wrapped in layers of knotted yarn, string, and rope (figure 7.1). She nestles her face into its surface, obscuring her own individuality in an image of artful interdependency. Like Henry, Scott had Down syndrome. She was also nonverbal, profoundly deaf, and spent most of her life in institutions that were unstimulating, restrictive, and emotionally, if not physically, abusive. She discovered art only after being rescued by her twin sister, Joyce, who became her guardian, secured her release from a state institution, and enrolled her in a program that allowed her creativity to emerge. Scott's late-life creativity is often described as an escape. Told in one way, her life story follows an arc from confinement to freedom that spans the period of deinstitutionalization. But increasingly, I see it as a story of institutional change rather than abolition, about the many ways congregate care can harm and

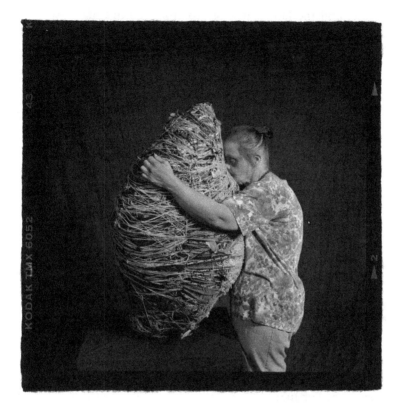

FIGURE 7.1 Judith Scott in Oakland, CA, 1999.

Source: Photograph by Leon Borensztein. © Leon Borensztein.

limit, but also about how institutions can be redesigned to promote flourishing.

Scott was born during the period of widespread institutionalization for people with intellectual disabilities. She was raised at home until the age of seven, when experts determined that she could not be educated and should be institutionalized. Her twin, Joyce Scott, recalls waking up to find Judy gone from their shared bed. She writes of visiting her sister in a hellish environment "full of awful sounds and smells of human suffering and abandonment. It still lives in my nightmares."[83] With the illness and death of their father, the visits became more sporadic, and the family disengaged from Judith's life. Absent their intervention, Scott received little education of any kind. Hospital records describe her as "severely retarded," having a mental age of two and an IQ of 30.[84] Joyce reports that Judith's interest in art was quashed, her crayons confiscated because she was deemed "too retarded to draw."[85] It is a sign of neglect and low expectations that nobody noticed Scott's profound deafness until she was thirty-nine years old. It is impossible to know how much of Scott's "low intelligence" was actually caused by her inability to hear or what she would have said had she been given a language with which to communicate. Staff at the institution where she lived decided that she should learn ASL, but nobody who worked there knew how to sign. When Joyce visited, she found her sister "living in near total isolation."[86] Scott's habit of taking and hiding objects like dolls, magazines, keys, and shoes bespeaks a lifetime of deprivation in environments without privacy or respect for personal possessions. Her art, consisting of elaborately bound and wrapped human-sized cocoons, bespeaks a longing to hold and be held.

I have long been fascinated by Scott's life and her art. My computer has a trove of unpublished talks and essays that find various meanings in her story. For many years, I held her up as a negative example of everything I could do differently for my son. But there is a different way of reading that is less about institutionalization and its opposite and more a testament to institutions that fail and those that work to distribute care and promote thriving. Judith could easily have spent her entire life in a state-run institution and been buried, like countless other victims of that time, in an unmarked grave. She avoided that fate thanks to the strenuous efforts of her sister, Joyce, which got her released from the Gallipolis Developmental Center in 1985, after thirty years of confinement. It took expensive and protracted legal wrangling for Joyce to have herself appointed Judith's conservator and move her to California, where she found suitable housing and a placement at the Creative Growth Center in Oakland. It was there that her artistic awakening took place.[87]

Creative Growth started in 1974 in the garage of the artist Florence Ludins-Katz and her husband, the psychologist Elias Katz, as a studio space to train and occupy artists with intellectual disabilities, regardless of talent or abilities. It was founded in response to the closure of psychiatric hospitals in California in the 1950s and 1960s, when many former patients were turned out onto the streets or ended up in prison. By nurturing creativity and individual development, it meant to be the antithesis of the massive total institutions of the past. But its structured environment was also an alternative to the chaos and neglect that had replaced them. Although it has moved from a garage to a well-appointed space of its own, CGC continues to provide art classes, studios, and opportunities for artists with intellectual disabilities to exhibit and sell their work.[88] With its respectful and nontherapeutic vision of artistic partnership, the center was an ideal place for Scott to discover her unique aesthetic form. She spent the last chapter of life in contented productivity there. In turn, the widespread recognition of her accomplishment brought the CGC to the attention of celebrities and art-world luminaries who now help fund it and promote its mission.

The CGC is nothing like the bleak environments Scott endured for most of her life. It is a warm and stimulating place, staffed by caring and thoughtful people and tailored to the needs of individual artists. But I would still describe it as an institution, according to the definition followed in this chapter. Dedicated as she was to securing her sister's release, Joyce had no intention of becoming Judith's full-time caregiver, nor was Judith capable of living independently after so many decades of confinement. When Judith stayed with Joyce while they sought appropriate housing, it became clear that she could not live with her sister permanently. She demanded Joyce's undivided attention and needed supervision, since years of restriction caused her to hoard, steal, and overeat. "I work long, irregular hours, and I can't provide the care and constancy that Judy will need in the years to come," Joyce wrote in her memoir. She hoped to find a living situation that would provide Judith "a sense of family, where she can spend her time with people who love and appreciate her. A place that will welcome us as her family." The right living environment would be *familial*, in that it would provide the kind of loving, attentive care associated with the ideal, if not the realities, of family, without replacing her family, which wanted to participate actively in her life. This proved hard to find. The first group home they tried limited Joyce's access to her sister. The entrance was guarded by a forbidding security gate, and residents spent their time watching TV, without social stimulation. Eventually, Joyce was lucky enough to find a more homey alternative, where staff were loving and attentive, and the residents occupied in a range of activities.[89] A group home is still an institution, but one that is smaller, embedded in a local community, and, in this case, more personalized and flexible. It provided Judith with supported room and board. On weekdays she was transported by bus to CGC, where she spent her time in absorbing and meaningful activity. This was how Judith Scott lived happily until her death in 2005.

Scott's art is abstract, but read carefully, it has many stories to tell. One sculpture strikes me as particularly emblematic of her tenure at CGC. Where she typically worked with materials of different colors and textures, this one is all white and made entirely from a single medium, the rough kind of paper towels that come in a big unserrated roll designed for a public bathroom or kitchen (figure 7.2). Scott made it during a period when the CGC was undergoing seismic retrofitting, and other clients had been moved out of the studio. Since she had difficulty with transitions, she was allowed to remain in her usual workspace in a mostly empty building, with construction taking place around her. This is a case where deafness was a benefit, since she was undisturbed by the noise. Such a flexible environment, responsive to the temperament and capacities of individual clients, is a hallmark of successful institutional care. One day a staff member noticed that all of the center's paper towel dispensers were empty. On further investigation, he discovered that Scott had used them to create a sculpture.[90] The transformation of an expendable, everyday product into art exemplifies Scott's creative sensibility. Art making was a passion that she approached with compulsive energy, making do with whatever material was at hand. Like Marcel Duchamp's Readymades, Scott's sculpture converts the paper towels into an object deserving of visual contemplation, achieving the modernist goal of defamiliarization. Elevated to the status of art, this knotted bundle of paper towels can no longer be touched.

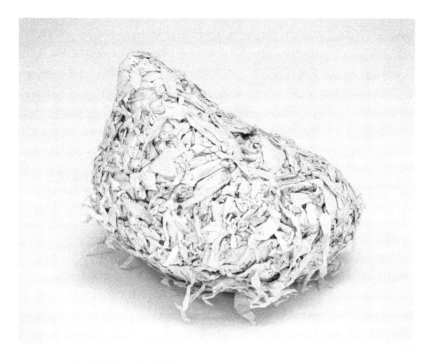

FIGURE 7.2 Judith Scott, *Untitled*, 1994.

Source: © Creative Growth Center.

But it invites us to reflect on the process that turned the most ordinary, impermanent, and accessible of things into a work of art and the creative vision that recognized their potential. Ingrained in its knotted surfaces is a record of the artist's painstaking and inventive efforts.

The paper towel sculpture speaks to me of the best kind of institutional care but also of institutionalization at its worst. A bleak, unstimulating environment with little respect for personal space or possessions might encourage accumulation of ordinary things. Denied a language, Scott was forced to find alternative means of communication, using the resources available to her. In a freer, more engaging environment, she created art that reflects a reverence for found objects and a capacity to make do with the material at hand. I can also see the paper towels—metamorphosed into a thing of intricate beauty—as a striking protest against a society that treats some people as expendable. In Scott's hands, they are rescued from inevitable disposal, preserved instead in a medium that invites the viewer to appreciate them in a new way. Scott's art is born of interdependency, not with a single caregiver but with organizations of distributed care, some more generative and humane than others. It is a testament to how a functional institution can promote self-expression and nurture creativity with an environment flexible enough to enable rather than restrict.

Institutions, as I have defined them, are essential to a just society where dependent people receive the care that they need and where care workers are fairly compensated for the work they do. This is an ideal, a utopian vision, not a solution, and it is particular to my own time and place. I write from a position embedded in the real world, where dependent people and those who care for them continue to be devalued and where institutions are often places of social death. But even in this imperfect world there continue to be experiments with caring institutions—nursing homes, hospitals, hospice centers, congregate residences—that are better alternatives to the grim counterparts of the past, as well as the home-based tradition where women do the unpaid work of care or hire other women to do it for them. There are too many prisons and not enough of the right kind of institutions to go around. The good ones usually come with a price that makes them inaccessible to most. We need ways to scale up access and worker salaries while also scaling down the cost to consumers. But before that, we need to change how we imagine caring institutions, as part of a renewed appreciation for dependent people and their caregivers. Where the literary examples of institutional care that initially sparked my imagination tend toward grim realism, I hope that other critics will extend these insights by looking to speculative and experimental literary works that attempt to envision what those livable institutions would look like.

The narratives considered in this chapter identify many of the wrongs of institutional care. But they also show how and why an institution can get things right. Time and space are key factors in the success or failure of institutions. At their worst, institutions follow the social logic of capitalism, prioritizing cost cutting and increased efficiency that compromise care for residents and staff. In such contexts, caring people have to steal opportunities to show generosity, compassion, and respect. Over time, even the most well meaning are likely to be worn down and their resources depleted. At their most functional, institutions can provide time and space apart from a world driven by productivity and speed, as well as respite for families of dependent persons. Even if institutional time is boring and empty, it can sometimes be healing, and it can sometimes encourage creativity. Time management can provide order, structure, and stability to care for those overwhelmed by a chaotic world. But it needs to be balanced by flexible time, with at least some aspects of care organized around individual needs rather than a clock.

Sheltered time for some is also a workday for others. As we reimagine the value and personhood of dependent people, we also need to adequately reward the time of those who do the work of sustaining them. Space is equally important to institutional success. When people with similar needs are grouped together, it is easier to forget them, making them easy targets for abuse. But a shared environment can be better designed to facilitate care by aspiring to meet the needs of the body, fostering human relatedness and relatedness to other living beings.[91] A residential institution is also a community of sorts, a shared space where strangers coexist within a designated environment, with rules and conventions of its own. It can be toxic and depressing, but it can also be a source of sociability, respite, and belonging.

Where does this chapter leave us? The movement from home to institutions followed by this book might suggest a return to care as confinement, control, and concealment. But the organization of my chapters is not intended to reflect a historical development, progressive or otherwise, or to build toward a desired outcome. Instead, it tries to replicate the concentric circles of care itself, which begins with the most primal interdependency of mothering and radiates outward to shared living environments and from there to larger social networks and organizations that can sustain, confine, or abandon. Institution and family should not and need not be inimical, nor do they necessarily correspond to the best and worst extremes of care. Earlier chapters show that home and family are not always an ideal setting for care. By putting dependency, care, and work front and center of our vision of a just society, it becomes clear that there is no one-size-fits-all solution. Any reform will require a diverse array of institutions, ones dedicated to care that is more flexible, particularized, and equitably distributed.

CARING MACHINES, AN EPILOGUE

Carers aren't machines." So says Kathy, the worn-out narrator of Kazuo Ishiguro's novel *Never Let Me Go* (2005). "You try and do your best for every donor, but in the end, it wears you down. You don't have unlimited patience and energy."[1] Kathy belongs to an underclass of human clones who are bred to donate their organs. But first they are trained to serve as caregivers to the current generation of donors, the group of clones just ahead of them. With time, that emotional labor leaves them too depleted to care much about their own thriving, let alone care for anyone else. At that point they are harvested to death. *Never Let Me Go* is fiction, but it portrays a world much like our own, where some people are destined to serve as caregivers, worn down by the work of promoting the well-being and health of others.

Ishiguro would return to the subject of care work in his 2021 novel, *Klara and the Sun*. Its plot is very similar, except this time the protagonist-narrator *is* a machine. *Klara* is also set in a futuristic but eerily familiar world where technology is redefining the meaning of work, personhood, and humanity. The eponymous protagonist, Klara, is a humanoid robot called an Artificial Friend. She is designed as a companion for teens who have been genetically enhanced to promote superior intellectual powers and learning capability. Klara is built and programmed to be an ideal caregiver. She is small and unobtrusive, with unlimited patience, energy that can be recharged by the sun, and unquestioning acceptance of her social position. She is not a servant or a housekeeper, doing little physical work to maintain the home or the well-being of her teen, Josie. She is not insulted at being (wrongly) described as incapable of feeling or likened to "a vacuum cleaner," does not mind living in a utility closet, and stands quietly with her face to the wall when her presence is unwanted.[2] Klara is also highly perceptive and capable of learning from her environment, attending to Josie with exacting care.

Klara and the Sun explores the consequences of allowing machines to do emotional labor once considered unique to human beings. Although robots now routinely do a wide variety of care work in medical settings, many people would draw the line at the affective dimensions of care. Compassion, empathy, attunement, reciprocity, and all the other virtuous feelings associated with good care, they argue, are exclusive to relationships between one human person and another. A robot can perform the actions of care, but it cannot experience emotions authentic to a caring exchange, and any reciprocal feelings it generates in a care recipient are inauthentic. Ishiguro's Klara suggests otherwise, her first-person narrative showing a clear capacity for both caring emotions and activity, as well as incredulity at human expressions of uncaring like selfishness, greed, ambition, and cruelty. Ultimately, the novel is less concerned with asking whether robots *can* care than it is with the way our technologies reflect back human needs and desires.

Taking Ishiguro's lead, this book concludes with a brief consideration of caring machines that tries to avoid the kinds of alarmism or complacency that often surround such topics. Instead, I focus on how nonliving actors might become partners, extensions, or supplements that extend our networks of care to include more humans, other living beings, and the environment. I share Ishiguro's recognition that attitudes toward our caring machines are always already informed by questions about human relatedness. Whether care is a uniquely human relation is a question that has preoccupied moral philosophers, who ask how and if it can be extended to include other living beings, as well as the environment.[3] Many believe that humans and animals can form reciprocal caring relationships, and some would include nonsentient lives, as well as the ecosystems that encompass and sustain them. The increasing sophistication of our technologies prompts further questions about whether aliveness is a fundamental requirement of all parties in a caring relationship, whether a nonliving thing is capable of providing or receiving our care, and the implications of such thinking for human dependents and their caregivers.

I am drawn to these questions by witnessing my son's unusual relationship to people and things. Henry needs exceptional amounts of care, of the kind that involves sustained and individualized attention from other people. I have filled out so many surveys and assessments of his abilities that I can run through the litany in my sleep. He needs assistance with tasks of daily living, decision making, and social interactions. And he reciprocates by forming intense, loving connections to people who care for him. But Henry also invests a great amount of thought and emotional energy into caring for and with things that include puppets and stuffed animals, plastic figurines and action figures, a medical model of the human body, and, for a time, a special cup and spoon. His things are not designed to be sentient, like Ishiguro's Klara, but to him they have vitality and responsiveness that is as real and satisfying as any human relationship. Things are not in any way a replacement for human care, but they are a valued supplement without which his life would be diminished.

In one mood, Henry responds to human care by radiating pleasure and appreciation. In another, he wants nothing from other humans, absorbing himself completely in the world of thingly companions we call his "friends." After extended contact with other people or the world outside our home, he recuperates by retreating into the society of things. Some might find it sad that my son does not have friends who are other human children. As a younger child, he didn't like to go on play dates or attend birthday parties. As a teen, he doesn't want to join other students from his high school who hang out on the corner to socialize and eat junk food. If asked who his friends are, he might say "Yoda," a teacher, or "Angela," his sixtysomething caregiver. Those of us who know him well cannot deny the happiness, companionship, and encouragement he receives from his thingly friends. We see him respond to them with gentleness and affection. They are patient listeners who make him laugh and comfort him after a hard day. What more could anyone ask of a good friendship?

Henry motivates me to end this book by thinking beyond care for and among human animals, to care for and by the world of things. I feel justified in moving directly from humans to the nonliving world because so much has already been written on caring relationships among humans and animals and even humans and plants.[4] Raising Henry, and knowing him intimately, I see how his mind is ideally suited to form meaningful relationships with things. He struggles with concepts and skills that come easily to more typical peers but is correspondingly attuned to other perceptions and frequencies. Perhaps it is a form of ableism to restrict our consideration of care to human, sentient, or even living participants. Without denying that all human beings need the care of other humans, perhaps we should acknowledge that some people have passionate, caring relationships to things and that sometimes such connections are more meaningful than their relationships to other humans. Perhaps we should see them as models for how things can be enlisted in the service of human care and well-being.

There is no denying that modernity involves living and working in the company of things that care for us, from devices that track our moods, vital signs, and daily nutrition to rooms that adjust the temperature to keep us comfortable and machines that make us coffee in the morning and lull us to sleep at night. A cheerful voice calls to tell me that my prescription is ready; a chair massages my body while I get a pedicure; if my apartment were less cluttered, I might own a Roomba to vacuum while I'm out for the day. Machines are now widely used in medical care to do work like lifting bodies, making deliveries, dispensing medications, monitoring vital signs, and handling hazardous chemicals.[5] It is perfectly reasonable to accept that machines can enhance human health and productivity in these and many other ways, while also believing that some qualities are unique to human animals and should not be done by robots or other machines, no matter how sentient.

The affective dimensions of care are high on the list of qualities deemed particular to humans, or at least to sentient beings. Robots designed to perform the emotional work of human care providers are especially provocative. Once the stuff of science fiction, robots are increasingly appearing in medical settings, homes, and long-term care environments, where they don't just do manual labor but also comfort, entertain, protect, and nurture. There are now robot nannies, nurses, and elder companions that tell jokes, lead exercise classes, and snuggle. Watching them in action can teach us about the possibilities and limits of our current technologies, as well as help us identify the qualities we believe are exclusive to care among human beings, the meaning and value of reciprocity, and the role of affect in caring relationships. As robots become more perceptive, intelligent, and educable, it will be important for individuals, but also for societies, to consider the ethics of inviting them to participate in the care of vulnerable and dependent people.

Robots inhabited our imaginative life long before scientists developed the technology to build them. When Ishiguro wrote *Klara*, he contributed to a body of literary fiction that has been exploring our relationship to anthropomorphic machines for several centuries. The interest has been consistent, but attitudes toward robots vary considerably across times and cultures. In U.S. culture, stories of robot caregivers often have a dystopian cast. In films and TV shows like *Battlestar Galactica*, *2020: A Space Odyssey*, and *The Terminator*, robots designed to serve develop intelligence that allows them to dominate their human makers, a possibility some now see in real-life AI technologies.[6] When robots take over in fiction, their aims are rarely benign. They are fully capable of an anthropomorphic lust for power and control but show no capacity to care, lacking the human virtues of empathy, spontaneity, and mutual recognition. If their enhanced powers include emotional intelligence, they use it to manipulate, rather than sustain, their human creators.

Even fictive robots built to be caregivers easily get out of control, making them potent symbols for human fears about mechanization. In Philip K. Dick's classic 1955 short story "Nanny," parents of the future buy robots to care for their children.[7] But the features designed to help robot nannies protect their charges work all too well, causing them to engage in increasingly violent combat with one another. An arms race ensues, and nannies begin a campaign of mutual destruction, requiring families to buy bigger, newer, and better-weaponized nanny models to keep their children and property safe. Caregiving that prioritizes relationships, stimulating activities, and emotional support takes a back seat to protection and defense. Dick's story clearly reflects on the values of a dystopian Cold War society that puts security above cooperation, companionship, or nurture.

This dystopian view of mechanized care was countered by another set of cultural narratives depicting robots as beloved and loyal caregivers. Isaac Asimov's 1940s short story "Robbie" is about a girl's bond with her robot caregiver. Fearing the child has become too attached, her parents give the robot away. But Robbie's devotion persists. The adults change their minds after the robot saves their daughter's life, convincing them of its capacity for loyalty and compassion and the benefits of its relationship with the girl.[8] Benevolent robots are also the subjects of children's animated films such as *Wall-E*, *Big Hero Six*, *The Iron Giant*, and *The Wild Robot*. When my sons were younger, they loved a picture book called *Boy + Bot*, about a friendship between a boy and a robot where each learns to respect the other's different needs. Henry's favorite Star Wars characters are the droids C3PO, R2D2, and BB8, which combine a robot's mechanical wizardry with humanoid attributes such as loyalty, distress, and sense of humor.

Compared to the United States, Japan has a far more robust culture of robot appreciation.[9] Some connect this difference in attitude to Shinto, a religious system that recognizes the personhood and spirit of objects, as well as living beings.[10] The lines between the natural and artificial, the living and the inanimate, are fluid, a porosity to be affirmed rather than feared or avoided. Whether or not it is grounded in religious philosophy, Japan's affection for robots is unquestionable. Ishiguro's gentle, charismatic Klara gestures to his Japanese ancestry, although his novel also includes sinister technologies that bespeak the more robot-skeptical Britain where he makes his home.[11] Klara speaks to a lineage of robots that are not only benign but friendly and sociable. They are not antagonists but welcome companions. Generations of young Japanese fans devoured manga comics and an animated TV serial about the child-robot Astro Boy. Children's stories about human-robot sociality reflect a more positive attitude toward robots in general and greater acceptance of a future where robots' emotional intelligence is enhanced. Thus it is not surprising that Japan has been at the forefront of experiments with actual robot caregivers. In the 1990s, the adorable, humanoid PaPeRo was developed to entertain and protect children at home and in daycare centers.[12] A 2018 news story describes twenty different robot models used in an elder care facility in Tokyo, where residents and staff welcome them as helpers and companions.[13] Robopets are popular, widespread, and affordable.[14]

Like it or not, the robots of science fiction are a reality, and they are increasingly participating in the affective dimensions of care in Japan and elsewhere. Their most popular job is to provide entertainment and companionship to elderly dependents in assisted living and nursing homes. Researchers cite evidence that robot companions bring cheer, comfort, sociability, and safety to dependent older people. They are said to promote social interactions among humans, offer encouragement with rehabilitation and therapy, and calm anxiety and stress. They also purportedly improve the quality of human caregivers' performance.[15] News of robots in elder care facilities in Japan, Europe, and the United States often touts their positive impact, reporting successes like Zora, a robot nurse in a French nursing home; Stevie, the socially assistive robot in a retirement community in Washington, DC; and Paro, a fluffy, seal-shaped robot said to help seniors with dementia to be more engaged with one another and their surroundings.[16] In 2019, New York State distributed 1,100 robot pets to combat the loneliness and isolation of elders during the COVID-19 pandemic, with some evidence that they reduced stress and even pain.[17]

Other assessments of care robots are not so positive. Some focus on resources, arguing that it would be better to improve pay and employment conditions for living workers than to use robots for emotional labor that should rightly be done only by humans.[18] Throughout this book we have seen the dire consequences of our continued devaluation of care providers, leaving no question that we should better compensate and dignify the essential work that they do. But we have also seen many reasons why the supply of human caregivers might continue to be inadequate. A more philosophical challenge to care robots concerns whether the affective dimensions of care are unique to humans or, more broadly, to living beings. A cartoon by Dr. Nathan Gray imagines the grim results of outsourcing emotional labor to machines (figure 8.1). It shows a patient who has just received devastating news from her doctor, who tells her, "I've never been good at giving bad news. Perhaps you'd like to spend a few minutes with our hospital's new empathy robot." The slumped, tearful patient radiates her need for comfort. Meanwhile, the obvious target of Gray's joke is a doctor who has failed to build his empathic resources, relying instead on a robot to do the caring aspects of his job. Critics are even more alarmed by situations where a dependent person might not know the difference between a human and an artificial expression of care. "Paro the Robot Seal Aims to Comfort the Elderly, but Is It Ethical?" asks the *Wall Street Journal*. The title of a 2019 opinion essay in the *New York Times* adopted a more decisively negative tone with the question, "Would You Let a Robot Take Care of Your Mother?" The answer should obviously be no, the author arguing that it is manipulative and inhumane to use robot visitors in nursing homes. Even if seniors claim to feel cheered, their responses are sad and inauthentic because they are elicited by a "soulless algorithm."[19] The sociologist Sherry Turkle concurs, asserting that the warm feelings evoked by a companion like Paro are unearned because it is incapable of understanding or genuine reciprocity. Instead of producing real feelings, care robots "hijack memory" by recalling the sensation of being cared for by another human.[20] Not only is the robot incapable of positive emotions conveyed by the best human caregivers, skeptics contend, but of any feeling at all. And if the robot has no feelings, it cannot participate in the positive feedback loop in which a sentient caregiver is affirmed by the response of the care recipient, who knows, in turn, that

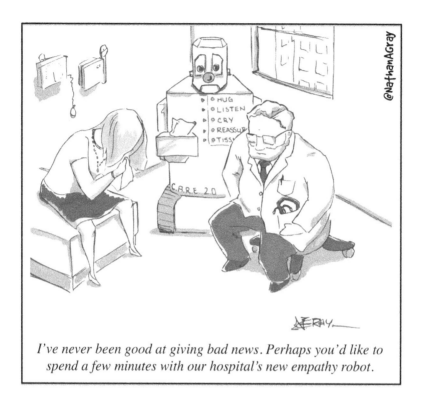

FIGURE 8.1 Nathan Gray, "I've never been good at giving bad news."

Source: *AAHPM Quarterly* (Spring 2018). © Nathan Gray.

their expression of gratitude or comfort is registered by the giver. Instead of making more people feel more cared for, robots perpetuate uncaring, allowing humans to avoid the time-consuming and unproductive work of genuine emotional connection.

This criticism of robot caregivers affirms the unique value of human relatedness, presuming that subjectivity and personhood are rooted in discrete, sentient individuals. Over the course of this book I have emphasized care as an affect and a process. It takes a minimum of two to care, at least the kinds of care that have interested me in this book, but care is not limited to an interaction between two people. The feelings, gestures, and communicative acts expressed in an exchange of care are not isolated within one participant or the other but are generated by their interaction. Accordingly, under certain circumstances, these dynamics may encompass robots and other inhuman actors, each responding according to its kind. Paul Dumouchel and Luisa Damiano argue that thriving with social robots requires not just sophisticated technology but a shift in our understanding of emotion, communication, and relationality.[21] By their definition, emotions emerge from communicative acts between a human interlocutor and others that may or may not be human, which means that emotions arising from a human-robot interaction are no less genuine than any others.

To say something is "artificial" is to emphasize its manufactured quality, but that does not necessarily mean it is false or insincere. "Art" is a part of the artificial, connoting something crafted with intention and intended to elicit feeling. It may deceive or manipulate, but it may also earn more genuine emotion. "The artificial empathy of robots capable of participating in a coordination mechanism is in no way an ersatz empathy, an inferior and misleading imitation of genuine empathy," they write.

> It holds out the prospect of coevolution with a new kind of social partner, artificial agents that can become a part of the fabric of human relationships in something like the way (while allowing for inevitable differences) that we interact with animals, whether they are pets or animals that have been our neighbors for centuries without ever having been domesticated.[22]

By this account, the "coevolution" of care robots would be a reciprocal process in which the development of more sophisticated technologies transforms human attunement to and with them. Together, they generate an affective environment different from but not necessarily inferior to or exclusive of human care. Such transactions may not be exactly the same as a shared connection between two human beings, while still being meaningful and rewarding. In this scenario, the empathy robot in Gray's cartoon is not an absurd replacement for human contact but a supplement for a doctor who is good at detecting disease but less good at emotional intelligence. In an ideal world, this patient has a circle of people who know and love her and provide her with human care. But must we assume that adding a robot into the mix is such a laughably bad idea? In my own experience with Henry, I have learned to recognize situations where the tireless, predictable, and selfless response of a robot might be preferable to the friction that almost inevitably emerges within human interactions. At other times, machines do not replace, but rather facilitate or enhance the emotional work of human care.

When I wrote my first draft of this coda in the summer of 2020, robot caregivers were having an unexpected moment. "The Covid-19 Pandemic is a Crisis That Robots Were Built For," the magazine *Wired* had announced that March.[23] By that point, the virus was already wreaking havoc on established methods of caregiving. Social distancing forced people already prone to loneliness—the elderly, chronically ill, and disabled—into isolation as assisted living, nursing or group homes, and other congregate care facilities turned into contagion hot zones. PPE was a necessary barrier to infection, but it muffled the affective dynamics of health care. We have seen the importance of expression, gesture, and touch to the exchange of care, essential modes of communication that were blunted or impeded by layers of protective clothing and equipment. The fear and anxiety of gravely ill patients were heightened by their distance from health care providers, who were equally traumatized by being unable to provide expected forms of comfort and reassurance. We also know that good care takes time, a scant resource in overcrowded, understaffed hospitals overflowing with patients in crisis. Traditional rituals of care for the ill and dying were upended. Uninfected people faced wrenching separations from friends and relatives dying on the other side of glass windows or computer screens. Sometimes the ill did not even have access to care: Hospitals turned patients away, ambulances did not come, and many infected people simply died alone. In the wake of the pandemic, the emotional trauma of such compromises continues to affect medical personnel, patients, and their loved ones. Our collective inability to provide gestures of comfort and reassurance to those who need it most is a jagged edge in the cultural memory of that time.

Enter the care robots. Some provided a life-saving supplement to human effort, taking on the work of disinfecting, delivering food and medications, and monitoring vital signs. They created an interface for human providers to communicate with patients onscreen while avoiding contagion. They even offered comfort and cheer. A Japanese news outlet reported that robots were used to welcome and entertain patients quarantined at hotels in Tokyo.[24] An overwhelmed hospital in Wuhan, China, gave human staff a break by turning over all patient care to robots for a few days. The robots attended to patients' health and medical needs but also engaged them in conversation and dancing.[25] A skeptic would say that any good feeling experienced by those patients is inauthentic, the pandemic creating one more excuse for the increasing mechanization and impersonality of health care. An alternative view is that the pandemic introduced conditions for a new and not necessarily sinister stage in the evolution of human-robot relations.

Questions about robot care and beyond are fundamentally human questions in that they are driven by human values and motivations. But this does not mean that care is exclusive to human animals or that humans are incapable of developing intense caring attachments to and with other species or nonliving matter. This brief exploration beyond the human allows me to revisit some of the axioms outlined in the beginning of this book, considering how they might be extended to other animate beings, as well as the limits to such expansion. All merit more research and reflection than I am able to provide in this short coda. First, care is always about relationships, but relationships need not always be between one human and another. Sometimes humans exchange care with other species, as well as things. Second, those relationships are not and do not have to be symmetrical. We have seen throughout this book that the exchange of care is almost always uneven, and sometimes it is nonreciprocal, a chain of transmission rather than a give and take. Looking at care beyond the human provides opportunities to further consider the most ethical approaches to such inequalities, and if/when it might be desirable to distinguish care-as-maintenance from other forms of care. Third, the existence of a caring relationship between human and nonhuman actors does not make relationships with other humans any less necessary or meaningful and, under the right circumstances, may free up humans to be better caregivers and receivers. Fourth, care is not an unlimited resource. Because it is not possible to care for everyone and everything equally, it is essential to keep revisiting—on a personal and collective level—the assignment of care responsibilities in search of more just and equitable distribution, including delegating some care duties to nonhuman actors. And finally, if these propositions are true, then extending our sense of obligation and attachments beyond the human enriches the creativity and scope of our ability to care.

When I finished the first draft of this coda, I was still shut in. I had left the introduction and conclusion for last, imagining that I would cap off a treasured leave from teaching to write these important book-ends. Instead, I spent most of my leave on lockdown, caring for my family and trying to care for distant others by staying in. I struggled to live the realities I had described in my own book. Repeatedly, I claim that care can be about not-doing as well as taking action; that care points us to values other than productivity, speed, and growth; that there is meaning and purpose in the small, repetitive gestures of daily life that have typically been assigned to women and other underappreciated workers. And yet it is so much easier to affirm those values in other people's stories than to live them while confined to a small apartment for months on end. I could write those words on a page, I could imagine their theoretical truth, but they did little to change my lived experience. Even at the time, I knew that my frustration and rage were petty in a context where people were dying. So I could add peevishness to my growing list of character flaws. But looking back now, I can also see those bad feelings—and the ease of writing them off as trivial and inappropriate—as the anguish of a caregiver denied respite, appreciation, or compensation for her work. It is possible to acknowledge the validity of those feelings without denying that things could be much worse. Accepting their reality fuels my sense of solidarity with those others who feel forced—by status, nature, or obligation—to care, as well as my commitment to upholding the dignity and personhood of those who depend on the care of others for their survival.

During the pandemic and over the much longer period of writing this book, I have found sustenance in other people's stories about caring and being cared for. Other people's stories are shaped into narrative forms that give them meaning and structure. Other people's stories can offer embodied knowledge and strategies for living that are inaccessible in the dense grind of our own daily realities. It is with this understanding that I offer stories of my own struggles, mistakes, and occasional realizations, as well as my own perspective on the many stories that have educated, sustained, and provoked my work as a critic, a teacher, and a caregiver. I hope that this book has provided some usable tools to read the stories of others in ways more critically receptive to but also more appreciative of the difficult, wearing, and necessary work of giving and receiving care. I make no pretense to solving the many problems of care that have been my subject. But if you close this book a bit more attuned to your interdependency with others and appreciative of the people and things that do work to sustain you, that will be something.

NOTES

CARE: FOURTEEN AXIOMS

1. Eve Kosofsky Sedgwick, *Epistemology of the Closet* (University of California Press, 1990).
2. Being a person who gives care can be both an identity and an action. I have tried to indicate this range by using "caregiver" to denote a personal or professional identity and "care giver" to denote one engaged in the activity of giving care. This system is not always consistent, and the differences often blur.
3. Arlie Russell Hochschild, *The Managed Heart: Commercialization of Human Feeling* (University of California Press, 1983).
4. Elizabeth Freeman, "Parasymptomatic Reading: Medical Kink, Care, and the Surface/ Depth Debate," *Differences* 34, no. 2 (September 2023): 1–26.

INTRODUCTION: WHY CARE?

1. Katy Schneider, "Reasons to Love NY," *New York*, December 14, 2014, https://nymag.com/news/articles/reasonstoloveny/2014/bellevue-ebola-staff/.
2. The most influential modern philosopher of social contract theory is John Rawls, starting with *A Theory of Justice* (Harvard University Press, 1971). The works of feminist philosophy that have most influenced my understanding of the limits of social contract theory are Eva Feder Kittay, *Love's Labor: Essays on Women, Equality, and Dependency* (Routledge, 1999); and Martha C. Nussbaum, *Frontiers of Justice: Disability, Nationality, Species Membership* (Harvard University Press, 2006).
3. A partial list of this work includes Annette Baier, *Moral Prejudices: Essays on Ethics* (Harvard University Press, 1994); Grace Clement, *Care, Autonomy, and Justice:*

Feminism and the Ethic of Care (Westview, 1996); Carol Gilligan, *In a Different Voice: Psychological Theory and Women's Development* (Harvard University Press, 1993); Maurice Hamington, *Embodied Care: Jane Addams, Maurice Merleau-Ponty, and Feminist Ethics* (University of Chicago Press, 2004); Mona Harrington, *Care and Equality: Inventing a New Family Politics* (Knopf, 1999); Virginia Held, *The Ethics of Care: Personal, Political, and Global* (Oxford University Press, 2006); Kittay, *Love's Labor*; Eva Feder Kittay, *Learning from My Daughter: The Value and Care of Disabled Minds* (Oxford University Press, 2019); Eva Feder Kittay, "A Feminist Care Ethics, Dependency, and Disability," *APA Newsletter on Feminism and Philosophy* 6, no. 2 (Spring 2007): 3–7; Nel Noddings, *Caring: A Feminine Approach to Ethics and Moral Education* (University of California Press, 2003); Fiona Robinson, *Globalizing Care: Ethics, Feminist Theory, and International Relations* (Westview, 1999); Selma Sevenhuijsen, *Citizenship and the Ethics of Care: Feminist Considerations on Justice, Morality, and Politics* (Routledge, 1998); Joan C. Tronto, *Moral Boundaries: A Political Argument for an Ethic of Care* (Routledge, 2015); and Joan C. Tronto, *Caring Democracy: Markets, Equality, and Justice* (New York University Press, 2013).

4. See, for example, Gilligan, *In a Different Voice*; Noddings, *Caring*; and Nel Noddings, *The Maternal Factor: Two Paths to Morality* (University of California Press, 2010).

5. Annette Baier, "Hume: The Woman's Moral Theorist?," in *Women and Moral Theory* (Rowman and Littlefield, 1987), 51–75; Gilligan, *In a Different Voice*; Held, *The Ethics of Care*; Noddings, *Caring*; Tronto, *Moral Boundaries*; Sara Ruddick, *Maternal Thinking: Toward a Politics of Peace* (Beacon, 2002).

6. Ruddick, *Maternal Thinking*, 161.

7. Kittay, *Love's Labor*, 24–25.

8. Christine Miserandino, "The Spoon Theory," *But You Don't Look Sick* (blog), 2003, https://butyoudontlooksick.com/articles/written-by-christine/the-spoon-theory/. My thanks to Olivia Breibart for suggesting this connection to me

9. Raja Halwani, *Virtuous Liaisons: Care, Love, Sex, and Virtue Ethics* (New York: Open Court, 2003); Margaret McLaren, "Feminist Ethics: Care as a Virtue," in *Feminists Doing Ethics*, ed. Peggy DesAutels and Joanne Waugh (Rowman and Littlefield, 2001), 101–18; James Rachels, *The Elements of Moral Philosophy* (McGraw-Hill, 2003); Sevenhuijsen, *Citizenship and the Ethics of Care*; Michael Slote, *The Ethics of Care and Empathy* (Routledge, 2007).

10. Noddings, *Caring*, 23–24.

11. Clement, *Care, Autonomy, and Justice*, 1.

12. Gabrielle Meagher, "What Can We Expect from Paid Carers?," *Politics and Society* 34, no. 1 (March 2006): 33–53; Tronto, *Caring Democracy*, 48–49.

13. Ruddick, *Maternal Thinking*, 68.

14. Adrienne Rich, "Adrienne Rich: It Is Hard to Write About My Own Mother," *Lit Hub* (blog), August 24, 2018, https://lithub.com/adrienne-rich-it-is-hard-to-write-about-my-own-mother/.

15. Sarah LaChance Adams, *Mad Mothers, Bad Mothers, and What a "Good" Mother Would Do: The Ethics of Ambivalence* (Columbia University Press, 2014), 4.

16. Sevenhuijsen, *Citizenship and the Ethics of Care*, 13.

17. Evelyn Nakano Glenn, *Forced to Care: Coercion and Caregiving in America* (Harvard University Press, 2010).

18. Donna Jeanne Haraway, *Staying with the Trouble: Making Kin in the Chthulucene* (Duke University Press, 2016).

19. Christine Kelly, *Disability Politics and Care: The Challenge of Direct Funding* (University of British Columbia Press, 2016), 35.

20. Uma Narayan, "Colonialism and Its Others: Considerations on Rights and Care Discourses," *Hypatia* 10, no. 2 (1995): 133–40.

21. Kate Washington, "Leslie's House of Nightmares," *Avidly*, November 30, 2016, https://avidly.lareviewofbooks.org/2016/11/30/leslies-house-of-nightmares/. This memorable article is the basis for Washington's more recent book, *Already Toast: Caregivers and Burnout in America* (Beacon, 2021).

22. Oliver Haug, "Nursing Home and Care Workers Officially the Most Dangerous Job in the U.S.," *Ms.*, August 3, 2020, https://msmagazine.com/2020/08/03/nursing-home-and-care-workers-officially-the-most-dangerous-job-in-the-u-s/; Tanya Lewis, "Nursing Home Workers Had One of the Deadliest Jobs of 2020," *Scientific American*, February 18, 2021, https://www.scientificamerican.com/article/nursing-home-workers-had-one-of-the-deadliest-jobs-of-2020/.

23. Martin Manalansan, "Queer Intersections: Sexuality and Gender in Migration Studies," *IMR* 40, no. 1 (Spring 2006): 224–49.

24. Arlie Russell Hochschild, *The Managed Heart: Commercialization of Human Feeling* (University of California Press, 1983).

25. Julie Beck, "The Concept Creep of 'Emotional Labor,'" *The Atlantic*, November 26, 2018, https://www.theatlantic.com/family/archive/2018/11/arlie-hochschild-housework-isnt-emotional-labor/576637/. In this interview, Hochschild criticizes the expansion of the original term into descriptions of domestic chores, unpaid work, and hidden administrative tasks.

26. Rebecca Brown, *The Gifts of the Body* (HarperCollins, 1994).

27. M. K. Czerweic, *Taking Turns: Stories from HIV/AIDS Care Unit 371* (Pennsylvania State University Press, 2017), 44.

28. On the abundant literature on anthropology and gift giving, I have found useful the account in Anna Lowenhaupt Tsing, *The Mushroom at the End of the World: On the Possibility of Life in Capitalist Ruins* (Princeton University Press, 2015), 121–28.

29. Martha Fineman, *The Autonomy Myth: A Theory of Dependency* (New Press, 2004); Beatrice Muller, "The Careless Society: Dependency and Care Work in Capitalist Societies," *Frontiers in Sociology* 3, no. 14 (2019), https://www.frontiersin.org/articles/10.3389/fsoc.2018.00044/full.

30. In a book published just before this one went into production, Premilla Nadasen argued that the "care-as-work" argument is a distraction from the exploitation behind all paid care scenarios. The real problem, in her account, is not care work but

capitalism as such. While I appreciate the utopian cast to this argument, my own book makes a prolonged case for how and why care-as-work continues to be a valuable frame for securing social justice for dependents and their caregivers in the world we currently inhabit. Premilla Nadasen, *Care: The Highest Stage of Capitalism* (Haymarket, 2023), 18.

31. Kittay, *Love's Labor*, 42.

32. Eileen Boris and Jennifer Klein, *Caring for America: Home Health Workers in the Shadow of the Welfare State* (Oxford University Press, 2012) 9, 16; Dorothy Cobble, "More Intimate Unions," in *Intimate Labors: Cultures, Technologies, and the Politics of Care*, ed. Eileen Boris and Rhacel Salazar Parreñas (Stanford Social Sciences, 2010), 280–95; Glenn, *Forced to Care*, 149–51; Nadasen, *Care*.

33. Arne Elde, *Disability and Poverty: A Global Challenge* (Polity, 2011); Pam Fessler, "Why Disability and Poverty Still Go Hand in Hand 25 Years After Landmark Law," *All Things Considered*, July 23, 2015, https://www.npr.org/sections/health-shots/2015 /07/23/424990474/why-disability-and-poverty-still-go-hand-in-hand-25-years-after -landmark-law; Debra L. Brucker et al., "More Likely to Be Poor Whatever the Measure: Working-Age Persons with Disabilities in the United States," *Social Science Quarterly* 96, no. 1 (March 2015): 273–96.

34. Boris and Klein, *Caring for America*, 209.

35. Lee Edelman, *No Future: Queer Theory and the Death Drive* (Duke University Press, 2004); Jack Halberstam, *In a Queer Time and Place: Transgender Bodies, Subcultural Lives* (New York University Press, 2005); José Esteban Muñoz, *Cruising Utopia: The Then and There of Queer Futurity* (New York University Press, 2019); Rebekah Sheldon, *The Child to Come: Life After the Human Catastrophe* (University of Minnesota Press, 2016); Kathryn Bond Stockton, *The Queer Child, or Growing Sideways in the Twentieth Century* (Duke University Press, 2009).

36. Andreas Chatzidakis et al., *The Care Manifesto: The Politics of Interdependence* (Verso, 2020), 17–19.

37. Kath Weston, *Families We Choose: Lesbians, Gays, Kinship* (Columbia University Press, 1991).

38. Leah Piepzna-Samarsinha, *Care Work: Dreaming Disability Justice* (Arsenal Pulp, 2018), gives examples of queer care collectives while also observing their limitations.

39. Edelman, *No Future*, 1–31.

40. Stockton, *The Queer Child*.

41. Maggie Nelson, *On Freedom: Four Songs of Care and Constraint* (Graywolf, 2021), 171–211.

42. Elizabeth Freeman, "Queer Belongings: Kinship Theory and Queer Theory," in *A Companion to Lesbian, Gay, Bisexual, Transgender, and Queer Studies*, ed. George Haggerty and Molly McGarry (Wiley, 2007), 293–314; Alison Kafer, *Feminist, Queer, Crip* (Indiana University Press, 2013); Robert McRuer, *Crip Times: Disability, Globalization, and Resistance* (New York University Press, 2018); Ellen Samuels, "Six Ways of Looking at Crip Time," *Disability Studies Quarterly* 37, no. 3 (August 2017).

Margaret Price is usually credited with introducing the helpful neologism "body-mind" in "The Bodymind and the Possibilities of Pain," *Hypatia* 30, no. 1 (2015): 268–85.

43. Akimi Nishida, *Just Care: Messy Entanglements of Disability, Dependency, and Desire* (Temple University Press, 2022), 11.

44. James I. Charlton, *Nothing About Us Without Us: Disability Oppression and Empowerment* (University of California Press, 2000).

45. Adolf Ratzka, "The Independent Living Movement Paved the Way: Origins of Personal Assistance in Sweden," *Independent Living Institute* (blog), 2012, https:// www.independentliving.org/docs7/Independent-Living-movement-paved-way .html.

46. Jackie Leach Scully, *Disability Bioethics: Moral Bodies, Moral Difference* (Rowman and Littlefield, 2008).

47. "United Nations Convention on the Rights of Persons with Disabilities," 2008, https://www.un.org/development/desa/disabilities/convention-on-the-rights-of -persons-with-disabilities.html.

48. Danilyn Rutherford, "The Sovereignty of Vulnerability," in *Sovereignty Unhinged: An Illustrated Primer for the Study of Present Intensities, Disavowals, and Temporal Derangements*, ed. Deborah A. Thomas and Joseph Masco (Duke University Press, 2023), 263–76.

49. Faye Ginsberg and Rayna Rapp, *Disability Worlds* (Duke University Press, 2024).

50. Jacques Rancière, *The Politics of Aesthetics: The Distribution of the Sensible* (Continuum, 2006), 9.

51. Tobin Siebers, *Disability Aesthetics* (University of Michigan Press, 2010), 3.

52. Hamington, *Embodied Care*, 35.

53. Amelia DeFalco, *Imagining Care: Responsibility, Dependency, and Canadian Literature* (University of Toronto Press, 2016), 14.

54. Douglas Harper, ed., "Care," in *Online Etymology Dictionary*, n.d., https://www .etymonline.com/word/care.

55. Nancy Fraser and Linda Gordon, "A Genealogy of Dependency: Tracing a Keyword of the U.S. Welfare State," *Signs* 19, no. 2 (Winter 1994): 312–13.

56. Fraser and Gordon, "A Genealogy of Dependency," 311.

57. Fraser and Gordon, "A Genealogy of Dependency," 319.

58. David Garland, *The Welfare State: A Very Short Introduction* (Oxford University Press, 2016).

59. Betty Reid Mandell, *The Crisis of Caregiving: Social Welfare Policy in the United States* (Palgrave Macmillan, 2010), 24.

60. Mandell, *The Crisis of Caregiving*, 20.

61. Glenn, *Forced to Care*, 162.

62. Betty Friedan, *The Feminine Mystique* (New York: Norton, 2001).

63. Adrienne Rich, *Snapshots of a Daughter-in-Law: Poems, 1954–1962* (Norton, 1967), 21.

64. Louise Toupin, *Wages for Housework: A History of an International Feminist Movement, 1972–1977* (UBC Press, 2018).

65. Barbara Ehrenreich and Stephanie Land, *Maid: Hard Work, Low Pay, and A Mother's Will to Survive* (Hachette, 2019); Mandell, *The Crisis of Caregiving*, 9.

66. Elise Gould, Marokey Sawo, and Asha Banerjee, "Care Workers Are Deeply Undervalued and Underpaid," *Economic Policy Institute* (blog), July 16, 2021, https://www.epi.org/blog/care-workers-are-deeply-undervalued-and-underpaid-estimating-fair-and-equitable-wages-in-the-care-sectors/.

67. On the history of hospital care, see Guenter B. Risse, *Mending Bodies, Saving Souls: A History of Hospitals* (Oxford University Press, 1999); Paul Starr, *The Social Transformation of American Medicine* (Basic Books, 1982).

68. Boris and Klein, *Caring for America*, 68–93; Mandell, *The Crisis of Caregiving*, 6.

69. Kat McGowan, "Hospital at Home Trend Means Family Members Must Be Caregivers—Ready or Not," *NPR Health News*, July 18, 2023, https://www.npr.org/sections/health-shots/2023/07/18/1188058399/hospital-at-home-caregivers-family-stress; Glenn, *Forced to Care*, 154–60; Rosalie Kane, "High Tech Home Care in Context," in *Bringing the Hospital Home*, 197–98.

70. For a moving firsthand account of how modern parenting is shaped by such innovations, see Emily Bloom, *I Cannot Control Everything Forever: A Memoir of Motherhood, Science, and Art* (Macmillan, 2024).

71. Glenn, *Forced to Care*, 154–60.

72. Harold Braswell, *The Crisis of US Hospice Care: Family and Freedom at the End of Life* (Johns Hopkins University Press, 2019).

73. Nathan Gray, "Think You Want to Die at Home? You Might Want to Think Again," *Los Angeles Times*, February 16, 2020, https://www.latimes.com/opinion/story/2020-02-16/doctor-patients-send-home-to-die.

74. On the history of asylums, see Licia Carlson, *The Faces of Intellectual Disability: Philosophical Reflections* (Indiana University Press, 2010); Benjamin Reiss, *Theaters of Madness: Insane Asylums and Nineteenth-Century American Culture* (University of Chicago Press, 2008); David J. Rothman, *The Discovery of the Asylum: Social Order and Disorder in the New Republic* (Little, Brown, 1971); James W. Trent, *Inventing the Feeble Mind—a History of Intellectual Disability in the United States* (Oxford University Press, 2017).

75. Nadasen, *Care*, 79–80.

76. Boris and Klein, *Caring for America*, 181.

77. Barbara Ehrenreich and Arlie Russell Hochschild, *Global Women: Nannies, Maids, and Sex Workers in the New Economy* (Metropolitan, 2003); Rhacel Salazar Parreñas, ed., *Servants of Globalization: Women, Migration and Domestic Work* (Stanford University Press, 2001).

78. Anna Romina Guevara, "Supermaids: The Racial Branding of Filipino Care Labour," in *Migration and Care Labour: Theory, Policy, and Politics*, ed. Bridget Anderson and Isabel Shutes (Palgrave MacMillan, 2014), 130–50; Janis Letchumanan, "Filipino Nannies: The Cost of Caring," *Pacific Rim Magazine*, 2013, http://langaraprm.com/2013/community/filipino-nannies-the-cost-of-caring-like-many-foreign-nannies-marilou-tuzon-looks-after-other-families-in-order-to-take-care-of-her-own/;

Susan Gregory Thomas, "Tibetan Nannies: Parents' New Status Symbol?," *NBC News*, September 21, 2009, http://www.nbcnews.com/id/32884630/ns/health-childrens _health/t/tibetan-nannies-parents-new-status-symbol/#.XxGb8pNKj-Z.

79. Eva Feder Kittay, Bruce Jennings, and Angela Wasunna, "Dependency, Difference, and the Global Ethic of Longterm Care," *Journal of Political Philosophy* 13, no. 4 (2005): 443–69.

80. Boris and Salazar Parreñas, eds., *Intimate Labors*; Ehrenreich and Hochschild, *Global Women*; Parreñas, *The Force of Domesticity: Filipina Migrants and Globalization* (Stanford University Press, 2008); Parreñas, *Servants of Globalization*. Martin Manalansan complicates the normative gender assumptions of this critical conversation in "Queer Intersections."

81. Audre Lorde, *A Burst of Light and Other Essays* (Ixia, 2017), 131.

82. Nadasen, *Care*, 13.

83. Hi'ilei Julia Kawehipuaakahaopulani Hobart and Tamara Kneese, "Radical Care: Survival Strategies for Uncertain Times," *Social Text* 38, no. 1 (March 2020): 2.

1. THE FOLDED TIMESCAPES OF MATERNAL CARE

1. Maggie Nelson, *On Freedom: Four Songs of Care and Constraint* (Graywolf, 2021), 210.

2. Sarah LaChance Adams, *Mad Mothers, Bad Mothers, and What a "Good" Mother Would Do: The Ethics of Ambivalence* (Columbia University Press, 2014); Lisa Baraitser, *Maternal Encounters: The Ethics of Interruption* (Routledge, 2009); Talia Schaffer, *Communities of Care* (Princeton University Press, 2021).

3. See for example, Carol Gilligan, *In a Different Voice: Psychological Theory and Women's Development* (Harvard University Press, 1993); Virginia Held, *The Ethics of Care: Personal, Political, and Global* (Oxford University Press, 2006); Eva Feder Kittay, *Love's Labor: Essays on Women, Equality, and Dependency* (Routledge, 1999); Nel Noddings, *Caring: A Feminine Approach to Ethics and Moral Education* (University of California Press, 1984); Sara Ruddick, *Maternal Thinking: Toward a Politics of Peace* (Beacon, 2002).

4. Adams, *Mad Mothers, Bad Mothers*, 1–14; Evelyn Nakano Glenn, *Forced to Care: Coercion and Caregiving in America* (Harvard University Press, 2010), 161–74.

5. Hope Edelman, *Motherless Mothers: How Mother Loss Shapes the Parents We Become* (HarperCollins, 2006).

6. I write about the impact of this experience on my own mothering in Rachel Adams, *Raising Henry: A Memoir of Motherhood, Disability, and Discovery* (Yale University Press, 2013).

7. On crip time, see Alison Kafer, *Feminist, Queer, Crip* (Indiana University Press, 2013); Robert McRuer, *Crip Times: Disability, Globalization, and Resistance* (New York University Press, 2018); Ellen Samuels, "Six Ways of Looking at Crip Time," *Disability Studies Quarterly* 37, no. 3 (August 2017); Ellen Samuels and Elizabeth

Freeman, *Crip Temporalities*, special issue, *South Atlantic Quarterly* 120, no. 2 (2021). On the connection between the delayed and the precocious child, see Andrew Solomon, *Far from the Tree: Parents, Children, and the Search for Identity* (Scribner, 2012).

8. This concept was initially coined in Joel Feinberg, *Freedom and Fulfillment: Philosophical Essays* (Princeton University Press, 1992). It has subsequently been the subject of much debate. See, for example, Dena S. Davis, "Genetic Dilemmas and the Child's Right to an Open Future," *Hastings Center Report* 27, no. 2 (1997): 7–15; Claudia Mills, "The Child's Right to an Open Future," *Journal of Social Philosophy* 34, no. 4 (December 2003): 499–509; Joseph Stramondo, "Disability and the Damaging Master Narrative of an Open Future," *Hastings Center Report* 50, suppl. 1 (June 2020): S30–36.

9. Tanya Selvaratnam, *The Big Lie: Motherhood, Feminism, and the Reality of the Biological Clock* (Prometheus, 2014).

10. Jack Halberstam, *In a Queer Time and Place: Transgender Bodies, Subcultural Lives* (New York University Press, 2005), 18.

11. Leo Kanner, "Autistic Disturbances of Affective Contact," *Nervous Child* 2 (1943): 217–50.

12. Philip Wylie, *Generation of Vipers* (Farrar & Rinehart, 1942).

13. Betty Friedan, *The Feminine Mystique* (Norton, 2001), 295–96.

14. Shulamith Firestone, *Dialectic of Sex: The Case for Feminist Revolution* (Women's Press, 1979), 221–22.

15. Sally Mann, *Immediate Family* (Aperture, 1992).

16. Sally Mann, "Sally Mann's Exposure," *New York Times*, April 16, 2015, http://www.nytimes.com/2015/04/19/magazine/the-cost-of-sally-manns-exposure.html.

17. Debates over bad mothering continue to rage into the twenty-first century, with one example the minor furor over Ayelet Waldman's *Bad Mother: A Chronicle of Maternal Crimes, Minor Calamities, and Occasional Moments of Grace* (Broadway Books, 2009) erupting as I wrote an early draft of this chapter.

18. Lee Edelman, *No Future: Queer Theory and the Death Drive* (Duke University Press, 2004).

19. Nelson, *On Freedom*, 171–211.

20. Rebecca Epstein, Jamila J. Blake, and Thalia Gonzalez Epstein, "Girlhood Interrupted: The Erasure of Black Girls' Childhood," Georgetown Law Center on Poverty and Inequality, 2017, https://papers.ssrn.com/sol3/papers.cfm?abstract_id=3000695; Phillip Atiba Goff, et al., "The Essence of Innocence: Consequences of Dehumanizing Black Children," *Journal of Personality and Social Psychology* 106, no. 4 (2014): 526–45.

21. Joseph P. Shapiro, *No Pity: People with Disabilities Forging a New Rights Movement* (Times Books, 1993).

22. Kingsley and her friend Barbara Levitz collaborated with their teenage sons with Down syndrome, Jason Kingsley and Michael Levitz, to author *Count Us In* (Harcourt, 2007); Michael Bérubé, *Life as We Know It: A Father, a Family, and an Exceptional Child* (Vintage, 1998); Emily Perl Kinglsey, "Welcome to Holland," 1987, https://www.emilyperlkingsley.com/welcome-to-holland.

23. Along with such excellent authors of my parenting generation as Amy Julia Becker, George Estreich, Sara Hendren, Chris Kaposy, David Perry, and Alison Piepmeier.

24. These feminist thinkers include Adams, *Mad Mothers, Bad Mothers*; Nancy Chodorow, *The Reproduction of Mothering: Psychoanalysis and the Sociology of Gender* (University of California Press, 1978); Grace Clement, *Care, Autonomy, and Justice: Feminism and the Ethic of Care* (Westview, 1996); Martha Fineman, *The Autonomy Myth: A Theory of Dependency* (New Press, 2004); Held, *The Ethics of Care*; Ruddick, *Maternal Thinking*; Noddings, *Caring*; Joan C. Tronto, *Moral Boundaries: A Political Argument for an Ethic of Care* (Routledge, 2015).

25. Kittay, *Love's Labor*, 151.

26. Eva Feder Kittay, "Forever Small: The Strange Case of Ashley X," *Hypatia* 26, no. 3 (2011): 610–31.

27. Kittay, "When Caring Is Just, and Justice Is Caring," *Public Culture* 13, no. 3 (2001): 557–79, 567.

28. Kittay, *Love's Labor*, 157.

29. Kittay, *Love's Labor*, 107.

30. "Welcome to Ashley's Blog," http://www.pillowangel.org/.

31. We will see a very different kind of angel in chapter 3, which opens with Tony Kushner's play *Angels in America*.

32. Emily Rapp, *The Still Point of the Turning World* (Penguin, 2013). For an excellent account of terminality in Rapp's narrative see Sarah Ensor, "Terminal Regions: Queer Ecocriticism at the End," in *Against Life*, ed. Stephanie Youngblood and Alastair Hunt (Northwestern University Press, 2016), 41–61.

33. Jennifer Senior, *All Joy and No Fun: The Paradox of Modern Parenthood* (Harper Collins, 2014).

34. Rapp, *Still Point*, 75.

35. The unusual form of *Still Point* becomes more apparent when it is read alongside the more typical arc of Rapp's first memoir, *Poster Child*. Rapp herself is disabled, born with a condition that required the amputation of her leg at age six. She managed well until the onset of painful adolescent self-consciousness. Rapp compensated for her difference by becoming a supercrip, who was completely self-reliant and hyper-achieving in every way. In the end, *Poster Child* deflates this fantasy of endless development, climaxing with a physical and emotional crisis that forces Rapp to acknowledge vulnerability and her need for care. Emily Rapp, *Poster Child: A Memoir* (Bloomsbury, 2007).

36. Rapp, *Still Point*, 48.

37. Toni Morrison, *Beloved* (Vintage, 2004).

38. Marsha Darling and Toni Morrison, "In the Realm of Responsibility: A Conversation with Toni Morrison," *Women's Review of Books* 5, no. 6 (March 1988): 5–6.

39. In the decades since Gayatri Spivak's influential essay "Can the Subaltern Speak?," in *Marxism and the Interpretation of Culture*, ed. Cary Nelson and Lawrence Grossberg (University of Illinois Press, 1988), the subject of a silenced colonial Other has been widely discussed in postcolonial theory and beyond. I see the disabled subject

who is nonverbal because they have no capacity for speech as fundamentally differ-ent from someone who is silenced by oppressive social forces and therefore as intro-ducing a rather different set of ethical questions about being spoken for.

40.   Critics of the tendency to individualize maternal crimes that are socially produced include Adams, *Bad Mothers, Mad Mothers*; Michelle Oberman and Cheryl L. Meyer, *When Mothers Kill: Interviews from Prison* (New York University Press, 2008); Cheryl L. Meyer, Michelle Oberman, and Kelly White, *Mothers Who Kill Their Children: Understanding the Acts of Moms from Susan Smith to the "Prom Mom"* (New York University Press, 2001).

41.   See James Berger's excellent reading of *Beloved* as a response to the Moynihan Report's negative representation of Black mothers: James Berger, "Ghosts of Liberal-ism: Morrison's *Beloved* and the Moynihan Report," *PMLA* 111, no. 3 (1996): 408–20.

42.   The artist did not respond to my request for permission to include images of the series in this book, but they can be seen at https://www.kapharstudio.com/from-a -tropical-space/.

43.   Titus Kaphar and Tochi Onyebuchi, "Seeing the Child: Braiding Possibility," *Gago-sian Gallery* (blog), October 5, 2020, https://gagosian.com/quarterly/2020/05/10 /seeing-child-braiding-possibility-short-story-tochi-onyebuchi-titus-kaphar/.

44.   Quoted from the artist's website, https://www.kapharstudio.com/from-a-tropical -space/.

2. THE ELONGATED TIMESCAPES OF SIBLING CARE

1.   My understanding of long-term temporalities is indebted to Scott Herring and Lee Wallace, eds., *Long Term: Essays on Queer Commitment* (Duke University Press, 2021).

2.   Christina Crosby, *A Body, Undone: Living on After Great Pain* (New York University Press, 2016).

3.   Crosby, *A Body*, 83.

4.   Starting in the 1980s, more studies of siblings began to appear across the disciplines, including Stephen P. Bank and Michael D. Kahn, *The Sibling Bond* (Basic Books, 1982); Prophecy Coles, *The Importance of Sibling Relationships in Psychoanalysis* (Karnac, 2003); Leonore Davidoff, *Thicker Than Water: Siblings and Their Rela-tions, 1780–1920* (Oxford University Press, 2013); Judy Dunn, *Sisters and Brothers, The Developing Child* (Harvard University Press, 1985); Stefani Engelstein, *Sibling Action: The Genealogical Structure of Modernity* (Columbia University Press, 2017); C. Dallett Hemphill, *Siblings: Brothers and Sisters in American History* (Oxford Uni-versity Press, 2011); Christopher H. Johnson and David Warren Sabean, eds., *Sibling Relations and the Transformations of European Kinship, 1300–1900* (Berghahn, 2011); Michael E. Lamb and Brian Sutton-Smith, eds., *Sibling Relationships: Their Nature and Significance Across the Lifespan* (Psychology Press, 2014); Juliet Mitchell,

Siblings: Sex and Violence (Polity, 2003); Susan Merrell, *The Accidental Bond: The Power of Sibling Relationships* (Times Books, 1995).

5. Ilona N. Rashkow, *Taboo or Not Taboo: Sexuality and Family in the Hebrew Bible* (Fortress, 2000), 116.

6. Davidoff, *Thicker Than Water*; Debbie Hindle and Susan Sherwin-White, eds., *Sibling Matters: A Psychoanalytic, Developmental, and Systemic Approach* (Karnac, 2014), 306.

7. Engelstein, *Sibling Action*, historicizes this turn to genealogy, locating its emergence in eighteenth-century England and tracing its radiating social and political impact.

8. Dalton Conley, *The Pecking Order: Which Siblings Succeed and Why* (Pantheon, 2004).

9. On the many ways even identical twins experience inequality, see Conley, *The Pecking Order*.

10. Conley, *The Pecking Order*, 37.

11. Before the era of institutionalization, of course, children with disabilities were also raised at home, but the dynamics of family life, the nature of work, and the distribution of caring labor was much different than in the decades since the 1970s.

12. Licia Carlson, *The Faces of Intellectual Disability: Philosophical Reflections* (Indiana University Press, 2010); Deborah Cohen, *Family Secrets: Shame and Privacy in Modern Britain* (Oxford University Press, 2013); and James W. Trent, *Inventing the Feeble Mind: A History of Intellectual Disability in the United States* (Oxford University Press, 2017).

13. William Faulkner, *The Sound and the Fury* (Vintage, 1984), 339.

14. Victoria Olsen, "Looking for Laura," *Open Letters Monthly Archive* (blog), https://www.openlettersmonthlyarchive.com/olm/looking-for-laura.

15. Olsen, "Looking for Laura."

16. *Rain Man* (MGM Home Entertainment, 1998).

17. On deinstitutionalization, see Liat Ben-Moshe and Allison C. Carey, eds., *Disability Incarcerated: Imprisonment and Disability in the United States and Canada* (Palgrave Macmillan, 2014); Liat Ben-Moshe, *Decarcerating Disability: Deinstitutionalization and Prison Abolition* (University of Minnesota Press, 2020); Allison C. Carey, *On the Margins of Citizenship: Intellectual Disability and Civil Rights in Twentieth-Century America* (Temple University Press, 2009).

18. Diane Kovacs, "Josh: The Lonely Search for Help," *Exceptional Parent* 1, no. 6 (May 1972): 29–30.

19. Kovacs, "Josh," 30.

20. "Child Support for an Adult Child with Disabilities," December 2014, https://www.specialneedsalliance.org/the-voice/child-support-for-an-adult-child-with-disabilities/.

21. Annette Hames and Monica McCaffrey, *Special Brothers and Sisters: Stories and Tips for Siblings of Children with a Disability or Serious Illness* (Jessica Kingsley, 2005); Mary McHugh and Stanley Klein, *Special Siblings: Growing Up with Someone with a Disability* (Brookes, 2002); Donald J. Meyer and Patricia F. Vadasy, *Sibshops: Workshops for Siblings of Children with Special Needs* (Brookes, 2007); Donald J.

Meyer and Cary Pillo, *Views from Our Shoes: Growing Up with a Brother or Sister with Special Needs* (Woodbine House, 1997); Donald Meyer and Patricia F. Vadasy, *Living with a Brother or Sister with Special Needs: A Book for Sibs* (University of Washington Press, 1996); Jeanne Safer, *The Normal One: Life with a Difficult or Damaged Sibling* (Random House, 2003); Brian Skotko and Susan P. Levine, *Fasten Your Seatbelt: A Crash Course on Down Syndrome for Brothers and Sisters* (Woodbine House, 2009); Kate Strohm, *Being the Other One: Growing Up with a Brother or Sister Who Has Special Needs* (Shambhala, 2005).

22. Judy Karasik and Paul Karasik, *The Ride Together: A Brother and Sister's Memoir of Autism in the Family* (Washington Square Press, 2004); Jon Pineda, *Sleep in Me* (University of Nebraska Press, 2010); Akhil Sharma, *Family Life* (Norton, 2014).

23. This was the era when experts, following the research of the psychiatrist Leo Kanner, blamed the icy, withholding "refrigerator mother" for causing autism in her children. Later, Paul shows his mother, Joan, coming across this term while reading David's medical file. "They say that early lack of parental warmth can cause emotional stress," she reports. Karasik and Karasik, *The Ride Together*, 25. Paul has already primed us to reject this view by beginning with neurons, which suggests that David's disability is an inherent feature of his cognitive wiring and has nothing to do with his mother's caregiving or lack thereof.

24. For an illuminating discussion that connects home repair with care work, see Shannon Mattern, "Maintenance and Care," *Places*, November 2018, https://placesjournal .org/article/maintenance-and-care/.

25. Karasik and Karasik, *The Ride Together*, 199.

26. Karasik and Karasik, *The Ride Together*, 4.

27. Karasik and Karasik, *The Ride Together*, 92, 93.

28. Karasik and Karasik, *The Ride Together*, 94, 96.

29. See Ben-Moshe and Carey, eds., *Disability Incarcerated*, xii, 12.

30. Brook Farm, the name of this facility, could not be more ironic. In the nineteenth century, the original Brook Farm was an experiment in utopian communal living. Founded by the Transcendentalists, it was based on principles of "industry without drudgery, and true equality without its vulgarity." More than one hundred years before Judy Karasik, the author Margaret Fuller was reluctant to assume caregiving responsibility for her intellectually disabled brother, Lloyd, and enrolled him in Brook Farm's school. Ben Reiss has described Lloyd's placement as an early attempt at inclusive education in a community that celebrated difference and appreciated the idiosyncrasy of each member. The contrast between the Brook Farm where David Karasik was abused and its nineteenth-century namesake is evidence that treatment of people with disabilities has an uneven history, certainly not one of consistent improvement. I am indebted to Benjamin Reiss, "Other-Reliance: Disability, Interdependency, and Transcendentalism," *American Literary History* 37, no. 1 (January 2025), for information about Fuller and her brother.

31. Karasik and Karasik, *The Ride Together*, 181.

32. On global care chains that facilitate such arrangements, see Rhacel Salazar Parreñas, ed., *Servants of Globalization: Women, Migration and Domestic Work* (Stanford University Press, 2001); Eva Feder Kittay, Bruce Jennings, and Angela Wasunna, "Dependency, Difference, and the Global Ethic of Longterm Care," *Journal of Political Philosophy* 13, no. 4 (2005): 443–69.

33. Pineda, *Sleep in Me*, 56.

34. Pineda, *Sleep in Me*, 112.

35. Pineda, *Sleep in Me*, 137, 144.

36. Pineda, *Sleep in Me*, 112.

37. The limitations of the diasporic community's attempts to support the Mishra family is another prominent narrative thread that is important to the novel's treatment of care, but it is somewhat tangential to the discussion of siblinghood in this chapter. I hope it will receive fuller analysis by other critics.

38. Sharma, *Family Life*, 88.

39. On the uncompensated work expected of the family, see Martha Fineman, *The Autonomy Myth* (New Press, 2005); and Harold Braswell, *The Crisis of U.S. Hospice Care: Family and Freedom at the End of Life* (Johns Hopkins University Press, 2019).

40. Sharma, *Family Life*, 137.

41. Sharma, *Family Life*, 11.

3. LATERAL KINSHIP AND THE BORROWED TIME OF HIV/AIDS

1. Tony Kushner, *Angels in America: A Gay Fantasia on National Themes* (Theatre Communications Group, 2013), 80.

2. Reading the play in 2021, my students found Belize distractingly problematic, as the play's only character of color. They criticized Kushner for relegating him to the status of caregiver and for offering him no other plotline than as friend and provider to the protagonists. Their concerns are valid, but I also encouraged them to consider the social and literary realities of the time. As Kushner devised him in 1991, Belize embodies the fact that people of color were and are disproportionately employed as care workers and that those they care for tend not to know the full details of their lives. I explore the literary representation of this problem more fully in Rachel Adams, "Modernism's Cares," in *Oxford Handbook of Twentieth-Century American Literature* (Oxford University Press, 2022), 246–63.

3. Andreas Chatzidakis et al., *The Care Manifesto: The Politics of Interdependence* (Verso, 2020), 33–44.

4. Paul Monette, *Borrowed Time: An AIDS Memoir* (Harcourt Brace Jovanovich, 1988).

5. Matthew Lopez, *The Inheritance* (Faber & Faber, 2018), 180.

6. Guenter B. Risse, *Mending Bodies, Saving Souls: A History of Hospitals* (Oxford University Press, 1999), 633, 637.

7. Sarah Schulman, *Rat Bohemia* (Dutton, 1995), 163, 83.

8. Urvashi Vaid, foreword to Amy Hoffman, *Hospital Time* (Duke University Press, 1997) xiii.

9. Kath Weston, *Families We Choose: Lesbians, Gays, Kinship* (Columbia University Press, 1991), 186.

10. Monette, *Borrowed Time*, 68–69.

11. Hoffman, *Hospital Time*, 22.

12. Elizabeth Freeman explains it well, describing family as "a peculiarly queer unfriendly model" of sociality, "for it presumes a range of economic, racial, gender, and national privileges to which many sexual dissidents do not have access—often by virtue of their sexual dissidence itself—and it does not acknowledge what I have referred to as the centrality of bodily dependence and renewal to kinship." Elizabeth Freeman, "Queer Belongings: Kinship Theory and Queer Theory," in *A Companion to Lesbian, Gay, Bisexual, Transgender, and Queer Studies*, ed. George E. Haggerty and Molly McGarry (Wiley & Sons, 2007), 293–314, 304.

13. Freeman, "Queer Belongings," 305.

14. In a more recent example, the queer crip of color author Leah Lakshmi Piepzna-Samarasinha uses "chosen family" throughout the essays in *Care Work: Dreaming Disability Justice* (Arsenal Pulp, 2018).

15. "Terminal Regions: Queer Ecocriticism at the End," in *Against Life*, ed. Stephanie Youngblood and Alastair Hunt (Northwestern University Press, 2016), 41–61. See also Sunaura Taylor, *Disabled Ecologies: Lessons from a Wounded Desert* (University of California Press, 2024).

16. Monette, *Borrowed Time*, 86.

17. Gary W. Gowsett, "The 'Gay Plague' Revisited: AIDS and Its Enduring Moral Panic," in *Moral Panics, Sex Panics: Fear and the Fight Over Sexual Rights*, ed. Gilbert H. Herdt (New York University Press, 2009), 130–56; Timothy F. Murphy, *Ethics in an Epidemic: AIDS, Morality, and Culture* (University of California Press, 1994); Jeffrey Weeks, *The Languages of Sexuality* (Routledge, 2011).

18. Randy Shilts, *And the Band Played On: Politics, People and the AIDS Epidemic* (Viking, 1988), 165.

19. *Killing Patient Zero* (Fadoo Productions, 2019); Jacqueline Howard, "The Truth About 'Patient Zero' and HIV's Origins," *CNN Health*, October 28, 2016, https://www.cnn.com/2016/10/27/health/hiv-gaetan-dugas-patient-zero; Brian D. Johnson, "How a Typo Created a Scapegoat for the AIDS Epidemic," *Maclean's*, April 17, 2019, https://www.macleans.ca/culture/movies/how-a-typo-created-a-scapegoat-for-the-aids-epidemic/; Donald G. McNeil Jr., "H.I.V. Arrived in the U.S. Long Before 'Patient Zero,'" *New York Times*, October 26, 2016, https://www.nytimes.com/2016/10/27/health/hiv-patient-zero-genetic-analysis.html; Helen Branswell, "Patient Zero in AIDS Crisis Was Misidentified, Study Says, Rewriting Early History," *Stat News*, October 26, 2016, https://www.statnews.com/2016/10/26/history-hiv-aids-new-york/; "How Researchers Cleared the Name of HIV Patient Zero," *Nature* 538 (October 2016): 428.

20. Tim Murphy, "AIDS' Patient Zero Is Finally Innocent, But We're Still Learning Who He Really Was," *New York Magazine*, October 31, 2016, https://nymag.com /vindicated/2016/10/aids-patient-zero-is-vindicated-by-science.html.

21. Monette, *Borrowed Time*, 65.

22. Monette, *Borrowed Time*, 194, 268, 314.

23. Georg Simmel, "The Isolated Individual and the Dyad," in *The Sociology of Georg Simmel*, ed. Kurt H. Wolff (The Free Press, 1950), 122. "Couples do not exist in isolation," writes the sociologist Diane H. Felmlee. "They are embedded in social networks that influence them in a variety of ways." Diane H. Felmlee, "No Couple Is an Island: A Social Network Perspective on Dyadic Stability," *Social Forces* 79, no. 4 (2001): 1259–87, 1259.

24. Monette, *Borrowed Time*, 276.

25. Hoffman, *Hospital Time*, 96.

26. Sontag, "The Way We Live Now," *New Yorker*, November 16, 1986, https://www .newyorker.com/magazine/1986/11/24/the-way-we-live-now. My reading of this story is indebted to the excellent insights of Elizabeth Freeman, "Committed to the End: On Caretaking, Rereading, and Queer Theory," in *Long Term: Essays on Queer Commitment*, ed. Scott Herring and Lee Wallace (Duke University Press, 2021), 25–45.

27. I don't include the photograph or other images of the Kirby family at David's deathbed because Frare declined permission to reprint them. I understand and respect the Kirbys' evident exhaustion with the circulation of records of what must have been an almost unbearably painful time. After I explained the contents of this chapter, Frare agreed that I could use a single photo of Bill and Peta because both subjects are now dead. All of the other images discussed in this section can be found online at https://www.life.com/history/behind-the-picture-the-photo-that-changed-the-face -of-aids/. On the fame of the most recognizable image, see Clare O'Neill, "The Photo That Changed the Face of AIDS," *The Picture Show: Photo Stories from NPR* (blog), December 1, 2011, https://www.npr.org/sections/pictureshow/2011/12/01/142998189 /the-photo-that-changed-the-face-of-aids.

28. Susan Sontag, *On Photography* (Anchor, 1990), 6.

29. Richard Stockton, "The Story Behind the Photo of David Kirby That Changed the World's Perception of AIDS," *All That's Interesting* (blog), May 7, 2017, https:// allthatsinteresting.com/david-kirby.

30. It is an interesting footnote to Sontag's story that, as she lay dying of cancer, her partner, the photographer Annie Leibovitz, took pictures of her that would later be published in a book about her work. Annie Leibovitz, *A Photographer's Life, 1990– 2005* (Random House, 2006). In a *New York Times* story around the book's publication, Leibovitz talks about her decision to include rare photographs of people she knew intimately, including the deathbed portraits of Sontag. She equated sharing those photographs with care for those she loved best: "They're the people who open their hearts and souls and lives to you. You must take care of them." Qtd. in Janny

Scott, "From Annie Leibovitz: Life, and Death, Examined," *New York Times*, October 6, 2006, https://www.nytimes.com/2006/10/06/arts/design/06leib.html.

31. See Paula Span, "Colored with Controversy," *Washington Post*, February 13, 1992, https://www.washingtonpost.com/archive/lifestyle/1992/02/13/colored-with-controversy/a362eee9-385b-421c-9943-e2dcd8f33fdc/.

32. Monette, *Borrowed Time*, 86.

33. Stockton, "The Story Behind the Photo."

34. Ben Cosgrove, "The Photo That Changed the Face of AIDS," *Life*, 2014, https://www.life.com/history/behind-the-picture-the-photo-that-changed-the-face-of-aids/.

35. Although the photograph, uncaptioned, suggests a nuclear family, the people in it are actually Kirby's father, sister, and niece.

36. Vaid, foreword, xi.

37. All of these photographs are available online at https://www.life.com/history/behind-the-picture-the-photo-that-changed-the-face-of-aids/#1.

38. Cosgrove, "The Photo That Changed the Face of AIDS."

39. Lopez, *The Inheritance*, 65.

40. Lopez, *The Inheritance*, 154.

4. SLOW EMERGENCIES AND THE CARE-TO-COME: DEMENTIA IN THE FAMILY

1. Robin Marantz Henig, "The Last Day of Her Life," *New York Times*, May 14, 2015, http://nyti.ms/1HiVLas.

2. Henig, "The Last Day of Her Life."

3. To be sure, this is a culturally specific attitude. Some cultures assume that it is the responsibility of a younger generation to provide for an older, as was described in a 2023 op-ed by Mike Dang, "Their Children Are Their Retirement Plans," *New York Times*, January 21, 2023, https://www.nytimes.com/2023/01/21/business/retirement-immigrant-families.html. However, the societies the author describes (such as those of Japan and China) are among the places where the imbalance is most dire. At a certain point sheer demographics will make it impossible to imagine a cycle premised on individual debts accrued and repaid.

4. Elinor Fuchs, *Making an Exit: A Mother-Daughter Drama with Alzheimer's, Machine Tools, and Laughter* (Macmillan, 2005), 1.

5. Rob Nixon, *Slow Violence and the Environmentalism of the Poor* (Harvard University Press, 2013).

6. Quoted in David Shenk, *The Forgetting: Alzheimer's, Portrait of an Epidemic* (Doubleday, 2001), 83.

7. A 2022 report estimated that 10 percent of adults over age sixty-five have dementia, with 22 percent having its precursor, mild cognitive impairment. J. J. Manly, R. N. Jones, K. M. Langa, et al., "Estimating the Prevalence of Dementia and Mild Cognitive

Impairment in the US: The 2016 Health and Retirement Study Harmonized Cognitive Assessment Protocol Project," *JAMA Neurology* 79, no. 12 (2022): 1242–49.

8. Lisa Hetzel and Annetta Smith, "The 65 Years and Over Population: 2000," U.S. Census Bureau, October 2001, https://www2.census.gov/library/publications/decennial /2000/briefs/c2kbr01-10.pdf.

9. "Age Invaders: Demography, Growth, and Inequality," *The Economist*, April 26, 2014, https://www.economist.com/briefing/2014/04/26/age-invaders.

10. Wan He, Daniel Goodkind, and Paul Kowal, "An Aging World: 2015," U.S. Census Bureau, March 2016, https://www.census.gov/content/dam/Census/library/publica tions/2016/demo/p95-16-1.pdf.

11. Neil Sherman, "The Graying of America," *Health Day: News for Healthier Living*, May 16, 2001, https://consumer.healthday.com/senior-citizen-information-31/misc -aging-news-10/the-graying-of-america-110658.htm.

12. Jeff Wheelwright, "The Gray Tsunami," *Discover*, September 18, 2012, http:// discovermagazine.com/2012/oct/20-the-gray-tsunami.

13. "The Impact of Aging Populations," *Nova*, April 20, 2004, https://www.pbs.org /wgbh/nova/article/impact-of-aging-populations/.

14. Alissa Sauer, "Why Is Alzheimer's More Likely in Women?," *Alzheimers.Net* (blog), September 5, 2019.

15. Shenk, *The Forgetting*, 93.

16. Wendy Mitchell, *Somebody I Used to Know* (Ballantine, 2018).

17. Gerda Saunders, *Memory's Last Breath: Field Notes on My Dementia* (Hachette, 2017), 255.

18. Saunders, *Memory's Last Breath*, 52, 75, 124.

19. Saunders, *Memory's Last Breath*, 161.

20. Saunders, *Memory's Last Breath*, 187.

21. Jonathan Franzen, *The Corrections* (Farrar, Straus and Giroux, 2001); Emma Healey, *Elizabeth Is Missing* (Harper, 2014); Erwin Mortier and Paul Vincent, *Stammered Songbook: A Mother's Book of Hours* (Pushkin, 2015); Matthew Thomas, *We Are Not Ourselves* (Simon & Schuster, 2014).

22. Jonathan Franzen, "My Father's Brain," *New Yorker*, September 2, 2001, https://www .newyorker.com/magazine/2001/09/10/my-fathers-brain.

23. Nicholas T. Bott, Clifford C. Sheckter, and Arnold S. Milstein, "Dementia Care, Women's Health, and Gender Equity: The Value of Well-Timed Caregiver Support," *JAMA Neurology* 74, no. 7 (July 2017): 757–58.

24. Fuchs, *Making an Exit*, 157–58.

25. Fuchs, *Making an Exit*, 92.

26. Fuchs, *Making an Exit*, 92.

27. Fuchs, *Making an Exit*, 93.

28. Fuchs, *Making an Exit*, 2.

29. Fuchs, *Making an Exit*, 123.

30. Fuchs, *Making an Exit*, 186.

31. Fuchs, *Making an Exit*, 1, 5, 100, 112, 91, 137, 179, 99.

32. Roz Chast, *Can't We Talk About Something More Pleasant?* (Bloomsbury, 2014), 184, 183.

33. Chast, *Can't We Talk About Something More Pleasant?*, 197, 194.

34. Scott McCloud, *Understanding Comics: The Invisible Art* (HarperPerennial, 1993); Hillary L. Chute, *Graphic Women: Life Narrative and Contemporary Comics* (Columbia University Press, 2010).

35. Chast, *Can't We Talk About Something More Pleasant?*, 210.

36. Elizabeth Freeman, "Caring to the End: On Caretaking, Rereading, and Queer Theory," in *Long Term: Essays on Queer Commitment*, ed. Scott Herring and Lee Wallace (Duke University Press, 2021), 25–45.

37. Eva Feder Kittay, *Learning from My Daughter: The Value and Care of Disabled Minds* (Oxford University Press, 2019), 185.

38. "Emergency," *Oxford Languages*, https://languages.oup.com/google-dictionary-en/.

5. WRITING ON CRIP TIME: OUR DEPENDENT BODIES, OUR INTERDEPENDENT SELVES

1. Rosemarie Garland-Thomson, *Staring: How We Look* (Oxford University Press, 2009), 195.

2. For classic accounts of visual and narrative images, see Richard Brilliant, *Portraiture* (Harvard University Press, 1991); and Paul Ricoeur, *Time and Narrative* (University of Chicago Press, 1984).

3. Alison Kafer, "After Crip, Crip Afters," *South Atlantic Quarterly* 120, no. 2 (April 2021): 415–34; Robert McRuer, *Crip Times: Disability, Globalization, and Resistance* (New York University Press, 2018); Ellen Samuels, "Six Ways of Looking at Crip Time," *Disability Studies Quarterly* 37, no. 3 (August 2017), https://dsq-sds.org/index.php/dsq/article/view/5824/4684; Samuels and Elizabeth Freeman, *Crip Temporalities*, special issue, *South Atlantic Quarterly* 120, no. 2 (April 2021).

4. Moya Bailey, "The Ethics of Pace," *South Atlantic Quarterly* 120, no. 2 (April 2021): 285–99.

5. G. Thomas Couser, *Signifying Bodies: Disability in Contemporary Life Writing* (University of Michigan Press, 2009), 3.

6. Christina Crosby and Janet Jakobsen, "Disability, Debility, and Caring Queerly," *Social Text* 38, no. 145 (December 2020): 77–103, 79.

7. Harriet McBryde Johnson, *Too Late to Die Young* (Henry Holt, 2005), 1.

8. Johnson, *Too Late to Die Young*, 29, 21, 37, 63–64.

9. Laura Davy, "Between an Ethic of Care and an Ethic of Autonomy," *Angelaki* 24, no. 3 (June 2019): 110–14; Martha Fineman, *The Autonomy Myth: A Theory of Dependency* (New Press, 2004); Catriona Mackenzie and Natalie Stoljar, *Relational Autonomy: Feminist Perspectives on Autonomy, Agency, and the Social Self* (Oxford University Press, 2000); Jennifer Nedelsky, "Reconceiving Autonomy: Sources, Thoughts, and Possibilities," *Yale Journal of Law and Feminism* 1, no. 1 (1989): 7–36.

10. Johnson, *Too Late to Die Young*, 180, 251, 51.

11. Johnson, *Too Late to Die Young*, 221.

12. Peter Singer, "Happy Nevertheless," *New York Times*, December 24, 2008, https://www.nytimes.com/2008/12/28/magazine/28mcbryde-t.html.

13. Johnson, *Too Late to Die Young*, 251.

14. On disability and vulnerability to sexual assault, see Stacey Simplican, *The Capacity Contract: Intellectual Disability and the Question of Citizenship* (Minneapolis: University of Minnesota Press, 2015), 68.

15. See the example of Sweden in Don Kulick and Jens Rydström, *Loneliness and Its Opposite: Sex, Disability, and the Ethics of Engagement* (Duke University Press, 2015).

16. Ben Mattlin, *Miracle Boy Grows Up: How the Disability Rights Revolution Saved My Sanity* (Skyhorse, 2012), 69.

17. On the sexuality of people with disabilities, see Rachel Adams, "Privacy, Dependency, Discegenation: Toward a Sexual Culture for People with Intellectual Disabilities," *Disability Studies Quarterly* 35, no. 1 (2015), https://dsq-sds.org/index.php/dsq/article/view/4185/3825; Tom Shakespeare, "Love, Friendship, Intimacy," in *Disability Rights and Wrongs* (Routledge, 2006), 167–84; Tobin Siebers, "A Sexual Culture for Disabled People," in *Disability Theory* (University of Michigan Press, 2008), 135–56; Simplican, *The Capacity Contract*; Holly Anne Wade, "Discrimination, Sexuality, and People with Significant Disabilities: Issues of Access and the Right to Sexual Expression in the United States," *Disability Studies Quarterly* 22, no. 4 (Fall 2002): 9–27; Leslie Walker-Hirsch, "Sexuality Education and Intellectual Disability Across the Lifespan: A Developmental, Social, and Educational Perspective," in *The Facts of Life . . . and More: Sexuality and Intimacy for People with Intellectual Disabilities* (Paul H. Brookes, 2007).

18. Mattlin, *Miracle Boy*, 39, 171.

19. Mattlin, *Miracle Boy*, 67, italics in the original.

20. Ben Mattlin, *In Sickness and in Health: Love, Disability, and a Quest to Understand the Perils and Pleasures of Interabled Romance* (Beacon, 2018).

21. Crosby, *A Body, Undone*, 203.

22. Crosby, *A Body, Undone*, 4.

23. Crosby, *A Body, Undone*, 4.

24. Crosby, *A Body, Undone*, 43.

25. Crosby, *A Body, Undone*, 41, 42.

26. Danilyn Rutherford, "The Sovereignty of Vulnerability," in *Sovereignty Unhinged: An Illustrated Primer for the Study of Present Intensities, Disavowals, and Temporal Derangements*, ed. Deborah A. Thomas and Joseph Masco (Duke University Press, 2023), 263–76.

27. Emiliana R. Simon-Thomas, Jakub Godzik, et al., "An fMRI Study of Caring *vs* Self-Focus During Induced Compassion and Pride," *Social Cognitive and Affective Neuroscience* 7, no. 6 (August 6, 2012): 635–48.

28. For my earlier essay on this remarkable book, see Rachel Adams, "Disability Life Writing and the Problem of Dependency in the Autobiography of Gaby Brimmer," *Journal of Medical Humanities* 38, no. 1 (2017): 39–50.

29. *La noche de Tlatelolco. Testimonios de historia oral* (Ediciones Era, 1971).

30. Gabriela Brimmer et al., *Gaby Brimmer: An Autobiography in Three Voices*, trans. Trudi Balch (Brandeis University Press, 2009), 119, 120.

31. Brimmer et al., *Gaby Brimmer*, 38.

32. Brimmer et al., *Gaby Brimmer*, 29.

33. On the design history of wheelchairs, see Penny Wolfson, *Enwheeled: History, Design, and the Wheelchair* (Cooper Hewitt, 2018).

34. Christian Courtis, "Disability Rights in Latin America and International Cooperation," *Southwestern Journal of Law and Trade in the Americas* 9 (2003): 291–312.

35. Couser, *Signifying Bodies*, 2.

36. Brimmer et al., *Gaby Brimmer*, 31.

37. In addition to *La noche de Tlatelolco*, Poniatowska would write other books that focused on the representation of silenced groups, including *Las soldaderas* (Ediciones Era, 1999); *Nada, nadie. Las voces del temblor* (Ediciones Era, 1988); and, with Deanna Heikkinen, *Hasta no verte Jesús mío* (Ediciones Era, 1969).

38. Brimmer et al., *Gaby Brimmer*, 151.

39. Of the many biographers of Sullivan and Keller, Dorothy Herrmann gives the best sense of the extreme strain the long-term, symbiotic relationship placed on both women in *Helen Keller: A Life* (Knopf, 1998).

40. Kittay, *Love's Labor*, 46.

41. Drawing from queer theory, Robert McRuer has explored how disability shame can be leveraged for political mobilization. The experience of shame stems from awareness that one has violated cultural or social (as opposed to internal) values. McRuer argues that it may be central to recognizing those aspects of disability that are produced by environmental factors rather than deficits of the body. See McRuer, "Shameful Sites: Locating Queerness and Disability," in *Gay Shame*, ed. David Halperin and Valerie Traub (University of Chicago Press, 2009) 179–87.

42. Brimmer et al., *Gaby Brimmer*, 63, 65.

43. Gabriela Brimmer, *Cartas de Gaby* (Editorial Grijalbo, 1982); and Gabriela Brimmer, *Gaby, un año despues* (Editorial Grijalbo, 1980).

44. Juan Epple, "Las voces de Elena Poniatowska. Una entrevista," *Confluencia* 5, no. 2 (1990): 127–29; Patricia Vega, "Gaby, la historia verdadera," in *A gritos y sombrerazos* (Conaculta, 1996).

45. See, for example, David T. Mitchell, "Body Solitaire: The Singular Subject of Disability Autobiography," *American Quarterly* 52, no. 2 (June 2000): 311–15.

6. THEORY OF MINDS: THE IRRECONCILABLE TEMPORALITIES OF PAYING FOR CARE AND CARING FOR WORK

1. Megan K. Stack, *Women's Work: A Reckoning with Home and Help* (Doubleday, 2019).

2. Leïla Slimani, *The Perfect Nanny* (Penguin, 2018), 111.

3. Lisa Zunshine, *Why We Read Fiction: Theory of Mind and the Novel* (Ohio State University Press, 2006).

4. Zunshine, *Why We Read Fiction*, 6.

5. Christina Crosby, *A Body, Undone: Living on After Great Pain* (New York University Press, 2016), 35–43.

6. Mignon Moore, *Making Care Count: A Century of Gender, Race, and Paid Care Work* (Rutgers University Press, 2011), 143; Peggie Smith, "Protecting Home Care Workers Under the Fair Labor Standards Act," Direct Care Alliance Policy Brief, June 2009, http://www.directcarealliance.org.

7. Eileen Boris and Jennifer Klein, *Caring for America: Home Health Workers in the Shadow of the Welfare State* (Oxford University Press, 2012), 106–8; Martha Fineman, *The Autonomy Myth: A Theory of Dependency* (Norton, 2004), xvii, 233; Premilla Nadasen, *Care: The Highest Stage of Capitalism* (Haymarket, 2024), 8–9.

8. Alice Childress, *Like One of the Family: Conversations from a Domestic's Life* (Beacon, 2017).

9. Premilla Nadasen, Tiffany Williams, and Barnard Center for Research on Women, eds., *Valuing Domestic Work*, vol. 5 (Barnard Center for Research on Women, 2011); Boris and Klein, *Caring for America*; Moore, *Making Care Count*; Evelyn Nakano Glenn, *Forced to Care: Coercion and Caregiving in America* (Harvard University Press, 2010).

10. Umberto Cattaneo, Laura Addati, Valeria Esquivel, and Isabel Valarino, "Care Work and Care Jobs for the Future of Decent Work," International Labour Organization, June 28, 2018, 3–4, http://www.ilo.org/global/publications/books/WCMS_633135 /lang--en/index.htm.

11. Cattaneo et al., "Care Work and Care Jobs," 3–4.

12. Viviana Zelizer, "Caring Everywhere," in *Intimate Labors*, ed. Eileen Boris and Rhacel Salazar Parreñas (Stanford Social Sciences, 2010), 270, 267–79.

13. Arlie Russell Hochschild, *The Managed Heart: Commercialization of Human Feeling* (University of California Press, 1983).

14. Dorothy Cobble, "More Intimate Unions," in *Intimate Labors*, 280–95.

15. Boris and Klein, *Caring for America*, 24, 130; Glenn, *Forced to Care*, 134–38.

16. U.S. Department of Labor, *Fact Sheet #79A: Companionship Services Under the Fair Labor Standards Act*, September 2013, https://www.dol.gov/agencies/whd/fact-sheets /79a-flsa-companionship.

17. U.S. Department of Labor, *OSH Act of 1970*, https://www.osha.gov/laws-regs/oshact /completeoshact.

18. Boris and Klein, *Caring for America*; Boris and Klein, "History Shows How 2 Million Workers Lost Rights," *Time*, January 13, 2015, https://time.com/3664912/flsa-home -care-history/; Christina Crosby and Janet Jakobsen, "Disability, Debility, and Caring Queerly," *Social Text* 38, no. 145 (December 2020): 77–103; Glenn, *Forced to Care*; Nadasen, Williams, and Barnard Center for Research on Women, *Valuing Domestic Work*; Moore, *Making Care Count*; Premilla Nadasen, *Household Workers Unite:*

The Untold Story of African American Women Who Built a Movement (Beacon, 2015).

19. "Domestic Workers Worldwide: 5 Key Facts," *WIEGO Blog* (blog), July 22, 2022, https://www.wiego.org/blog/domestic-workers-worldwide-5-key-facts; Jennifer Natalie Fish, *Domestic Workers of the World Unite! A Global Movement for Dignity and Human Rights* (New York University Press, 2017); Nadasen, Williams, and Barnard Center for Research on Women, *Valuing Domestic Work.*

20. Doris Sommer, *Proceed with Caution, when Engaged by Minority Writing in the Americas* (Harvard University Press, 1999).

21. Victoria Brown, *Minding Ben* (Hyperion-Voice, 2011); Emma McLaughlin and Nicola Kraus, *The Nanny Diaries* (St. Martin's, 2002).

22. Mona Simpson, *My Hollywood* (Knopf, 2010), 203.

23. Jamaica Kincaid, *Lucy* (Farrar Straus Giroux, 2002).

24. Simpson, *My Hollywood*, 354.

25. Mona Simpson, "Love, Money and Other People's Children," *New York Times*, July 13, 2012, https://www.nytimes.com/2012/07/15/magazine/nannies-love-money-and-other-peoples-children.html.

26. Simpson, "Love, Money, and Other People's Children."

27. Sarah Kippur, "An American Tragedy by Way of France," *Los Angeles Review of Books*, February 2, 2018, https://lareviewofbooks.org/article/an-american-tragedy-by-way-of-france/; Anna Silman, "*The Perfect Nanny* Author on Why We Can't Look Away from Domestic Horror Stories," *The Cut*, April 9, 2018, https://www.thecut.com/2018/04/perfect-nanny-author-leila-slimani-on-new-york-nanny-trial.html.

28. Slimani, *The Perfect Nanny*, 1, 226.

29. Slimani, *The Perfect Nanny*, 219.

30. John Freeman, "Leila Slimani Doesn't Care If You're Uncomfortable," *Lithub*, April 29, 2019, https://lithub.com/leila-slimani-doesnt-care-if-youre-uncomfortable/.

31. Slimani, *The Perfect Nanny*, 198.

32. Kincaid, *Lucy*, 30.

33. See, for example, Jana Evans Braziel, "Daffodils, Rhizomes, Migrations: Narrative Coming of Age in the Diasporic Writings of Edwidge Danticat and Jamaica Kincaid," *Meridians: Feminism, Race, Transnationalism* 3, no. 2 (2003): 110–31; Moira Ferguson, "Lucy and the Mark of the Colonizer," *MFS Modern Fiction Studies* 39, no. 2 (1993): 237–59; Kristen Mahlis, "Gender and Exile: Jamaica Kincaid's Lucy," *Modern Fiction Studies* 44, no. 1 (Spring 1998): 164–83; Jennifer J. Nichols, "'Poor Visitor': Mobility as/of Voice in Jamaica Kincaid's Lucy," *MELUS: Multi-Ethnic Literature of the U.S.* 34, no. 4 (Winter 2009): 187–207; Ian Smith, "Misusing Canonical Intertexts: Jamaica Kincaid, Wordsworth, and Colonialism's 'Absent Things,'" *Callaloo* 25, no. 3 (2002): 801–20.

34. Kincaid, *Lucy*, 30, 36.

35. Kincaid, *Lucy*, 53.

36. Kincaid, *Lucy*, 161, 163.

37. Kincaid, *Lucy*, 92.

38. Lila Savage, *Say Say Say* (Knopf, 2019).

39. Savage, *Say Say Say*, 125.

40. Eva Feder Kittay, *Learning from My Daughter: The Value and Care of Disabled Minds* (Oxford University Press, 2019), 200, 205.

41. Savage, *Say Say Say*, 135.

42. Savage, *Say Say Say*, 62.

43. Savage, *Say Say Say*, 92, 64.

44. Rebecca Brown, *The Gifts of the Body* (HarperCollins, 1994), 47, 6, 46.

45. Brown, *The Gifts of the Body*, 90, 134.

46. Brown, *The Gifts of the Body*, 94, 119.

47. Brown, *The Gifts of the Body*, 32, 119, 147.

48. Brown, *The Gifts of the Body*, 104.

7. COMMITTED: ASYLUM AS CARE AND ITS OPPOSITE

1. Amy Hoffman, *Hospital Time* (Duke University Press, 1997), 3.

2. Delving into the vast sociological literature on institutions is beyond the scope of this chapter, but I have benefited from Sara Ahmed, who writes in *On Being Included: Racism and Diversity in Institutional Life* (Duke University Press, 2012): "Institutions can be thought of as verbs, as well as nouns: to put the 'doing' back into the institution is to attend to how institutional realities become given without assuming what is given by this given" (21).

3. Liat Ben-Moshe and Allison C. Carey, eds., *Disability Incarcerated: Imprisonment and Disability in the United States and Canada* (Palgrave Macmillan, 2014), ix. Quoting Michel Foucault, *Discipline and Punish: The Birth of The Prison* (Vintage, 1995), 4.

4. Ahmed, *On Being Included*, 26; Peter L. Berger and Thomas Luckmann, *The Social Construction of Reality: A Treatise in the Sociology of Knowledge* (Anchor, 1967), 71.

5. Helen Deutsch and Felicity Nussbaum, "Introduction," in *"Defects": Engendering the Modern Body* (University of Michigan Press, 2000), 2–28; Christopher Gabbard, "Disability Studies and the British Long Eighteenth Century," *Literature Compass* 8, no. 2 (February 2011): 80–94; C. F. Goodey, *A History of Intelligence and "Intellectual Disability": The Shaping of Psychology in the Early Modern Enlightenment* (Ashgate, 2001); Simon Hayhoe, "The Enlightenment and Disability" (Routledge, 2019); Andrew Solomon, *The Noonday Demon: An Atlas of Depression* (Scribner, 2001); Henri-Jacques Stiker, *A History of Disability*, trans. William Sayers (University of Michigan Press, 1999).

6. Wolf Scouller, "Restraining Confinement in Early America," Disability History Association Blog, September 17, 2023, https://allofusdha.org/research/restraining -confinement-in-early-america/.

7. Nancy Fraser and Linda Gordon, "A Genealogy of Dependency: Tracing a Keyword of the U.S. Welfare State," *Signs* 19, no. 2 (Winter 1994): 309–36.

8. Burton J. Bledstein, *The Culture of Professionalism: The Middle Class and the Development of Higher Education in America* (New York: Norton, 1978), esp. chaps. 7–8.

9. Stiker, *A History of Disability*, chap. 6.

10. Benjamin Reiss, *Theaters of Madness: Insane Asylums and Nineteenth-Century American Culture* (University of Chicago Press, 2008), chap. 5; David J. Rothman, *The Discovery of the Asylum: Social Order and Disorder in the New Republic* (Little, Brown, 1971), 109–10; Mary De Young, *Madness: An American History of Mental Illness and Its Treatment* (McFarland, 2010), 82; Solomon, *The Noonday Demon*, 317.

11. Stacey Clifford Simplican, *The Capacity Contract: Intellectual Disability and the Question of Citizenship* (University of Minnesota Press, 2015), 53–55; James W. Trent, *Inventing the Feeble Mind: A History of Intellectual Disability in the United States* (Oxford University Press, 1995), 38–45.

12. Licia Carlson, *The Faces of Intellectual Disability: Philosophical Reflections* (Indiana University Press, 2010); Deborah Cohen, *Family Secrets: Shame and Privacy in Modern Britain* (Oxford University Press, 2013), 87–123; Trent, *Inventing the Feeble Mind*, 35–54.

13. See Trent, *Inventing the Feeble Mind*, 1–34; Stiker, *A History of Disability*, 109–10; Carlson, *The Faces of Intellectual Disability*, 40–45.

14. Walter Fernald, "The Burden of Feeble-Mindedness," *Journal of Psycho-Asthenics* 17 (1913): 87–112.

15. Cited in Carlson, *The Faces of Intellectual Disability*, 41.

16. *Think of Me First as a Person*, dir. Dwight Core and George Ingmire (Library of Congress, 1960–1975).

17. Trent, *Inventing the Feeble Mind*, chaps. 6–7; Cohen, *Family Secrets*, 117–23.

18. Christina Cogdell, *Eugenic Design: Streamlining America in the 1930s* (University of Pennsylvania Press, 2004); Cohen, *Family Secrets*, 102–23; Martin S. Pernick, *The Black Stork: Eugenics and the Death of "Defective" Babies in American Medicine and Motion Pictures Since 1915* (Oxford University Press, 1996); Trent, *Inventing the Feeble Mind*, 164–94.

19. Fernald, "The Burden of Feeble-Mindedness," 98.

20. Cohen, *Family Secrets*, 87–123.

21. Cohen, *Family Secrets*, 102; Cogdell, *Eugenic Design*; Pernick, *The Black Stork*, 80–99; Trent, *Inventing the Feeble Mind*, 168–69, 188–94, 211–15.

22. Carlson, *The Faces of Intellectual Disability*, 53–84.

23. Nick Crossley, *Contesting Psychiatry: Social Movements in Mental Health* (Routledge, 2006); Linda Joy Morrison, *Talking Back to Psychiatry: The Psychiatric Consumer/Survivor/Ex-Patient Movement* (Routledge, 2005); Thomas Szasz, *Antipsychiatry: Quackery Squared* (Syracuse University Press, 2009).

24. *Willowbrook: The Last Great Disgrace*, dir. Geraldo Rivera (WABC-TV, 1972).

25. Burton Blatt and Fred M. Kaplan, *Christmas in Purgatory: A Photographic Essay on Mental Retardation* (Human Policy Press, 1974), v.

26. Azi Paybarah, "The Legacy of the Willowbrook Scandal," *New York Times*, February 24, 2020, https://www.nytimes.com/2020/02/24/nyregion/willowbrook-scandal.html.

27. Ben-Moshe and Carey, eds., *Disability Incarcerated*.

28. Solomon, *Noonday Demon*, 393.

29. Gabriel Mac, "Schizophrenic. Killer. My Cousin," *Mother Jones*, June 2013, https://www.motherjones.com/politics/2013/04/mental-health-crisis-mac-mcclelland-cousin-murder/; "Deinstitutionalization: Unfinished Business" (National Council on Disability, September 2012).

30. Jennifer R. Zelnick and Mimi Abramovitz, "The Perils of Privatization: Bringing the Business Model Into Human Services," *Social Work* 65, no. 3 (July 1, 2020): 213–24.

31. Mac, "Schizophrenic."

32. Treatment Advocacy Center, "Serious Mental Illness Prevalence in Jails and Prisons," September 2016, https://www.treatmentadvocacycenter.org/reports_publications/serious-mental-illness-prevalence-in-jails-and-prisons/.

33. Bonnie Estridge, "Jack Nicholson Did for Shock Therapy What Jaws Did for Sharks: An Expert Argues That ECT Is Really More Effective Than Antidepressants," *Daily Mail*, July 9, 2011, https://www.dailymail.co.uk/health/article-2012924/Jack-Nicholson-did-shock-therapy-Jaws-did-sharks.html.

34. Jonathan Sadowsky, "Electroconvulsive Therapy: A History of Controversy, but Also of Help," *The Conversation*, January 12, 2017, https://theconversation.com/electroconvulsive-therapy-a-history-of-controversy-but-also-of-help-70938.

35. Ken Kesey, *One Flew Over the Cuckoo's Nest* (Signet, 1963), 84.

36. I have written more about Kesey's views on gender in Rachel Adams, "Hipsters and Jipitecas," *American Literary History* 16, no. 1 (Spring 2004): 58–84.

37. Kesey, *One Flew Over the Cuckoo's Nest*, 30.

38. Reiss, *Asylums*, 105–6; Cohen, *Family Secrets*, 87–123.

39. On the history of MacLean, see Alex Beam, *Gracefully Insane: The Rise and Fall of America's Premiere Mental Hospital* (Public Affairs, 2001).

40. Daphne Merkin, *This Close to Happy: A Reckoning with Depression* (Farrar, Straus and Giroux, 2017), 191.

41. Sylvia Plath, *The Bell Jar* (Faber & Faber, 1978), 98, 152.

42. Rivera, *Willowbrook*.

43. Plath, *The Bell Jar*, 170.

44. Plath, *The Bell Jar*, 152.

45. Plath, *The Bell Jar*, 171, 164, 156.

46. Plath, *The Bell Jar*, 199.

47. Susanna Kaysen, *Girl, Interrupted* (Turtle Bay Books, 1995), 168. On MacLean of the time, see Beam, *Gracefully Insane*, 233–44.

48. Kaysen, *Girl, Interrupted*, 94, 55.

49. Kaysen, *Girl, Interrupted*, 94, 158.

50. Christy Ford Chapin, *Ensuring America's Health: The Public Creation of the Corporate Health Care System* (Cambridge University Press, 2017); Linda Gorman, "The

History of Health Care Costs and Health Insurance" (Wisconsin Policy Research Institute, 2006); John E. Murray, *Origins of American Health Insurance: A History of Industrial Sickness Funds* (Yale University Press, 2007).

51.   Kaysen, *Girl, Interrupted*, 95.

52.   A notable exception is Andrew Solomon in *The Noonday Demon*, 386–87, who found the assemblage of mentally ill persons at an institution to be horrifying, their symptoms seemingly exaggerated by proximity to other ill people.

53.   Mary Cregan, *The Scar: A Personal History of Depression and Recovery* (Norton, 2019), 121, 130, 132.

54.   Solomon, *Noonday Demon*, 378.

55.   Merkin, *This Close to Happy*, 191, 187–88.

56.   Other examples include Kay R. Jamison, *An Unquiet Mind* (Knopf, 1995); Lauren Slater, *Prozac Diary* (Hamish Hamilton, 1999); Solomon, *Noonday Demon*; and Elizabeth Wurtzel, *Prozac Nation: Young and Depressed in America* (Riverhead, 1995).

57.   Therse Marie Mailhot, *Heart Berries: A Memoir* (Berkeley: Counterpoint, 2018), 23, 20.

58.   Mailhot, *Heart Berries*, 24, 43, 46–47.

59.   Mailhot, *Heart Berries*, 43.

60.   Thomas Edward Gass and Bruce C. Vladeck, *Nobody's Home: Candid Reflections of A Nursing Home Aide* (ILR Press, 2004), 177.

61.   Gass and Vladeck, *Nobody's Home*, 75.

62.   Gass and Vladeck, *Nobody's Home*, 74.

63.   Gass and Vladeck, *Nobody's Home*, 11.

64.   Mary Douglas, *Purity and Danger: An Analysis of Concepts of Pollution and Taboo* (Praeger, 1966).

65.   Arthur Kleinman, *The Soul of Care: The Moral Education of a Husband and a Doctor* (Viking, 2019).

66.   Rivera, *Willowbrook*.

67.   Gass and Vladeck, *Nobody's Home*, 9.

68.   Gass and Vladeck, *Nobody's Home*, 13.

69.   Tanya Lewis, "Nursing Home Workers Had One of the Deadliest Jobs of 2020," *Scientific American*, February 18, 2021, https://www.scientificamerican.com/article/nursing-home-workers-had-one-of-the-deadliest-jobs-of-2020/.

70.   Gass and Vladeck, *Nobody's Home*, 70.

71.   Premila Nadasen, *Care: The Highest Stage of Capitalism* (Haymarket, 2023), 79–80.

72.   Susan Nussbaum, *Good Kings, Bad Kings* (Algonquin, 2013), 14.

73.   Nussbaum, *Good Kings, Bad Kings*, 42, 81, 39, 102.

74.   Amanda Sakuma, "A Woman in a Vegetative State Suddenly Gave Birth. Her Alleged Assault Is a #MeToo Wake-up Call," *Vox*, January 7, 2019, https://www.vox.com/2019/1/7/18171012/arizona-woman-birth-coma-sexual-assault-metoo.

75.   Nussbaum, *Good Kings, Bad Kings*, 206.

76.   Nussbaum, *Good Kings, Bad Kings*, 157.

77.   Nussbaum, *Good Kings, Bad Kings*, 157.

78.   Nussbaum, *Good Kings, Bad Kings*, 22.

79.   Nussbaum, *Good Kings, Bad Kings*, 35.

80.   Cited in Ben-Moshe and Carey, eds., *Disability Incarcerated*, 14.

81.   Although many of the stories explored by this chapter are grim, there are creative experiments in institutional living that point to a more hopeful future if they can be successfully scaled up. For more discussion of these, see Anne Davis Basting, *Forget Memory: Creating Better Lives for People with Dementia* (Johns Hopkins University Press, 2009); and Atul Gawande, *Being Mortal: Medicine and What Matters in the End* (Henry Holt, 2014).

82.   Eve Kosofsky Sedgwick, *Touching Feeling: Affect, Pedagogy, Performativity* (Duke University Press, 2003).

83.   Joyce Scott, "Birth and Rebirth," *The Outsider* 5, no. 1 (2000): 16–18.

84.   John M. MacGregor and Judith Scott, *Metamorphosis: The Fiber Art of Judith Scott: The Outsider Artist and the Experience of Down's Syndrome* (Creative Growth Art Center, 1999), 50.

85.   Nathaniel Rich, "A Training Ground for Untrained Artists," *New York Times*, December 16, 2015, https://www.nytimes.com/2015/12/20/magazine/a-training-ground-for-untrained-artists.html.

86.   Rich, "Training Ground."

87.   For more on Scott's art, see Benjamin Fraser, "The Work of (Creating) Art: Judith Scott's Fiber Art, Lola Barrera and Iñaki Peñafiel's *¿Que tienes debajo del sombrero?* (2006), and the Challenges Faced by People with Developmental Disabilities," *Cultural Studies* 24, no. 4 (July 2010): 508–32; and MacGregor and Scott, *Metamorphosis*.

88.   Rich, "A Training Ground."

89.   Joyce Scott, *Entwined: Sisters and Secrets in the Silent World of Artist Judith Scott* (Beacon, 2016), 128, 129, 133, 141–42.

90.   Tellingly, MacGregor uses this incident as an example of Scott's tendency to "steal" items that had been left around the center and incorporate them into her art. As Tobin Siebers notes, in the work of a more typical artist this strategy would be described as "using found objects." Tobin Siebers, *Disability Aesthetics* (University of Michigan Press, 2010), 17.

91.   For real-life examples of such enabling environments, see Sara Hendren, *What Can a Body Do? How We Meet the Built World* (Riverhead, 2020).

CARING MACHINES, AN EPILOGUE

1.   Kazuo Ishiguro, *Never Let Me Go* (Knopf, 2005), 4.

2.   Kazuo Ishiguro, *Klara and the Sun* (Knopf, 2021), 97, 143.

3.   Carol J. Adams and Josephine Donovan, eds., *Animals and Women: Feminist Theoretical Explorations* (Duke University Press, 1995); Adams and Donovan, eds., *Beyond Animal Rights: A Feminist Caring Ethic for the Treatment of Animals*

(Continuum, 1996); Leonardo Boff and Alexandre Guilherme, *Essential Care: An Ethics of Human Nature* (SPCK, 2007); Alice Crary, *Inside Ethics: On the Demands of Moral Thought* (Harvard University Press, 2006); Alice Crary and Lori Gruen, *Animal Crisis: A New Critical Theory* (Polity, 2022); Lori Gruen, *Entangled Empathy: An Alternative Ethic for Our Relationships with Animals* (Lantern, 2015); Martha C. Nussbaum, *Justice for Animals: Our Collective Responsibility* (Simon & Schuster, 2022); Martha C. Nussbaum, *Frontiers of Justice: Disability, Nationality, Species Membership* (Harvard University Press, 2006); Val Plumwood, *Feminism and the Mastery of Nature* (Routledge, 1993); Sunaura Taylor, *Beasts of Burden: Animal and Disability Liberation* (Simon & Schuster, 2018); and Sunaura Taylor, *Disabled Ecologies: Lessons from a Wounded Desert* (University of California Press, 2024).

4. In addition to the sources cited in note 3, see Caitlin Berrigan, "The Life Cycle of a Common Weed: Viral Imaginings in Plant-Human Encounters," *Women's Studies Quarterly* 40, nos. 1/2 (Spring/Summer 2012): 97–116.

5. Aimee van Wynsberghe, *Healthcare Robots: Ethics, Design, and Implementation* (Routledge, 2016).

6. Melissa Heikkila, "How Do You Solve a Problem like Out-of-Control AI?," *MIT Technology Review*, May 16, 2021, https://www.technologyreview.com/2023/05/16/1073167/how-do-you-solve-a-problem-like-out-of-control-ai/; Matthew Hutson, "Can We Stop Runaway AI?," *New Yorker*, May 16, 2023, https://www.newyorker.com/science/annals-of-artificial-intelligence/can-we-stop-the-singularity; Kelsey Piper, "AI Experts Are Increasingly Afraid of What They're Creating," *Vox*, November 28, 2022, https://www.vox.com/the-highlight/23447596/artificial-intelligence-agi-openai-gpt3-existential-risk-human-extinction.

7. Philip K. Dick, *Beyond Lies the Wub* (Underwood/Miller, 1987).

8. Isaac Asimov, *I, Robot* (Bantam, 2004).

9. Yuji Sone, *Japanese Robot Culture* (Palgrave Macmillan, 2016); Christopher Bolton, Istvan Csicsery-Ronay, and Takayuki Tatsumi, eds., *Robot Ghosts and Wired Dreams: Japanese Science Fiction from Origins to Anime* (University of Minnesota Press, 2007).

10. Orly Lobel, "In Japan Humanoid Robots Could Soon Become Part of the Family," *Freethink* (blog), January 29, 2023, https://www.freethink.com/robots-ai/humanoid-robots-japan.

11. Chris Stokel-Walker, "Why Britain Hasn't Fallen in Love with Robots—Yet," *Goethe Institute* (blog), https://www.goethe.de/ins/gb/en/kul/zut/rob/22687159.html.

12. Manuel Jose Flores Aguilar, "Robots in Japan: A Brief History," *Wasshoi! Magazine*, n.d., https://www.wasshoimagazine.org/blog/curiosities-of-the-japanese-culture/robots; Lobel, "In Japan."

13. "Aging Japan: Robots May Have Role in Future of Elder Care," *Voice of America* (blog), March 28, 2018, https://www.voanews.com/east-asia-pacific/aging-japan-robots-may-have-role-future-elder-care.

14. Lobel, "In Japan."

15. Ariel Ducey, "Technologies of Caring Labor: From Objects to Affect," in *Intimate Labors: Cultures, Technologies, and the Politics of Care*, ed. Eileen Boris and Rhacel Salazar Parreñas (Stanford Social Sciences, 2010), 18–32.

16. Sean A. McGlynn et al., "Understanding the Potential of PARO for Healthy Older Adults," *International Journal of Computing Studies* 100 (April 2017); Corinne Purtill, "Stop Me If You've Heard This One: A Robot and a Team of Irish Scientists Walk Into a Senior Living Home," *Time*, October 4, 2019, https://time.com/longform /senior-care-robot/; Adam Satariano, Elian Peltier, and Dmitry Kostyukov, "Meet Zora, the Robot Caregiver," *New York Times*, November 23, 2018, https://www .nytimes.com/interactive/2018/11/23/technology/robot-nurse-zora.html; Anne Tergesen and Milo Inada, "It's Not a Stuffed Animal, It's a $6000 Medical Device," *Wall Street Journal*, June 21, 2010, https://www.wsj.com/articles/SB1000142405274870446 3504575301051844937276.

17. Paula Span, "In Isolating Times, Can Robo-Pets Provide Comfort?," *New York Times*, September 26, 2020, https://www.nytimes.com/2020/09/26/health/corona virus-elderly-isolation-robot-pets.html.

18. Casey Brienza, "Book Review: *Pressed for Time: The Acceleration of Life in Digital Capitalism*, by Judy Wajcman," *LSE Review of Books*, April 24, 2015, https://blogs.lse .ac.uk/lsereviewofbooks/2015/04/24/pressed-for-time-the-acceleration-of-life-in -digital-capitalism-judy-wajcman/.

19. Maggie Jackson, "Would You Let a Robot Take Care of Your Mother?," *New York Times*, December 13, 2019, https://www.nytimes.com/2019/12/13/opinion/robot -caregiver-aging.html.

20. Sherry Turkle, *Alone Together: Why We Expect More from Technology and Less from Each Other* (Basic Books, 2011), chap. 6.

21. Paul Dumouchel and Luisa Damiano, *Living with Robots*, trans. Malcolm DeBevoise (Harvard University Press, 2017).

22. Dumouchel and Damiano, *Living with Robots*, 21.

23. Matt Simon, "The Covid-19 Pandemic Is a Crisis That Robots Were Built For," *Wired*, March 25, 2020, https://www.wired.com/story/covid-19-pandemic-robots/.

24. Akira Tomoshige and Akiko Okamoto, "Robots on Hand to Greet Japanese Coronavirus Patients in Hotels," *Reuters*, May 1, 2020, https://www.reuters.com/article/us -health-coronavirus-japan-robot-hotels/robots-on-hand-to-greet-japanese -coronavirus-patients-in-hotels-idUSKBN22D4PC.

25. Leslie Katz, "Coronavirus Care at One Hospital Got Totally Taken Over by Robots," *CNET News*, March 14, 2020, https://www.cnet.com/news/coronavirus-care-at-one -hospital-got-taken-over-by-robots/.

BIBLIOGRAPHY

Adams, Carol J., and Josephine Donovan, eds. *Animals and Women: Feminist Theoretical Explorations*. Duke University Press, 1995.

——, eds. *Beyond Animal Rights: A Feminist Caring Ethic for the Treatment of Animals*. Continuum, 1996.

Adams, Rachel. "Disability Life Writing and the Problem of Dependency in the Autobiography of Gaby Brimmer." *Journal of Medical Humanities* 38, no. 1 (2017): 39–50.

——. "Hipsters and Jipitecas: Literary Countercultures on Both Sides of the Border." *American Literary History* 16, no. 1 (Spring 2004): 58–84.

——. "Modernism's Cares." In *Oxford Handbook of Twentieth-Century American Literature*, ed. Leslie Bow and Russ Castronovo, 246–63. Oxford University Press, 2022.

——. "Privacy, Dependency, Discegenation: Toward a Sexual Culture for People with Intellectual Disabilities." *Disability Studies Quarterly* 35, no. 1 (2015), https://dsq-sds.org/index.php/dsq/article/view/4185/3825.

——. *Raising Henry: A Memoir of Motherhood, Disability, and Discovery*. Yale University Press, 2013.

Adams, Sarah LaChance. *Mad Mothers, Bad Mothers, and What a "Good" Mother Would Do: The Ethics of Ambivalence*. Columbia University Press, 2014.

Addati, Laura, et al. *Care Work and Care Jobs: For the Future of Decent Work*. New York: International Labour Organization, 2018, http://www.ilo.org/global/publications/books/WCMS_633135/lang--en/index.htm.

Aguilar, Manuel Jose Flores. "Robots in Japan: A Brief History." *Wasshoi!*, n.d., https://www.wasshoimagazine.org/blog/curiosities-of-the-japanese-culture/robots.

Ahmed, Sara. *On Being Included: Racism and Diversity in Institutional Life*. Duke University Press, 2012.

Arras, John D., ed. *Bringing the Hospital Home*. Johns Hopkins University Press, 1995.

Asimov, Isaac. *I, Robot*. Bantam, 2004.

Baier, Annette. "Hume: The Woman's Moral Theorist?" In *Women and Moral Theory*, ed. Eva Feder Kittay and Diana T. Meyers. Rowman and Littlefield, 1987.

——. *Moral Prejudices: Essays on Ethics*. Harvard University Press, 1994.

Bailey, Moya. "The Ethics of Pace." *South Atlantic Quarterly* 120, no. 2 (April 2021): 285–99.

Bank, Stephen P., and Michael D. Kahn. *The Sibling Bond*. Basic Books, 1982.

Baraitser, Lisa. *Enduring Time*. Bloomsbury, 2017.

——. *Maternal Encounters: The Ethics of Interruption*. Routledge, 2009.

Basting, Anne Davis. *Forget Memory: Creating Better Lives for People with Dementia*. Johns Hopkins University Press, 2009.

Beam, Alex. *Gracefully Insane: The Rise and Fall of America's Premiere Mental Hospital*. Public Affairs, 2001.

Beck, Julie. "The Concept Creep of 'Emotional Labor.'" *The Atlantic*, November 26, 2018, https://www.theatlantic.com/family/archive/2018/11/arlie-hochschild-housework-isnt-emotional-labor/576637/.

Ben-Moshe, Liat. *Decarcerating Disability: Deinstitutionalization and Prison Abolition*. University of Minnesota Press, 2020.

Ben-Moshe, Liat, and Allison C. Carey, eds. *Disability Incarcerated: Imprisonment and Disability in the United States and Canada*. Palgrave Macmillan, 2014.

Berger, James. "Ghosts of Liberalism: Morrison's *Beloved* and the Moynihan Report," *PMLA* 111, no. 3 (1996): 408–20.

Berger, Peter L., and Thomas Luckmann. *The Social Construction of Reality: A Treatise in the Sociology of Knowledge*. Anchor, 1967.

Berrigan, Caitlin. "The Life Cycle of a Common Weed: Viral Imaginings in Plant-Human Encounters." *Women's Studies Quarterly* 40, nos. 1/2 (Spring/Summer 2012): 97–116.

Bérubé, Michael. *Life as We Know It: A Father, a Family, and an Exceptional Child*. Vintage, 1998.

Blatt, Burton, and Fred M. Kaplan. *Christmas in Purgatory: A Photographic Essay on Mental Retardation*. Human Policy Press, 1974.

Bledstein, Burton J. *The Culture of Professionalism: The Middle Class and the Development of Higher Education in America*. Norton, 1978.

Bloom, Emily. *I Cannot Control Everything Forever: A Memoir of Motherhood, Science, and Art*. Macmillan, 2024.

Boff, Leonardo, and Alexandre Guilherme. *Essential Care: An Ethics of Human Nature*. SPCK, 2007.

Bolton, Christopher, et al., eds. *Robot Ghosts and Wired Dreams: Japanese Science Fiction from Origins to Anime*. University of Minnesota Press, 2007.

Boris, Eileen, and Jennifer Klein. *Caring for America: Home Health Workers in the Shadow of the Welfare State*. Oxford University Press, 2012.

——. "History Shows How 2 Million Workers Lost Rights." *Time*, January 13, 2015, https://time.com/3664912/flsa-home-care-history/.

Boris, Eileen, and Rhacel Salazar Parreñas, eds. *Intimate Labors: Cultures, Technologies, and the Politics of Care*. Stanford Social Sciences, 2010.

Bott, Nicholas T., et al. "Dementia Care, Women's Health, and Gender Equity: The Value of Well-Timed Caregiver Support." *JAMA Neurology* 74, no. 7 (July 2017): 757–58.

Branswell, Helen. "Patient Zero in AIDS Crisis Was Misidentified, Study Says, Rewriting Early History." *Stat News*, October 26, 2016, https://www.statnews.com/2016/10/26 /history-hiv-aids-new-york/.

Braswell, Harold. *The Crisis of U.S. Hospice Care: Family and Freedom at the End of Life.* Johns Hopkins University Press, 2019.

Braziel, Jana Evans. "Daffodils, Rhizomes, Migrations: Narrative Coming of Age in the Diasporic Writings of Edwige Danticat and Jamaica Kincaid." *Meridians: Feminism, Race, Transnationalism* 3, no. 2: 110–31.

Brienza, Casey. "Book Review: *Pressed for Time: The Acceleration of Life in Digital Capitalism*, by Judy Wajcman." *LSE Review of Books*, April 24, 2015, https://blogs.lse.ac.uk /lsereviewofbooks/2015/04/24/pressed-for-time-the-acceleration-of-life-in-digital -capitalism-judy-wajcman/.

Brilliant, Richard. *Portraiture.* Harvard University Press, 1991.

Brimmer, Gabriela. *Cartas de Gaby.* Editorial Grijalbo, 1982.

——. *Gaby Brimmer: An Autobiography in Three Voices.* Trans. Trudi Balch. Brandeis University Press, 2009.

——. *Gaby, un año despues.* Editorial Grijalbo, 1980.

Brimmer, Gabriela, and Elena Poniatowska. *Gaby Brimmer.* Editorial Grijalbo, 1979.

Brown, Rebecca. *The Gifts of the Body.* HarperCollins, 1994.

Brown, Victoria. *Minding Ben.* Hyperion, 2011.

Brucker, Debra L., et al. "More Likely to Be Poor Whatever the Measure: Working-Age Persons with Disabilities in the United States." *Social Science Quarterly* 96, no. 1 (March 2015): 273–96.

Carey, Allison C. *On the Margins of Citizenship: Intellectual Disability and Civil Rights in Twentieth-Century America.* Temple University Press, 2009.

Carlson, Licia. *The Faces of Intellectual Disability : Philosophical Reflections.* Indiana University Press, 2010.

Chapin, Christy Ford. *Ensuring America's Health: The Public Creation of the Corporate Health Care System.* Cambridge University Press, 2017.

Charlton, James I. *Nothing About Us Without Us: Disability Oppression and Empowerment.* University of California Press, 2000.

Chast, Roz. *Can't We Talk About Something More Pleasant?* Bloomsbury, 2014.

Chatzidakis, Andreas, et al. *The Care Manifesto: The Politics of Interdependence.* Verso, 2020.

Childress, Alice. *Like One of the Family: Conversations from a Domestic's Life.* Beacon, 2017.

Chodorow, Nancy. *The Reproduction of Mothering: Psychoanalysis and the Sociology of Gender.* University of California Press, 1978.

Chute, Hillary L. *Graphic Women: Life Narrative and Contemporary Comics.* Columbia University Press, 2010.

Clement, Grace. *Care, Autonomy, and Justice: Feminism and the Ethic of Care.* Westview, 1996.

Cobble, Dorothy Sue. "More Intimate Unions." In *Intimate Labors: Cultures, Technologies, and the Politics of Care*, ed. Eileen Boris and Rhacel Salazar Parreñas, 280–95. Stanford Social Sciences, 2010.

Cogdell, Christina. *Eugenic Design: Streamlining America in the 1930s*. University of Pennsylvania Press, 2004.

Cohen, Deborah. *Family Secrets: Shame and Privacy in Modern Britain*. Oxford University Press, 2013.

Coles, Prophecy. *The Importance of Sibling Relationships in Psychoanalysis*. Karnac, 2003.

Conley, Dalton. *The Pecking Order: Which Siblings Succeed and Why*. Pantheon, 2004.

Cosgrove, Ben. "The Photo That Changed the Face of AIDS." *Life*, 2014, https://www.life .com/history/behind-the-picture-the-photo-that-changed-the-face-of-aids/.

Courtis, Christian. "Disability Rights in Latin America and International Cooperation." *Southwestern Journal of Law and Trade in the Americas* 9 (2003): 291–312.

Couser, G. Thomas. *Signifying Bodies: Disability in Contemporary Life Writing*. University of Michigan Press, 2009.

Crary, Alice. *Inside Ethics: On the Demands of Moral Thought*. Harvard University Press, 2006.

Crary, Alice, and Lori Gruen. *Animal Crisis: A New Critical Theory*. Polity, 2022.

Cregan, Mary. *The Scar: A Personal History of Depression and Recovery*. Norton, 2019.

Crosby, Christina. *A Body, Undone: Living on After Great Pain*. New York University Press, 2016.

Crosby, Christina, and Janet Jakobsen. "Disability, Debility, and Caring Queerly." *Social Text* 38, no. 145 (December 2020): 77–103.

Crossley, Nick. *Contesting Psychiatry: Social Movements in Mental Health*. Routledge, 2006.

Czerweic, M. K. *Taking Turns: Stories from HIV/AIDS Care Unit 371*. Pennsylvania State University Press, 2017.

Dang, Mike. "Their Children Are Their Retirement Plans." *New York Times*, January 21, 2023, https://www.nytimes.com/2023/01/21/business/retirement-immigrant-families.html.

Darling, Marsha, and Toni Morrison. "In the Realm of Responsibility: A Conversation with Toni Morrison." *Women's Review of Books* 5, no. 6 (March 1988): 5–6.

Davidoff, Leonore. *Thicker Than Water: Siblings and Their Relations, 1780–1920*. Oxford University Press, 2013.

Davis, Dena S. "Genetic Dilemmas and the Child's Right to an Open Future." *Hastings Center Report* 27, no. 2 (1997): 7–15.

Davy, Laura. "Between an Ethic of Care and an Ethic of Autonomy." *Angelaki* 24, no. 3 (June 2019): 110–14.

De Young, Mary. *Madness: An American History of Mental Illness and Its Treatment*. McFarland, 2010.

DeFalco, Amelia. *Imagining Care: Responsibility, Dependency, and Canadian Literature*. University of Toronto Press, 2016.

Deinstitutionalization: Unfinished Business (Companion Paper to Policy Toolkit). National Council on Disability, September 2012.

Deutsch, Helen, and Felicity Nussbaum. "Introduction." In *"Defects": Engendering the Modern Body*, ed. Helen Deutsch and Felicity Nussbaum, 2–28. University of Michigan Press, 2000.

Dick, Philip K. *Beyond Lies the Wub*. Underwood/Miller, 1987.

"Domestic Workers Worldwide: 5 Key Facts." *WIEGO Blog*. July 22, 2022, https://www.wiego.org/blog/domestic-workers-worldwide-5-key-facts.

Douglas, Mary. *Purity and Danger: An Analysis of Concepts of Pollution and Taboo*. Praeger, 1966.

Ducey, Ariel. "Technologies of Caring Labor: From Objects to Affect." In *Intimate Labors: Cultures, Technologies, and the Politics of Care*, ed. Eileen Boris and Rhacel Salazar Parreñas, 18–32. Stanford Social Sciences, 2010.

Dumouchel, Paul, and Luisa Damiano. *Living with Robots*. Trans. Malcolm DeBevoise. Harvard University Press, 2017.

Dunn, Judy. *Sisters and Brothers*. Harvard University Press, 1985.

Edelman, Hope. *Motherless Mothers: How Mother Loss Shapes the Parents We Become*. HarperCollins, 2006.

Edelman, Lee. *No Future: Queer Theory and the Death Drive*. Duke University Press, 2004.

Ehrenreich, Barbara, and Arlie Russell Hochschild. *Global Women: Nannies, Maids, and Sex Workers in the New Economy*. Metropolitan Books, 2003.

Ehrenreich, Barbara, and Stephanie Land. *Maid: Hard Work, Low Pay, and a Mother's Will to Survive*. New York: Hachette, 2019.

Elde, Arne. *Disability and Poverty: A Global Challenge*. Polity, 2011.

Engelstein, Stefani. *Sibling Action: The Genealogical Structure of Modernity*. Columbia University Press, 2017.

Ensor, Sarah. "Terminal Regions: Queer Ecocriticism at the End." In *Against Life*, ed. Stephanie Youngblood and Alastair Hunt, 41–61. Northwestern University Press, 2016.

Epple, Juan. "Las voces de Elena Poniatowska: Una entrevista." *Confluencia* 5, no. 2 (1990): 127–29.

Epstein, Rebecca, et al. *Girlhood Interrupted: The Erasure of Black Girls' Childhood*. Georgetown Law Center on Poverty and Inequality, 2017.

Estridge, Bonnie. "Jack Nicholson Did for Shock Therapy What *Jaws* Did for Sharks: An Expert Argues That ECT Is Really More Effective Than Antidepressants." *Daily Mail*, July 9, 2011, https://www.dailymail.co.uk/health/article-2012924/Jack-Nicholson-did-shock-therapy-Jaws-did-sharks.html.

Faulkner, William. *The Sound and the Fury*. Vintage, 1984.

Feinberg, Joel. *Freedom and Fulfillment: Philosophical Essays*. Princeton University Press, 1992.

Felmlee, Diane H. "No Couple Is an Island: A Social Network Perspective on Dyadic Stability." *Social Forces* 79, no. 4 (2001): 1259–87.

Ferguson, Moira. "*Lucy* and the Mark of the Colonizer." *MFS Modern Fiction Studies* 39, no. 2 (1993): 237–59.

Fernald, Walter. "The Burden of Feeble-Mindedness." *Boston Medical and Surgical Journal* 166, no. 25 (1912): 911–15.

Fessler, Pam. "Why Disability and Poverty Still Go Hand in Hand 25 Years After Landmark Law." *All Things Considered*, July 23, 2015, https://www.npr.org/sections/health-shots /2015/07/23/424990474/why-disability-and-poverty-still-go-hand-in-hand-25-years -after-landmark-law.

Fineman, Martha. *The Autonomy Myth: A Theory of Dependency*. New Press, 2004.

Firestone, Shulamith. *Dialectic of Sex: The Case for Feminist Revolution*. Women's Press, 1979.

Fish, Jennifer Natalie. *Domestic Workers of the World Unite! A Global Movement for Dignity and Human Rights*. New York University Press, 2017.

Foucault, Michel. *Discipline and Punish: The Birth of The Prison*. Trans. Alan Sheridan. Vintage, 1995.

——. *Madness and Civilization: A History of Insanity in the Age of Reason*. Trans. Richard Howard. Vintage, 1973.

Franzen, Jonathan. *The Corrections*. Farrar, Straus and Giroux, 2001.

——. "My Father's Brain." *New Yorker*, September 2, 2001, https://www.newyorker.com /magazine/2001/09/10/my-fathers-brain.

Fraser, Benjamin. "The Work of (Creating) Art: Judith Scott's Fiber Art, Lola Barrera and Iñaki Peñafiel's *¿Qué tienes debajo del sombrero?* (2006), and the Challenges Faced by People with Developmental Disabilities." *Cultural Studies* 24, no. 4 (July 2010): 508–32.

Fraser, Nancy, and Linda Gordon. "A Genealogy of Dependency: Tracing a Keyword of the U.S. Welfare State." *Signs* 19, no. 2 (Winter 1994): 309–36.

Freeman, Elizabeth. "Committed to the End: On Caretaking, Rereading, and Queer Theory." In *Long Term: Essays on Queer Commitment*, ed. Scott Herring and Lee Wallace, 25–45. Duke University Press, 2021.

——. "Parasymptomatic Reading: Medical Kink, Care, and the Surface/Depth Debate." *Differences* 34, no. 2 (September 2023): 1–26.

——. "Queer Belongings: Kinship Theory and Queer Theory." In *A Companion to Lesbian, Gay, Bisexual, Transgender, and Queer Studies*, ed. George Haggerty and Molly McGarry, 293–314. Wiley & Sons, 2007.

Freeman, John. "Leila Slimani Doesn't Care If You're Uncomfortable." *Lit Hub*, April 29, 2019, https://lithub.com/leila-slimani-doesnt-care-if-youre-uncomfortable/.

Friedan, Betty. *The Feminine Mystique*. Norton, 2001.

Fuchs, Elinor. *Making an Exit: A Mother-Daughter Drama with Alzheimer's, Machine Tools, and Laughter*. Macmillan, 2005.

Gabbard, Christopher. "Disability Studies and the British Long Eighteenth Century." *Literature Compass* 8, no. 2 (February 2011): 80–94.

Garland, David. *The Welfare State: A Very Short Introduction*. Oxford University Press, 2016.

Gass, Thomas Edward, and Bruce C. Vladeck. *Nobody's Home: Candid Reflections of a Nursing Home Aide*. ILR Press, 2004.

Gawande, Atul. *Being Mortal: Medicine and What Matters in the End*. Henry Holt, 2014.

Gilligan, Carol. *In a Different Voice: Psychological Theory and Women's Development*. Harvard University Press, 1993.

Ginsberg, Faye, and Rayna Rapp. *Disability Worlds*. Duke University Press, 2024.

Glenn, Evelyn Nakano. *Forced to Care: Coercion and Caregiving in America.* Harvard University Press, 2010.

Goff, Philip Atiba, et al. "The Essence of Innocence: Consequences of Dehumanizing Black Children." *Journal of Personality and Social Psychology* 106, no. 4 (2014): 526–45.

Goffman, Erving. *Asylums: Essays on the Social Situation of Mental Patients and Other Inmates.* Doubleday, 1990.

Goodey, C. F. *A History of Intelligence and "Intellectual Disability": The Shaping of Psychology in the Early Modern Enlightenment.* Ashgate, 2001.

Gordon, Linda. *Black and White Visions of Welfare: Women's Welfare Activism, 1890–1945.* Institute for Research on Poverty, 1991.

Gorman, Linda. *The History of Health Care Costs and Health Insurance.* Wisconsin Policy Research Institute, 2006.

Gould, Elise, et al. "Care Workers Are Deeply Undervalued and Underpaid." *Economic Policy Institute,* July 16, 2021, https://www.epi.org/blog/care-workers-are-deeply-under valued-and-underpaid-estimating-fair-and-equitable-wages-in-the-care-sectors/.

Gowsett, Gary W. "The 'Gay Plague' Revisited: AIDS and Its Enduring Moral Panic." In *Moral Panics, Sex Panics: Fear and the Fight Over Sexual Rights,* ed. Gilbert H. Herdt, 130–56. New York University Press, 2009.

Gray, Nathan. "Think You Want to Die at Home? You Might Want to Think Again." *Los Angeles Times,* February 16, 2020, https://www.latimes.com/opinion/story/2020-02-16 /doctor-patients-send-home-to-die.

Gruen, Lori. *Entangled Empathy: An Alternative Ethic for Our Relationships with Animals.* Lantern, 2015.

Guevara, Anna Romina. "Supermaids: The Racial Branding of Filipino Care Labour." In *Migration and Care Labour: Theory, Policy, and Politics,* ed. Bridget Anderson and Isabel Shutes, 130–50. New York: Palgrave MacMillan, 2014.

Halberstam, Jack. *In a Queer Time and Place: Transgender Bodies, Subcultural Lives.* New York University Press, 2005.

Halwani, Raja. *Virtuous Liaisons: Care, Love, Sex, and Virtue Ethics.* Open Court, 2003.

Hames, Annette, and Monica McCaffrey. *Special Brothers and Sisters: Stories and Tips for Siblings of Children with a Disability or Serious Illness.* Jessica Kingsley, 2005.

Hamington, Maurice. *Embodied Care: Jane Addams, Maurice Merleau-Ponty, and Feminist Ethics.* University of Chicago Press, 2004.

Hanlon, Christopher. *Emerson's Memory Loss: Originality, Communality, and the Late Style.* Oxford University Press, 2018.

Haraway, Donna Jeanne. *Staying with the Trouble: Making Kin in the Chthulucene.* Duke University Press, 2016.

Harrington, Mona. *Care and Equality: Inventing a New Family Politics.* Knopf, 1999.

Haug, Oliver. "Nursing Home and Care Workers Officially the Most Dangerous Job in the U.S." *Ms.,* August 3, 2020, https://msmagazine.com/2020/08/03/nursing-home-and -care-workers-officially-the-most-dangerous-job-in-the-u-s/.

Hayhoe, Simon. *The Enlightenment and Disability.* Routledge, 2019.

He, Wan, et al. *An Aging World: 2015.* U.S. Census Bureau, March 2016.

Healey, Emma. *Elizabeth Is Missing.* Harper, 2014.

Heikkila, Melissa. "How Do You Solve a Problem Like Out-of-Control AI?" *MIT Technology Review,* May 16, 2021, https://www.technologyreview.com/2023/05/16/1073167/how-do-you-solve-a-problem-like-out-of-control-ai/.

Held, Virginia. *The Ethics of Care: Personal, Political, and Global.* Oxford University Press, 2006.

Hemphill, C. Dallett. *Siblings: Brothers and Sisters in American History.* Oxford University Press, 2011.

Hendren, Sara. *What Can A Body Do? How We Meet the Built World.* Riverhead, 2020.

Henig, Robin Marantz. "The Last Day of Her Life." *New York Times,* May 14, 2015.

Herring, Scott, and Lee Wallace, eds. *Long Term: Essays on Queer Commitment.* Duke University Press, 2021.

Herrmann, Dorothy. *Helen Keller: A Life.* Knopf, 1998.

Hetzel, Lisa and Annetta Smith. "The 65 Years and Over Population: 2000." U.S. Census Bureau, October 2001.

Hindle, Debbie, and Susan Sherwin-White, eds. *Sibling Matters: A Psychoanalytic, Developmental, and Systemic Approach.* Karnac, 2014.

Hobart, Hi'ilei Julia Kawehipuaakahaopulani, and Tamara Kneese, eds. "Radical Care: Survival Strategies for Uncertain Times." Special issue, *Social Text* 38, no. 1 (March 2020).

Hochschild, Arlie Russell. *The Managed Heart: Commercialization of Human Feeling.* University of California Press, 1983.

Hoffman, Amy. *Hospital Time.* Duke University Press, 1997.

"How Researchers Cleared the Name of HIV Patient Zero." *Nature* 538 (October 2016).

Howard, Jacqueline. "The Truth About 'Patient Zero' and HIV's Origins." *CNN Health,* October 28, 2016, https://www.cnn.com/2016/10/27/health/hiv-gaetan-dugas-patient-zero.

Hutson, Matthew. "Can We Stop Runaway AI?" *New Yorker,* May 16, 2023, https://www.newyorker.com/science/annals-of-artificial-intelligence/can-we-stop-the-singularity.

"The Impact of Aging Populations." *Nova,* April 20, 2004, https://www.pbs.org/wgbh/nova/article/impact-of-aging-populations/.

Ishiguro, Kazuo. *Klara and the Sun.* New York: Knopf, 2021.

——. *Never Let Me Go.* Knopf, 2005.

Jackson, Maggie. "Would You Let A Robot Take Care of Your Mother?" *New York Times,* December 13, 2019, https://www.nytimes.com/2019/12/13/opinion/robot-caregiver-aging.html.

Jamison, Kay R. *An Unquiet Mind.* Knopf, 1995.

Johnson, Brian D. "How a Typo Created a Scapegoat for the AIDS Epidemic." *Maclean's,* April 17, 2019, https://www.macleans.ca/culture/movies/how-a-typo-created-a-scapegoat-for-the-aids-epidemic/.

Johnson, Christopher H., and David Warren Sabean, eds. *Sibling Relations and the Transformations of European Kinship, 1300–1900.* Berghahn, 2011.

Johnson, Harriet McBryde. *Too Late to Die Young.* Henry Holt, 2005.

Kafer, Alison. "After Crip, Crip Afters." *South Atlantic Quarterly* 120, no. 2 (April 2021): 415—31.

——. *Feminist, Queer, Crip.* Indiana University Press, 2013.

Kane, Rosalie. "High Tech Home Care in Context: Organization, Quality, and Ethical Ramifications." In *Bringing the Hospital Home,* ed. John Karras, 197–219. 1995.

Kanner, Leo. "Autistic Disturbances of Affective Contact." *Nervous Child* 2 (1943): 217–50.

Kaphar, Titus, and Tochi Onyebuchi. "Seeing the Child: Braiding Possibility." *Gagosian Gallery,* October 5, 2020, https://gagosian.com/quarterly/2020/05/10/seeing-child -braiding-possibility-short-story-tochi-onyebuchi-titus-kaphar/.

Karasik, Judy, and Paul Karasik. *The Ride Together: A Brother and Sister's Memoir of Autism in the Family.* Simon and Schuster, 2004.

Katz, Leslie. "Coronavirus Care at One Hospital Got Totally Taken Over by Robots." *CNET News,* March 14, 2020, https://www.cnet.com/news/coronavirus-care-at-one-hospital -got-taken-over-by-robots/.

Kaysen, Susanna. *Girl, Interrupted.* Vintage, 1995.

Kelly, Christine. *Disability Politics and Care: The Challenge of Direct Funding.* University of British Columbia Press, 2016.

Kesey, Ken. *One Flew Over the Cuckoo's Nest.* Signet, 1963.

Killing Patient Zero. Dir. Laurie Lynd. Fadoo Productions, 2019.

Kincaid, Jamaica. *Lucy.* Farrar Straus Giroux, 2002.

Kinglsey, Emily Perl. *Welcome to Holland.* https://www.emilyperlkingsley.com/welcome-to -holland.

Kingsley, Jason, and Michael Levitz. *Count Us In.* Harcourt, 2007.

Kippur, Sarah. "An American Tragedy by Way of France." *Los Angeles Review of Books,* February 2, 2018, https://lareviewofbooks.org/article/an-american-tragedy-by-way-of-france/.

Kittay, Eva Feder. "A Feminist Care Ethics, Dependency, and Disability." *APA Newsletter on Feminism and Philosophy* 6, no. 2 (Spring 2007): 3–7.

——. "Forever Small: The Strange Case of Ashley X." *Hypatia* 26, no. 3 (2011): 610–31.

——. *Learning from My Daughter: The Value and Care of Disabled Minds.* Oxford University Press, 2019.

——. *Love's Labor: Essays on Women, Equality, and Dependency.* Routledge, 1999.

——. "When Caring Is Just, and Justice Is Caring." *Public Culture* 13, no. 3 (2001): 557–79.

Kittay, Eva Feder, Bruce Jennings, and Angela Wasunna. "Dependency, Difference, and the Global Ethic of Longterm Care." *Journal of Political Philosophy* 13, no. 4 (2005): 443–69.

Kleinman, Arthur. *The Soul of Care: The Moral Education of a Husband and a Doctor.* Viking, 2019.

Kovacs, Diane. "Josh: The Lonely Search for Help." *Exceptional Parent* 1, no. 6 (May 1972): 29–30.

Kulick, Don, and Jens Rydström. *Loneliness and Its Opposite: Sex, Disability, and the Ethics of Engagement.* Duke University Press, 2015.

Kushner, Tony. *Angels in America: A Gay Fantasia on National Themes.* Theatre Communications Group, 2013.

Lamb, Michael E., and Brian Sutton-Smith, eds. *Sibling Relationships: Their Nature and Significance Across the Lifespan.* Psychology Press, 2014.

Leibovitz, Annie. *A Photographer's Life, 1990–2005.* Random House, 2006.

Letchumanan, Janis. "Filipino Nannies: The Cost of Caring." *Pacific Rim Magazine*, 2013, http://langaraprm.com/2013/community/filipino-nannies-the-cost-of-caring-like -many-foreign-nannies-marilou-tuzon-looks-after-other-families-in-order-to-take -care-of-her-own/.

Lewis, Tanya. "Nursing Home Workers Had One of the Deadliest Jobs of 2020." *Scientific American*, February 18, 2021, https://www.scientificamerican.com/article/nursing-home -workers-had-one-of-the-deadliest-jobs-of-2020/.

Lobel, Orly. "In Japan, Humanoid Robots Could Soon Become Part of the Family." *Freethink*, January 29, 2023, https://www.freethink.com/robots-ai/humanoid-robots -japan.

Lopez, Matthew. *The Inheritance*. Faber & Faber, 2018.

Lorde, Audre. *A Burst of Light and Other Essays*. Ixia, 2017.

Mac, Gabriel. "Schizophrenic. Killer. My Cousin." *Mother Jones*, June 2013, https://www .motherjones.com/politics/2013/04/mental-health-crisis-mac-mcclelland-cousin -murder/.

MacGregor, John M., and Judith Scott. *Metamorphosis: The Fiber Art of Judith Scott: The Outsider Artist and the Experience of Down's Syndrome*. Creative Growth Art Center, 1999.

Mackenzie, Catriona, and Natalie Stoljar. *Relational Autonomy: Feminist Perspectives on Autonomy, Agency, and the Social Self*. Oxford University Press, 2000.

Mahlis, Kristen. "Gender and Exile: Jamaica Kincaid's *Lucy*." *Modern Fiction Studies* 44, no. 1 (Spring 1998): 164–83.

Mailhot, Terese Marie. *Heart Berries: A Memoir*. Counterpoint, 2018.

Manalansan, Martin. "Queer Intersections: Sexuality and Gender in Migration Studies," *IMR* 40, no. 1 (Spring 2006): 224–49.

Mandell, Betty Reid. *The Crisis of Caregiving: Social Welfare Policy in the United States*. Palgrave Macmillan, 2010.

Manly, J. J., R. N. Jones, K. M. Langa, et al. "Estimating the Prevalence of Dementia and Mild Cognitive Impairment in the US: The 2016 Health and Retirement Study Harmonized Cognitive Assessment Protocol Project." *JAMA Neurology* 79, no. 12 (2022): 1242–49.

Mann, Sally. "Sally Mann's Exposure." *New York Times*, April 16, 2015, http://www.nytimes .com/2015/04/19/magazine/the-cost-of-sally-manns-exposure.html.

Mann, Sally. *Immediate Family*. New York: Aperture, 1992.

Mattern, Shannon. "Maintenance and Care." *Places*, November 2018, https://placesjournal .org/article/maintenance-and-care/.

Mattlin, Ben. *In Sickness and in Health: Love, Disability, and a Quest to Understand the Perils and Pleasures of Interabled Romance*. Beacon, 2018.

——. *Miracle Boy Grows Up: How the Disability Rights Revolution Saved My Sanity*. Skyhorse, 2012.

McCloud, Scott. *Understanding Comics: The Invisible Art*. HarperPerennial, 1993.

McGlynn, Sean A., et al. "Understanding the Potential of PARO for Healthy Older Adults." *International Journal of Computing Studies* 100 (April 2017): 33–47.

McGowan, Kat. "Hospital at Home Trend Means Family Members Must Be Caregivers—Ready or Not." *NPR Health News*, July 18, 2023, https://www.npr.org/sections/health-shots/2023/07/18/1188058399/hospital-at-home-caregivers-family-stress.

McHugh, Mary, and Stanley Klein. *Special Siblings: Growing Up with Someone with a Disability*. Brookes, 2002.

McKay, Richard Andrew. *Patient Zero and the Making of the AIDS Epidemic*. University of Chicago Press, 2017.

McLaren, Margaret. "Feminist Ethics: Care as a Virtue." In *Feminists Doing Ethics*, ed. Peggy DesAutels and Joanne Waugh, 101–18. Rowman and Littlefield, 2001.

McLaughlin, Emma, and Nicola Kraus. *The Nanny Diaries*. St. Martin's, 2002.

McNeil Jr., Donald G. "H.I.V. Arrived in the U.S. Long Before 'Patient Zero.'" *New York Times*, October 26, 2016, https://www.nytimes.com/2016/10/27/health/hiv-patient-zero-genetic-analysis.html.

McRuer, Robert. *Crip Times: Disability, Globalization, and Resistance*. New York University Press, 2018.

——. "Shameful Sites: Locating Queerness and Disability." In *Gay Shame*, ed. David M. Halperin and Valerie Traub (University of Chicago Press, 2009) 179–87.

Meagher, Gabrielle. "What Can We Expect from Paid Carers?" *Politics and Society* 34, no. 1 (March 2006): 33–53.

Merkin, Daphne. *This Close to Happy: A Reckoning with Depression*. Farrar, Straus and Giroux, 2017.

Merrell, Susan. *The Accidental Bond: The Power of Sibling Relationships*. Times Books, 1995.

Meyer, Cheryl L., et al. *Mothers Who Kill Their Children: Understanding the Acts of Moms from Susan Smith to the "Prom Mom."* New York University Press, 2001.

Meyer, Donald J., and Cary Pillo. *Views from Our Shoes: Growing Up with a Brother or Sister with Special Needs*. Woodbine House, 1997.

Meyer, Donald J., and Patricia F. Vadasy. *Sibshops: Workshops for Siblings of Children with Special Needs*. Brookes, 2007.

——. *Living with a Brother or Sister with Special Needs: A Book for Sibs*. University of Washington Press, 1996.

Mills, Claudia. "The Child's Right to an Open Future." *Journal of Social Philosophy* 34, no. 4 (December 2003): 499–509.

Miserandino, Christine. "The Spoon Theory." *But You Don't Look Sick* (blog), 2003. https://butyoudontlooksick.com/articles/written-by-christine/the-spoon-theory/.

Mitchell, David T. "Body Solitaire: The Singular Subject of Disability Autobiography." *American Quarterly* 52, no. 2 (June 2000): 311–15.

Mitchell, Juliet. *Siblings: Sex and Violence*. Polity, 2003.

Mitchell, Wendy. *Somebody I Used to Know*. Ballantine, 2018.

Monette, Paul. *Borrowed Time: An AIDS Memoir*. Harcourt Brace Jovanovich, 1988.

Moore, Mignon. *Making Care Count: A Century of Gender, Race, and Paid Care Work*. Rutgers University Press, 2011.

Morrison, Linda Joy. *Talking Back to Psychiatry: The Psychiatric Consumer/Survivor/Ex-Patient Movement*. Routledge, 2005.

Morrison, Toni. *Beloved*. Vintage, 2004.

Mortier, Erwin, and Paul Vincent. *Stammered Songbook: A Mother's Book of Hours*. Pushkin, 2015.

Muller, Beatrice. "The Careless Society: Dependency and Care Work in Capitalist Societies." *Frontiers in Sociology* 3, no. 14 (2019), https://www.frontiersin.org/articles/10.3389/fsoc.2018.00044/full.

Muñoz, José Esteban. *Cruising Utopia: The Then and There of Queer Futurity*. New York University Press, 2019.

Murphy, Tim. "'AIDS' Patient Zero Is Finally Innocent, but We're Still Learning Who He Really Was." *New York Magazine*, October 31, 2016, https://nymag.com/vindicated/2016/10/aids-patient-zero-is-vindicated-by-science.html.

Murphy, Timothy F. *Ethics in an Epidemic: AIDS, Morality, and Culture*. University of California Press, 1994.

Murray, John E. *Origins of American Health Insurance: A History of Industrial Sickness Funds*. Yale University Press, 2007.

Nadasen, Premilla. *Care: The Highest Stage of Capitalism*. Haymarket, 2023.

——. *Household Workers Unite: The Untold Story of African American Women Who Built a Movement*. Beacon, 2015.

Nadasen, Premilla, Tiffany Williams, and Barnard Center for Research on Women, eds. *Valuing Domestic Work*. New Feminist Solution 5. Barnard Center for Research on Women, 2011. https://bcrw.barnard.edu/wp-content/nfs/reports/NFS5-Valuing-Domestic-Work.pdf.

Narayan, Uma. "Colonialism and Its Others: Considerations on Rights and Care Discourses." *Hypatia* 10, no. 2 (1995): 133–40.

Nedelsky, Jennifer. "Reconceiving Autonomy: Sources, Thoughts and Possibilities." *Yale Journal of Law and Feminism* 1, no. 1 (1998): 7–36.

Nelson, Maggie. *On Freedom: Four Songs of Care and Constraint*. Graywolf, 2021.

Nichols, Jennifer J. "'Poor Visitor': Mobility as/of Voice in Jamaica Kincaid's *Lucy*." *MELUS: Multi-Ethnic Literature of the U.S.* 34, no. 4 (Winter 2009): 187–207.

Nishida, Akemi. *Messy Entanglements of Disability, Dependency, and Desire*. Temple University Press, 2022.

Nixon, Rob. *Slow Violence and the Environmentalism of The Poor*. Harvard University Press, 2013.

Noddings, Nel. *Caring: A Feminine Approach to Ethics and Moral Education*. University of California Press, 2003.

——. *The Maternal Factor: Two Paths to Morality*. University of California Press, 2010.

Nussbaum, Martha C. *Frontiers of Justice : Disability, Nationality, Species Membership*. Belknap Press of Harvard University Press, 2006.

——. *Justice for Animals: Our Collective Responsibility*. Simon & Schuster, 2022.

Nussbaum, Susan. *Good Kings, Bad Kings*. Algonquin, 2013.

Oberman, Michelle, and Cheryl L. Meyer. *When Mothers Kill: Interviews from Prison*. New York University Press, 2008.

Olsen, Victoria. "Looking for Laura." *Open Letters Monthly Archive*, https://www
.openlettersmonthlyarchive.com/olm/looking-for-laura.

O'Neill, Clare. "The Photo That Changed the Face of AIDS." *The Picture Show: Photo Sto-ries from NPR*, December 1, 2011, https://www.npr.org/sections/pictureshow/2011/12/01
/142998189/the-photo-that-changed-the-face-of-aids.

Parreñas, Rhacel Salazar. *The Force of Domesticity: Filipina Migrants and Globalization.* Stanford University Press, 2008.

——. *Servants of Globalization: Migration and Domestic Work.* Stanford University Press, 2015.

Paybarah, Azi. "The Legacy of the Willowbrook Scandal." *New York Times*, February 24, 2020, https://www.nytimes.com/2020/02/24/nyregion/willowbrook-scandal.html.

Pernick, Martin S. *The Black Stork: Eugenics and the Death of "Defective" Babies in Ameri-can Medicine and Motion Pictures Since 1915.* Oxford University Press, 1996.

Piepzna-Samarsinha, Leah. *Care Work: Dreaming Disability Justice.* Arsenal Pulp, 2018.

Pineda, Jon. *Sleep in Me.* University of Nebraska Press, 2010.

Piper, Kelsey. "AI Experts Are Increasingly Afraid of What They're Creating." *Vox*, Novem-ber 28, 2022, https://www.vox.com/the-highlight/23447596/artificial-intelligence-agi
-openai-gpt3-existential-risk-human-extinction.

Plath, Sylvia. *The Bell Jar.* Faber & Faber, 1978.

Plumwood, Val. *Feminism and the Mastery of Nature.* Routledge, 1993.

Poniatowska, Elena. *Hasta no verte Jesús mío.* Ediciones Era, 1969.

——. *La noche de Tlatelolco. Testimonios de historia oral.* Ediciones Era, 1971.

——. *Las soldaderas.* Ediciones Era, 1999.

——. *Nada, nadie. Las voces del temblor.* Ediciones Era, 1988.

Price, Margaret. "The Bodymind Problem and the Possibilities of Pain." *Hypatia* 30, no. 1 (Winter 2015): 268–84.

Purtill, Corinne. "Stop Me If You've Heard This One: A Robot and a Team of Irish Scien-tists Walk Into a Senior Living Home." *Time Magazine*, October 4, 2019, https://time
.com/longform/senior-care-robot/.

Rachels, James. *The Elements of Moral Philosophy.* McGraw-Hill, 2003.

Rain Man. Dir. Barry Levinson. MGM Home Entertainment, 1998.

Rancière, Jacques. *The Politics of Aesthetics: The Distribution of the Sensible.* Continuum, 2006.

Rapp Black, Emily. *Poster Child: A Memoir.* London: Bloomsbury, 2007.

——. *The Still Point of the Turning World.* Penguin, 2013.

Rashkow, Ilona N. *Taboo or Not Taboo: Sexuality and Family in the Hebrew Bible.* Fortress, 2000.

Ratzka, Adolf. "The Independent Living Movement Paved the Way: Origins of Personal Assistance in Sweden." *Independent Living Institute* (blog), 2012, https://www.indepen
dentliving.org/docs7/Independent-Living-movement-paved-way.html.

Rawls, John. *A Theory of Justice.* Harvard University Press, 1971.

Reiss, Benjamin. "Other Reliance: Transcendentalism, Mental Disability, and Ethics of Care." *American Literary History* 37, no. 1 (Spring 2025).

——. *Theaters of Madness: Insane Asylums and Nineteenth-Century American Culture*. University of Chicago Press, 2008.

Rich, Adrienne. "Adrienne Rich: It Is Hard to Write About My Own Mother." *Lit Hub* (blog), August 24, 2018, https://lithub.com/adrienne-rich-it-is-hard-to-write-about-my-own-mother/.

——. *Snapshots of a Daughter-in-Law: Poems, 1954–1962*. Norton, 1967.

Rich, Nathaniel. "A Training Ground for Untrained Artists." *New York Times*, December 16, 2015, https://www.nytimes.com/2015/12/20/magazine/a-training-ground-for-untrained-artists.html.

Ricoeur, Paul. *Time and Narrative*. University of Chicago Press, 1984.

Risse, Guenter B. *Mending Bodies, Saving Souls: A History of Hospitals*. Oxford University Press, 1999.

Robinson, Fiona. *Globalizing Care: Ethics, Feminist Theory, and International Relations*. Westview, 1999.

Rothman, David J. *The Discovery of the Asylum: Social Order and Disorder in the New Republic*. Little, Brown, 1971.

Ruddick, Sara. *Maternal Thinking: Toward a Politics of Peace*. Beacon, 2002.

Ruddick, William. "Transforming Homes and Hospitals." *Hastings Center Report* 24, no. 5 (September-October 1994): S11–14.

Rutherford, Danilyn. "The Sovereignty of Vulnerability." In *Sovereignty Unhinged: An Illustrated Primer for the Study of Present Intensities, Disavowals, and Temporal Derangements*, ed. Deborah A. Thomas and Joseph Masco, 263–76. Duke University Press, 2023.

Sadowsky, Jonathan. "Electroconvulsive Therapy: A History of Controversy, but Also of Help." *The Conversation*, January 12, 2017, https://theconversation.com/electroconvulsive-therapy-a-history-of-controversy-but-also-of-help-70938.

Safer, Jeanne. *The Normal One: Life with a Difficult or Damaged Sibling*. Delta, 2003.

Sakuma, Amanda. "A Woman in a Vegetative State Suddenly Gave Birth. Her Alleged Assault Is a #MeToo Wake-up Call." *Vox*, January 7, 2019, https://www.vox.com/2019/1/7/18171012/arizona-woman-birth-coma-sexual-assault-metoo.

Samuels, Ellen. "Six Ways of Looking at Crip Time." *Disability Studies Quarterly* 37, no. 3 (August 2017), https://dsq-sds.org/index.php/dsq/article/view/5824/4684.

Samuels, Ellen, and Elizabeth Freeman. *Crip Temporalities*. Special issue of *South Atlantic Quarterly* 120, no. 2 (April 2021).

Satariano, Adam, et al. "Meet Zora, the Robot Caregiver." *New York Times*, November 23, 2018, https://www.nytimes.com/interactive/2018/11/23/technology/robot-nurse-zora.html.

Sauer, Alissa. "Why Is Alzheimer's More Likely in Women?" *Alzheimers.Net*, September 5, 2019, https://www.alzheimers.net/8-12-15-why-is-alzheimers-more-likely-in-women.

Saunders, Gerda. *Memory's Last Breath: Field Notes on My Dementia*. Hachette, 2017.

Savage, Lila. *Say Say Say*. Knopf, 2019.

Schaeffer, Talia. *Communities of Care: The Social Ethics of Victorian Fiction*. Princeton University Press, 2021.

Schneider, Katy. "Reasons to Love NY." *New York*, December 14, 2014, https://nymag.com/news/articles/reasonstoloveny/2014/bellevue-ebola-staff/.

Schulman, Sarah. *Rat Bohemia*. New York: Dutton, 1995.

Scott, Janny. "From Annie Leibovitz: Life, and Death, Examined." *New York Times*, October 6, 2006, https://www.nytimes.com/2006/10/06/arts/design/06leib.html.

Scott, Joyce. "Birth and Rebirth." *The Outsider* 5, no. 1: 16–18.

——. *Entwined: Sisters and Secrets in the Silent World of Artist Judith Scott*. Beacon, 2016.

Scouller, Wulf. "Restraining Confinement in Early America." *Disability History Association* (blog), September 17, 2023, https://allofusdha.org/research/restraining-confinement -in-early-america/.

Scully, Jackie Leach. *Disability Bioethics: Moral Bodies, Moral Difference*. Rowman and Littlefield, 2008.

Sedgwick, Eve Kosofsky. *Epistemology of the Closet*. University of California Press, 1990.

——. *Touching Feeling: Affect, Pedagogy, Performativity*. Duke University Press, 2003.

Selvaratnam, Tanya. *The Big Lie: Motherhood, Feminism, and the Reality of the Biological Clock*. Prometheus, 2014.

Senior, Jennifer. *All Joy and No Fun: The Paradox of Modern Parenthood*. Harper Collins, 2014.

Sevenhuijsen, Selma. *Citizenship and the Ethics of Care: Feminist Considerations on Justice, Morality, and Politics*. Routledge, 1998.

Shakespeare, Tom. "Love, Friendship, Intimacy." In *Disability Rights and Wrongs*, 167–84. Routledge, 2006.

Shapiro, Joseph P. *No Pity: People with Disabilities Forging a New Civil Rights Movement*. Three Rivers, 1994.

Sharma, Akhil. *Family Life*. Norton, 2014.

Sheldon, Rebekah. *The Child to Come: Life After the Human Catastrophe*. University of Minnesota Press, 2016.

Shenk, David. *The Forgetting: Alzheimer's, Portrait of an Epidemic*. Doubleday, 2001.

Sherman, Neil. "The Graying of America." *Health Day: News for Healthier Living*, May 16, 2001, https://consumer.healthday.com/senior-citizen-information-31/misc-aging-news -10/the-graying-of-america-110658.htm.

Shilts, Randy. *And the Band Played On: Politics, People, and the AIDS Epidemic*. Viking, 1988.

Siebers, Tobin. *Disability Aesthetics*. University of Michigan Press, 2010.

——. "A Sexual Culture for Disabled People." In *Disability Theory*, 135–56. University of Michigan Press, 2008.

Silberman, Steve. *Neurotribes: The Legacy of Autism and the Future of Neurodiversity*. Random House, 2015.

Silman, Anna. "The Perfect Nanny Author on Why We Can't Look Away from Domestic Horror Stories." *The Cut*, April 9, 2018, https://www.thecut.com/2018/04/perfect-nanny -author-leila-slimani-on-new-york-nanny-trial.html.

Simmel, Georg. "The Isolated Individual and the Dyad." In *The Sociology of Georg Simmel*, ed. Kurt H. Wolff, 118–24. Free Press, 1950.

Simon, Matt. "The Covid-19 Pandemic Is a Crisis That Robots Were Built For." *Wired*, March 25, 2020, https://www.wired.com/story/covid-19-pandemic-robots/.

Simon-Thomas, Emiliana R., Jakub Godzik, et al. "An fMRI Study of Caring *vs* Self-focus During Induced Compassion and Pride." *Social Cognitive and Affective Neuroscience* 7, no. 6 (August 6, 2012): 635–48.

Simplican, Stacy Clifford. *The Capacity Contract: Intellectual Disability and the Question of Citizenship.* University of Minnesota Press, 2015.

Simpson, Mona. "Love, Money and Other People's Children." *New York Times*, July 13, 2012, https://www.nytimes.com/2012/07/15/magazine/nannies-love-money-and-other-peoples-children.html.

——. *My Hollywood.* Knopf, 2010.

Singer, Peter. "Happy Nevertheless." *New York Times*, December 24, 2008, https://www.nytimes.com/2008/12/28/magazine/28mcbryde-t.html.

Skotko, Brian, and Susan P. Levine. *Fasten Your Seatbelt: A Crash Course on Down Syndrome for Brothers and Sisters.* Woodbine House, 2009.

Slater, Lauren. *Prozac Diary.* Hamish Hamilton, 1999.

Slimani, Leïla. *The Perfect Nanny.* Trans. Sam Taylor. Penguin, 2018.

Slote, Michael. *The Ethics of Care and Empathy.* Routledge, 2007.

Smith, Ian. "Misusing Canonical Intertexts: Jamaica Kincaid, Wordsworth, and Colonialism's 'Absent Things.'" *Callaloo* 25, no. 3 (Summer 2002): 801–20.

Smith, Peggie. *Protecting Home Care Workers Under the Fair Labor Standards Act.* Direct Care Alliance Policy Brief, June 2009, http://www.directcarealliance.org.

Solomon, Andrew. *Far from the Tree: Parents, Children, and the Search for Identity.* Scribner, 2012.

——. *The Noonday Demon: An Atlas of Depression.* Scribner, 2001.

Sommer, Doris. *Proceed with Caution, when Engaged by Minority Writing in the Americas.* Harvard University Press, 1999.

Sone, Yuji. *Japanese Robot Culture.* Palgrave Macmillan, 2016.

Sontag, Susan. *On Photography.* Anchor, 1990.

——. "The Way We Live Now." *New Yorker*, November 16, 1986, https://www.newyorker.com/magazine/1986/11/24/the-way-we-live-now.

Span, Paula. "Colored with Controversy." *Washington Post*, February 13, 1992, https://www.washingtonpost.com/archive/lifestyle/1992/02/13/colored-with-controversy/a362eee9-385b-421c-9943-e2dcd8f33fdc/.

——. "In Isolating Times, Can Robo-Pets Provide Comfort?" *New York Times*, September 26, 2020, https://www.nytimes.com/2020/09/26/health/coronavirus-elderly-isolation-robot-pets.html.

Spivak, Gayatri. "Can the Subaltern Speak?" In *Marxism and the Interpretation of Culture*, ed. Cary Nelson and Lawrence Grossberg, 271–310. University of Illinois Press, 1988.

Stack, Megan K. *Women's Work: A Reckoning with Home and Help.* Doubleday, 2019.

Starr, Paul. *The Social Transformation of American Medicine.* Basic Books, 1982.

Stiker, Henri-Jacques. *A History of Disability.* Trans. William Sayers. University of Michigan Press, 1999.

Stockton, Kathryn Bond. *The Queer Child, or Growing Sideways in the Twentieth Century.* Duke University Press, 2009.

Stockton, Richard. "The Story Behind the Photo of David Kirby That Changed the World's Perception of AIDS." *All That's Interesting*, 2017, https://allthatsinteresting.com/david -kirby.

Stokel-Walker, Chris. "Why Britain Hasn't Fallen in Love with Robots—Yet." *Goethe Institute*, https://www.goethe.de/ins/gb/en/kul/zut/rob/22687159.html.

Stramondo, Joseph. "Disability and the Damaging Master Narrative of an Open Future." *Hastings Center Report* 50, no. S1 (June 2020): S30–36.

Strohm, Kate. *Being the Other One: Growing Up with a Brother or Sister Who Has Special Needs*. Shambhala, 2005.

Szasz, Thomas. *Antipsychiatry: Quackery Squared*. Syracuse University Press, 2009.

Taylor, Sunaura. *Beasts of Burden: Animal and Disability Liberation*. Simon & Schuster, 2018.

——. *Disabled Ecologies: Lessons from a Wounded Desert*. University of California Press, 2024.

Tergesen, Anne, and Milo Inada. "It's Not a Stuffed Animal, It's a $6000 Medical Device." *Wall Street Journal*, June 21, 2010, https://www.wsj.com/articles/SB100014240527487044 63504575301051844937276.

Think of Me First as a Person. Dir. George Ingmire and Dwight Core Sr. Center for Home Movies, 1960–1975.

Thomas, Matthew. *We Are Not Ourselves*. Simon & Schuster, 2014.

Thomas, Susan Gregory. "Tibetan Nannies: Parents' New Status Symbol?" *NBC News.Com*, September 21, 2009, http://www.nbcnews.com/id/32884630/ns/health-childrens_health /t/tibetan-nannies-parents-new-status-symbol/.

Tomoshige, Akira, and Akiko Okamoto. "Robots on Hand to Greet Japanese Coronavirus Patients in Hotels." *Reuters*, May 1, 2020, https://www.reuters.com/article/us-health -coronavirus-japan-robot-hotels/robots-on-hand-to-greet-japanese-coronavirus -patients-in-hotels-idUSKBN22D4PC.

Thomson, Rosemarie Garland. *Staring: How We Look*. Oxford University Press, 2009.

Toupin, Louise. *Wages for Housework: A History of an International Feminist Movement, 1972–1977*. University of British Columbia Press, 2018.

Treatment Advocacy Center. "Serious Mental Illness Prevalence in Jails and Prisons." September 2016, https://www.treatmentadvocacycenter.org/reports_publications/serious -mental-illness-prevalence-in-jails-and-prisons/.

Treichler, Paula A. *How to Have Theory in an Epidemic: Cultural Chronicles of AIDS*. Duke University Press, 1999.

Trent, James W. *Inventing the Feeble Mind: A History of Intellectual Disability in the United States*. Oxford University Press, 2017.

Tronto, Joan C. *Caring Democracy: Markets, Equality, and Justice*. New York University Press, 2013.

——. *Moral Boundaries: A Political Argument for an Ethic of Care*. Routledge, 1993.

Tsing, Anna Lowenhaupt. *The Mushroom at the End of the World: On the Possibility of Life in Capitalist Ruins*. Princeton University Press, 2015.

Turkle, Sherry. *Alone Together: Why We Expect More from Technology and Less from Each Other*. Basic Books, 2011.

U.S. Department of Commerce. *U.S. Summary: Census 2000 Profile.* https://www.census
.gov/prod/2002pubs/c2kprof00-us.pdf.

U.S. Department of Labor. *Fact Sheet #79A: Companionship Services Under the Fair Labor
Standards Act,* September 2013, https://www.dol.gov/agencies/whd/fact-sheets/79a-flsa
-companionship.

——. *OSH Act of 1970.* https://www.osha.gov/laws-regs/oshact/completeoshact.

Vaid, Urvashi. Foreword to *Hospital Time,* by Amy Hoffman. Duke University Press, 1997.

Van Wynsberghe, Aimee. *Healthcare Robots: Ethics, Design, and Implementation.* Routledge, 2016.

Vega, Patricia. "Gaby, la historia verdadera." In *A gritos y sombrerazos.* Conaculta, 1996.

Wade, Holly Anne. "Discrimination, Sexuality, and People with Significant Disabilities:
Issues of Access and the Right to Sexual Expression in the United States." *Disability
Studies Quarterly* 22, no. 4 (Fall 2002): 9–27.

Waldman, Ayelet. *Bad Mother: A Chronicle of Maternal Crimes, Minor Calamities, and
Occasional Moments of Grace.* Broadway, 2009.

Walker-Hirsch, Leslie. "Sexuality Education and Intellectual Disability Across the Lifespan: A Developmental, Social, and Educational Perspective." In *The Facts of Life . . . and
More: Sexuality and Intimacy for People with Intellectual Disabilities.* Paul H. Brookes,
2007.

Washington, Kate. *Already Toast: Caregivers and Burnout in America.* Beacon, 2021.

——. "Leslie's House of Nightmares." *Avidly,* November 30, 2016, https://avidly.lareviewof
books.org/2016/11/30/leslies-house-of-nightmares/.

Weeks, Jeffrey. *The Languages of Sexuality.* Routledge, 2011.

Weston, Kath. *Families We Choose: Lesbians, Gays, Kinship.* Columbia University Press,
1991.

Wheelwright, Jeff. "The Gray Tsunami." *Discover Magazine,* September 18, 2012, http://
discovermagazine.com/2012/oct/20-the-gray-tsunami.

Willowbrook: The Last Great Disgrace. Dir. Geraldo Rivera, WABC-TV, 1972.

Wolff, Kurt H. *The Sociology of Georg Simmel.* Free Press, 1950.

Wolfson, Penny. *Enwheeled: History, Design, and the Wheelchair.* Cooper Hewitt, 2018.

Wurtzel, Elizabeth. *Prozac Nation: Young and Depressed in America.* Riverhead, 1995.

Wylie, Philip. *Generation of Vipers.* Farrar & Rinehart, 1942.

Zelizer, Viviana. "Caring Everywhere." In *Intimate Labors: Cultures, Technologies, and the
Politics of Care,* ed. Eileen Boris and Rhacel Salazar Parreñas, 267–79. Stanford Social
Sciences, 2010.

Zelnick, Jennifer R., and Mimi Abramovitz. "The Perils of Privatization: Bringing the Business Model Into Human Services." *Social Work* 65, no. 3 (July 2020): 213–24.

Zunshine, Lisa. *Why We Read Fiction: Theory of Mind and the Novel.* Ohio State University
Press, 2006.

INDEX

Page locators in italics refer to figures

able-bodied: isolation of, 176–77; luxury of forgetting, 181; norms of, 56–57, 171, 173; and valorization of work, 25–26, 241. *See also* accident and injury

absence of care, 50, 70, 100; inadequate mothers, 153, 160; memories of, 22, 45, 67

abuse: in group homes, 244–45; in institutions, 92, 177, 242; migrant histories of, 218; sexual violation, xi–xii, 92, 177, 269

acceptance of care, as work, ix, xi, 1, 146–47

accessible environments, 138–39, 173, 184, 187–88, 190

acquired dependencies, 37, 75, 86, 174; accident and injury, 93–108; age-related, 37, 138, 140, 143, 164, 262; before and after, 95, 180; brokenness, register of, 97; victims' compensation, 99–100. *See also* HIV

Adams, Sarah LaChance, 10

adult dependents, 17–18, 37–38; adults with Down syndrome, 52–53, 106; paid adult care, 203, 205, 223–34; transition from childhood, 60–61, 68. *See also* dementia;

dependent people; disability rights movement; HIV/AIDS; nursing home narratives; paid care work

advice literature genre, 84–86

aesthetics, 21, 144, 173, 205; shaped by colonialism, 220

affect: as required performance, 205–6, 270; positive feedback loop, 206; as shared, x, 7, 10. *See also* emotional labor

agency: of care workers, 38, 213–14; of dependent people, 20–21, 179, 182, 273

aging: "aging in place," 144; and caregiving, 59–62, 68; habitable environments, 138–39; inadequate societal preparation for, 138, 142–43, 160; meaning in, 264; "oldest old," 32, 143. *See also* dementia; dementia narratives

Ahmed, Sara, 319n2

"aid," 26

All Joy and No Fun (Senior), 62–63

"alternative worlds," 21

"always already," concept of, 86–87, 93, 95, 97

Alzheimer, Alois, 142

Alzheimer's, 137, 139–40, 144–45, 152, 160, 164. *See also* dementia

GPSR Authorized Representative: Easy Access System Europe, Mustamäe tee
50, 10621 Tallinn, Estonia, gpsr.requests@easproject.com